Law and Ethics in Nursing and Health Care

Judith Hendrick
Senior Lecturer in Law
Oxford Brookes University

First published in 2000 by:
Stanley Thornes (Publishers) Ltd

Reprinted in 2001 by:
Nelson Thornes Ltd
Delta Place
27 Bath Road
CHELTENHAM
GL53 7TH
United Kingdom

02 03 04 05 06 / 12 11 10 9 8 7 6 5 4 3

A catalogue record for this book is available from the British Library

ISBN 0 7487 3321 3

Page make-up by Acorn Bookwork

Printed and bound in Spain by GraphyCems

For Josie, Eve, Miriam and Michael, with love.

'In a civilised life, law floats in a sea of ethics'.
Earl Warren (1891–1974), American Chief Justice,
New York Times 12 November 1962.

Contents

LIST OF CASES

Key
AC = Law Reports, Appeal Cases
All ER = All England Law Reports
BMLR = Butterworths Medico-Legal Reports
Crim LR = Criminal Law Review
EHRR = European Human Rights Reports
FLR = Family Law Reports
KB = Law Reports, King's Bench
Med LR = Medical Law Reports
QB = Law Reports, Queen's Bench Division
Sol J = Solicitors Journal
WLR = Weekly Law Reports
Note: Bracketed page numbers refer to instances where there are references to cases in the text; unbracketed page numbers refer to text in which the cases are actually described.

LIST OF STATUTES

PREFACE

That nurses should study ethics is widely accepted and its inclusion in nurse education is now commonplace. The burgeoning literature on health-care law for nurses is a more recent development but not surprising given that the subject area is now firmly established as a distinct and important discipline within law itself. In fact the subject has developed so rapidly in the last decade that legal texts need to be constantly updated to keep pace with the huge rise in medical case law and the increasing complexity of the subject. Much less common, but also now beginning to proliferate, are nursing texts that combine law and ethics. Again, this development is not surprising as it reflects the recognition that to study law or ethics as isolated phenomena is distorting when in practice they are so interdependent. This, of course, has always been the case but, given the speed of technological developments in medicine and changes in nursing practice the legal and ethical dilemmas nurses now routinely face are inherently more complex than in the past. Thus life and death decisions, access to health care, issues of consent, confidentiality, responsibility and accountability are, if not more pressing than they once were, then at the very least more open to public scrutiny and legal challenge. As a consequence it has become more important than ever to understand the moral values that inform the law and to question its role in controlling and regulating health care. Yet this process is a discomforting one since it reveals the law's limitations and its inability always to come up with the 'right' answer. The failure of the law to live up to its expectations and provide acceptable answers to the new legal and ethical questions that contemporary practice raises is particularly disconcerting at a time when patients and clients see recourse to the law and involvement of the courts as a solution to their grievances.

But despite the limits of the law there can be little doubt that it has an important role to play in modern nursing practice. What is less clear is precisely what that role is. Hence although it may be self-evident that law and ethics are interconnected, that in itself tells us little about the nature of the relationship between them. That the relationship is a complex one in which the distinctions are often blurred explains perhaps why almost all the texts that do consider the legal and ethical implications of nursing practice fail to draw explicit comparisons, leaving it to the reader to reach his/her own conclusions as to how and why they may differ. The approach taken in this book is different. In describing the law and the moral considerations that have informed its development, it attempts to tease out their differences and similarities, and explore and explain them. It uses practical examples to highlight the comparisons between them and to help nurses make the transition between an academic approach and what really happens or what the law says should happen in practice. Each chapter therefore begins (after a short introduction) with some hypothetical case studies. These introduce readers to some of the scenarios they may have to face. A theoretical discussion then follows, which looks at each topic from a legal and ethical perspective. At the end of the chapter the case studies are answered in such a way that the differences and similarities between the law and ethics are highlighted.

In a book of this length it is not, of course, possible to provide a comprehensive analysis of either law or ethics. The book aims to offer the reader an introduction to thinking about the kinds of questions that the author has so often been asked: What's wrong with the law? Why does it do this or fail to do that? How can it allow that to happen? How can that be the right thing to do?

The law is stated as at February 2000 and applies to England and Wales.

Judith Hendrick
Oxford, April 2000

1 AN INTRODUCTION TO LAW AND ETHICS

WHAT IS LAW?

It is very difficult to think of any aspect of everyday life that is not regulated by law. Law affects almost everything we do, setting standards of behaviour even in the most 'private' areas of our lives. Indeed, the range of subjects controlled in one way or other by the law is quite extraordinary and it takes some imagination, if not ingenuity, to identify any activity that is not in some way legally regulated. Most people would therefore expect there to be laws regulating family and commercial life, property transactions and medical and nursing practice. However, laws protecting bats from disturbance or catering for the welfare of breeding ospreys and laws governing the provision of exits from village halls may be less well known (Simpson, 1988). But despite the pervasiveness of law a universal definition remains as elusive as when the question 'What is law?' was first asked some 2500 years ago. That said, a good starting point is to describe the law in very simple terms: in other words, as a rule or a body of rules. A rule has been described as 'a general norm mandating or guiding conduct or action in types of situation or circumstance' (Twining and Miers, 1991, p. 131). Rules can both guide and serve as standards for behaviour. But all rules, whether they are legal, moral, ethical or social, have the same basic characteristics: they are general and so apply to everybody or a specific class; they are normative or prescriptive, meaning that they set standards of how things ought or ought not to be, rather than how they are; and finally they lay down standards of behaviour with which we must comply if the rule affects us. To be ascribed the status of law, however, several other conditions must be met. First, the rules must be reasonably definite, consistent and understandable. Rules that are so vague or imprecise that no-one knows how to comply with them are arguably not legal at all. Secondly, they must be openly promulgated and not retroactive, i.e. everybody who is affected by them must know what they are in advance. Thirdly, they must be recognized and enforced by the courts. As McLeod (1996, p. 3) observes, the law is 'those rules which the law will enforce'.

One of the most influential legal philosophers of his time who defined law in terms of rules was H. L. A. Hart (1907–92). In his seminal book *The Concept of Law* (1961; Hart, 1994) he distinguished between primary and secondary rules. Primary rules were those that any society needed in order to survive – for example, those that prohibited violence, theft, murder and fraud. According to Hart a simple society could survive with only these basic primary rules but the more complex it became the more it would require what he described as secondary rules. Secondary rules consisted of three types:

- **rules of adjudication**, which gave officials the authority to decide disputes and to impose sanctions;

- **rules of change**, which dealt with how new rules could be made;
- **rules of recognition**, which spelt out which of the many rules that govern society would actually have legal force.

The idea that law can be defined in terms of rules is popular but has been much criticized. One major criticism is that many who write about the institutions and processes involved in the administration of justice talk of a legal system. As a legal system the law is associated with government and so includes Parliament, the courts, the judiciary, the legal profession, the police and the bureaucracy that services the system. But, as White (1999, p. 14) observes, this suggests a planned, coherent and complete set of structures following well-defined rules, whereas in practice the English legal system is far from systematic. Similarly, law is also often described as a process in which case legislative and judicial processes are emphasized, i.e. how the law is made, whether by Parliament or the judges (Farrar and Dugdale, 1990).

But for many writers the key to the nature of law lies in the tasks it performs, i.e. what it actually does. This approach focuses on law in its social context, namely the role it plays as a social institution in relation to other processes and phenomena in society such as politics and economics. Yet to talk about law having a purpose is in one sense misleading because law is an abstraction, a set of rules and principles. In itself it therefore has no mind of its own (Atiyah, 1995). Rather, it is those who make and enforce the law who have purposes that they wish the law to achieve. Often the purposes of the law-makers, at least on a general level, are very clear. For example, the intention behind the Abortion Act 1967 was to radically reform the law on abortion. With this kind of legislation it is not difficult to ascribe to the law itself the purposes that are actually held by the law-makers. But sometimes it is much harder to do this, especially when an Act of Parliament is very complex or a particular section is badly drafted. The difficulty in saying what are the purposes of the law is summed up by Atiyah when he describes the multilayered process by which the law develops:

> *the common law, or even statute law, once encrusted with interpretative case law, is not the work of a single mind, or even of a small number of minds. Much of the common law is the work of generation after generation of judges, layer upon layer of juristic interpretation and commentary and classification.*   Atiyah (1995, p18)

But notwithstanding that 'the law' is not an independent institution with purposes of its own, it nevertheless can be said to have some very general functions. These are:

- **To maintain public order.** This function is often expressed in the cliché 'law and order'. It is performed by prohibiting and prosecuting deviant behaviour, i.e. criminalizing it.
- **To facilitate co-operative action.** This is achieved by recognizing certain basic interests – such as the right to own property and personal freedom.
- **To constitute and control the principal organs of power.** This is a process

that involves defining who has the right to exercise power in society and regulating political life (Farrar and Dugdale, 1990).

A similar approach to the social functions of law is taken by the American legal writer Karl Llewellyn (1893–1962). Llewellyn was a 'rule sceptic' who dismissed rules as 'pretty playthings'. He believed that the basic functions of law were twofold, namely to aid the survival of the community and to pursue justice, efficacy and a richer life. To fulfil these functions there were a number of 'law-jobs', which the institution of the law had to do. In his view no society could function effectively or even survive unless these jobs were performed. They were, in other words, fundamental to every community or social organization irrespective of its size because group life is 'potentially conflictual, potentially chaotic, and potentially destructive' (Adams and Brownsword, 1996, p. 11). They include establishing mechanisms and procedures for preventing and resolving disputes; regulating group life (by e.g. giving effect to private arrangements such as family, contract and property law); encouraging social cohesion; and allocating authority within the group. Although these jobs are common to all societies the way they are carried out will, of course, vary from society to society.

Finally a brief word about justice. In one sense the whole of the law can be said to be concerned with justice. Judges are appointed to do justice according to the law whether they administer criminal or civil law (Raphael, 1994). Achieving justice can thus be described as one of the most basic aims or functions of the law. Yet the scope of justice is much wider than law, even though the two are often referred to as if they were synonymous. Superficially, this coupling might not seem inappropriate in so far as a law that does not aspire to 'do justice' hardly merits the label 'law' at all. Also, notions of justice can be used as a measure for testing the law, in the sense that a court that reaches its decision by applying accepted standards of legal reasoning can be said to have done justice according to the law.

But tying law and justice together is problematic for several reasons. One is that ideas of justice are so variable that there is unlikely ever to be an agreed set of 'just aims' that can be identified as those to which the law must aspire. Another is that, however well-intentioned a legal rule might be in itself, it might nonetheless lead to an unjust outcome in a particular case – for example, when laws against terrorism result in the imprisonment of innocent people. Finally, conflating law and justice is misleading because it implies that the law is more committed to achieving justice than any other institution in society.

WHAT MAKES THE LAW VALID? – THE RELATIONSHIP BETWEEN LAW AND MORALITY

If the link between law and justice is thus not all that clear, it becomes important to ask another question: What makes the law valid? This is a question that raises fundamental issues about the 'proper' relationship between law and morality. It is also one that has long divided two of the strongest traditions in legal philosophy: legal positivism and natural law doctrine.

There are several different versions of **natural law** and its supporters include the Greek philosopher Aristotle and the medieval scholar St Thomas Aquinas. But all theorists adopting this approach believe that law should reflect morality – in other words, that it should have some moral content and that it should embody basic human rights, which governments should respect. Central to the doctrine is the view that natural law is a kind of higher law that stands above and apart from the activities of human law-makers. It is stronger than any statute or other 'man-made' law because it reflects absolute values and ideals, which are universal. As such it represents a basic moral code (although its content may well differ according to the specific natural law stance taken), which can be used to test the morality of human laws and which can be understood by everyone simply by use of their reason. Most importantly, human laws that conflict with natural law are regarded as invalid – for example, many of the laws passed by Nazi Germany. In short, they are wrong and unjust and therefore not 'law' at all (Elliott and Quinn, 1998).

A very different approach is taken by **legal positivists**. Legal positivism has its roots in the writings of Jeremy Bentham (1748–1832), a very influential legal reformer and social critic who was so appalled by the lack of professionalism of the legal profession that he refused to become a lawyer like his father. Bentham objected to the way 18th century lawyers justified particular laws and legal institutions by reference to natural law and natural rights – which he dismissed as 'nonsense on stilts'. For him, property rights (and the laws that protected them) did not predate society but were a product of it. As such, they were no more natural than any other rights that a particular society might chose to protect by law. Laws were, in other words a human creation, made by humans for humans, and there was nothing sacred and mysterious about them.

There are many variations of legal positivism. All, however, consider the question: 'What is the law'? to be separate from the question: 'What should the law be?' The law can thus be separated from what is just or morally right. The main elements of the positivist approach consist of the following principles:

- Law is essentially a command by a legislative or other body. It is therefore the creation of human beings (and so can be made or unmade when they wish) and does not derive its validity from any superior order.
- There is no necessary connection between law and morality in the sense that law is 'value-neutral' and so can still be valid despite being 'bad'. Whether a 'bad' law should be obeyed is, of course, another matter.
- Law and legal concepts can be understood by 'scientific' enquiry, i.e. one that is objective and pure.

The different approaches taken by the naturalist and positivist schools of philosophy are linked to another long-standing debate about the relationship between law and morality, in particular whether the law should follow and enforce morality. The most recent airing of this debate was triggered by the publication in the late 1950s of the Wolfenden Report, which recommended that homosexuality and prostitution should be legalized, with some restrictions. That the law has always enforced some morality is, of course, self evident. Thus most people would agree that to survive every society must have basic rules restricting violence, theft, deception, and so on. As a consequence laws that prohibit such behaviour do uphold moral positions but are largely uncontroversial. But what about sexual morality, euthanasia and abortion? The diversity of modern society make it unlikely that there will be much of a consensus on where the legal boundaries should be drawn on these and similar issues. It was not surprising therefore that the report was so hotly debated.

The Wolfenden Committee argued that there were some areas of behaviour that should be left to individual morality and should be beyond the scrutiny of the law. Lord Devlin was one of its sternest critics. He believed that morals and religion were inextricably linked and in his book *The Enforcement of Morals* (1965) he argued very strongly that society – which is made up of people with a shared, common public morality – had not only the right but also the duty to pass judgement on moral matters. As a consequence it also had the right and the duty to use the law to punish acts that the 'right-minded man' considered morally wrong. In fact, society must condemn such activities since its very existence depended on the enforcement of its public morality, without which it would disintegrate. His views are well summed up in the much quoted passage: 'the suppression of vice is as much the law's business as the suppression of subversive activities' (Devlin, 1965, p. 13).

Devlin's views were controversial, even though he acknowledged that different societies had different moralities and insisted that the law should only concern itself with the minimum necessary for the preservation of society, so that as far as possible privacy should be respected. Nevertheless, he did believe that behaviour that caused a real feeling of reprobation should not be tolerated and that there were no theoretical limits to the State's right to legislate against immorality. Not surprisingly Devlin's thesis prompted much debate. Many supported his view that the Committee's recommendations were too liberal. Others rejected his conservative approach for failing to keep up with the times.

One of his main opponents was H. L. A. Hart. Hart opposed what he called Devlin's 'legal moralism', i.e. the view that general agreement among the members of society that conduct is immoral is a ground for legally prohibiting it (Harris, 1997). Hart's starting point in his essay 'Law, Liberty and Morality' (1968) was the 'harm principle' identified by John Stuart Mill (1806–73). Briefly, that principle asserts that law should not be used to uphold morality but should only seek to prevent harm to others. This meant that people should largely be left to make their own choices and do what they like as long as they do not harm anyone else. Hart's concern was to protect the liberty of the individual. Nevertheless, he did concede that, given every society's limited resources, it must have rules against violence, theft and deception since minimum forms of protection for persons, property and promises were indispensable to any social grouping. Furthermore he accepted that society could act paternalistically to prevent people doing themselves physical harm. However, he denied that any society needed to have a shared morality beyond these very basic rules. Moreover, even supposing that agreement could be reached on moral issues – which he doubted was ever possible – he did not accept that society's survival depended on preserving and enforcing them.

CLASSIFICATION OF LAW

The law is usually classified into public and private law, and into civil and criminal law.

Public law

This comprises the criminal law and the constitutional and administrative rules governing how public bodies such as local authorities, the courts, civil service, the police and other public institutions operate. It thus includes the law relating to the provision of health services and the legal rules that are designed to protect the civil liberties and rights of citizens and enable them to question how public law agencies such as health authorities and NHS trusts exercise their powers and statutory duties.

Private law

Private law deals with the legal relationship between private individuals and organizations. It has several functions. These include regulating the provision of health care and providing a system of compensation for the victims of malpractice. It also creates rights and duties and other liabilities arising from 'private' arrangements such as property and commercial transactions.

Civil law

Actions in civil law are typically based on a claim that a remedy – usually money paid as damages – be recovered from another party. Civil law comprises a very large area, including every division of private law and all of public law except the criminal law. Those sections of civil law most likely to involve nurses are as follows.

Tort law

A tort is a civil wrong recognized by the law that arises independently of any agreement between the parties. The word comes from the Latin *tortus* meaning 'twisted' or 'wrong'. It includes many different types of action, such as trespass, negligence, defamation, breach of statutory duty and nuisance. One of the main aims of tort law is to provide compensation when someone is harmed – physically or economically – by another. Consent-related claims – such as battery (i.e. trespass to the person) – and those arising from allegations of professional malpractice (i.e. medical negligence) are examples of tort actions that might involve nurses.

Contract law

Put simply, contract law is all about agreements and promises. However, not all agreements are legally enforceable, since what counts as a binding agreement for legal purposes is often very different from our everyday understanding of the term. Agreements are legally binding (which means that you can be sued for breaking them) only if both parties have 'paid' some kind of price, meaning that they have given something of value in return for their promise. Employment disputes are contract-based, as are those that involve private patients. Contract law may also be relevant should a victim of a drug-induced injury want to sue the manufacturer or seller of a harmful drug.

Family law

This branch of the law deals with legal relationships within the family and so includes divorce, domestic violence and most disputes about the care and upbringing of children. Child-centred disputes typically focus on the exercise and scope of parental responsibility but are likely to involve nurses only when they concern health care – controversial medical treatment, for example, or disputes about consent, i.e. when life-saving surgery for a young child is refused by his/her parents.

Criminal law

Although criminal law may well be the branch of the law that attracts most attention it is in practice the least likely to involve nurses in their everyday dealings with patients. Basically it includes any behaviour (an act or omission) that the state considers harmful or disruptive and so hopes to prevent by punishing offenders. In some cases there is an overlap between criminal and civil law. For example, treating a patient without consent is a civil wrong and a crime. A nurse whose negligent behaviour harms a patient may therefore be sued and face criminal charges. Criminal prosecutions are almost always brought by the state but private prosecutions are not unknown.

The court system

Only a relatively small proportion of medical disputes are dealt with in the courts since the vast majority are resolved through various complaints procedures. But despite their very minor role the courts are still regarded as the focal point of the English legal system. The court system can be classified in a number of ways.

Criminal and civil courts

Generally, civil courts deal with civil disputes and criminal courts with criminal cases, although there are some courts that hear both civil and criminal cases. Whether the court is exercising its civil or criminal jurisdiction, however, it has three main functions. The first is to investigate the facts; the second is to identify and formulate the relevant legal issues and rules, which involves applying the law to the facts; the third is to reach a decision, i.e. to decide 'what the law is' or 'what the law ought to be'.

European Court of Human Rights
(Strasbourg)

HOUSE OF LORDS

- Hears appeals from Court of Appeal
  and the Divisional Court of Queen's
  Bench

COURT OF APPEAL: CRIMINAL DIVISION

- Hears appeals against conviction and
  sentence
- Is not bound to follow previous
  decisions if this would cause injustice

HIGH COURT: QUEEN'S BENCH DIVISION

- Deals with criminal appeals and judicial
  review of inferior courts

CROWN COURT

- Bound by all courts above it
- Does not create binding precedents
- Tries most serious criminal offences on
  indictment with a jury
- Hears appeals from magistrates'
  criminal cases

MAGISTRATES' COURT

- Hears summary trials (i.e. magistrates
  decide the verdict and the sentence)
- Acting as youth courts tries young
  offenders

Figure 1.1   Criminal courts

EUROPEAN COURT OF
JUSTICE (LUXEMBOURG)

- Supervises uniform application
  of community law
- Hears disputes between member
  states and proceedings against
  EC institutions

EUROPEAN COURT
OF HUMAN RIGHTS

- Hears cases brought by
  individuals alleging breach of
  the Convention of Human
  Rights and Fundamental
  Freedoms

HOUSE OF LORDS

- Highest superior appeal court
- Decisions bind all lower courts
- Decisions can be overruled by
  legislation or subsequent decisions
  of the House itself

COURT OF APPEAL CIVIL DIVISION

- Superior court hearing appeals from
  mainly High Court and County Court
- Decisions bind all lower courts
- Usually follows its own previous
  decisions

HIGH COURT

CHANCERY DIVISION

- Superior court hearing
  disputes about financial and
  property matters
- Can produce binding
  precedents for inferior courts

QUEEN'S BENCH DIVISION

- Largest Division and superior
  court dealing with complicated
  civil disputes such as tort (medical
  negligence) and contract
- Can produce precedents for
  inferior courts

FAMILY DIVISION

- Superior court hearing all
  types of case about the family,
  including disputes about
  children's medical treatment
- Can produce binding
  precedents for inferior courts

DIVISIONAL COURT

As a divisional court the Queen's Bench Division deals with criminal appeals and judicial review (a procedure
for overseeing decisions of public bodies and officials). The Chancery Divisional Court hears appeals from
County Court (in bankruptcy cases) and the Family Divisional Court hears appeals from magistrates' courts in
family proceedings.

COUNTY COURTS

- Inferior court with limited
  jurisdiction, which hears less
  serious civil disputes including
  some family cases
- Bound by decisions of all
  superior courts
- Own decisions not officially
  reported and have no binding
  force

MAGISTRATES' COURT

- Inferior court with limited civil
  jurisdiction, e.g. licensing and
  hearings under the Children
  Act 1989

Note also:
1. *Coroner's Court*, which investigates unexplained deaths and holds inquests to establish how, where and when the deceased
died.
2. *Tribunals*, which provide a system of adjudication that is less formal and more accessible than courts; examples include
employment, mental health tribunals and domestic tribunals.

Figure 1.2   Civil courts

First-instance and appeal courts

Courts can be either first-instance ones, where cases are heard for the first time, or appeal courts. Some courts hear cases both at first instance and on appeal. An appeal system is necessary not just because judges can make mistakes (about facts or the law) but because the law needs constantly to develop to reflect social and other changes in society. The appeal courts have considerable powers to review, adapt and create new law.

The courts

House of Lords

This is the highest appeal court. It hears both civil and criminal appeals. Although very few cases reach the House of Lords its decisions are very important since they bind every other court in the system. It is not bound by its own previous decisions but only very rarely overrules them. One such example is *R v. R* [1992] 1 AC 599, when the House of Lords overruled a centuries-old rule that rape within marriage was not a crime.

Court of Appeal

The Court of Appeal plays a major role in the development of the law, as it hears far more appeals than the House of Lords. As a result it has considerable influence over the pace and nature of legal reform because its decisions are binding on all courts below it in the hierarchy, i.e. all courts except the House of Lords. The Court of Appeal has two divisions. One hears civil appeals and the other deals with criminal appeals. It is bound by decisions of the House of Lords. The civil division is usually bound by its own decisions except in a few rare circumstances. The criminal division follows its own previous decisions unless this would cause injustice.

High Court

This court has three divisions. All divisions hear cases for the first time as well as having an appellate jurisdiction. As a court of first instance the Queen's Bench Division is the largest and busiest. It deals with major civil disputes such as tort claims (i.e. medical negligence cases). The Family Division hears all aspects of family law including those involving children, such as disputed medical treatment. The Chancery Division deals with financial and property matters. High Court decisions bind lower courts.

Crown Court

This court tries the most serious criminal cases 'on indictment', i.e. with a jury. It also hears appeals from the magistrates' courts. The Crown Court is bound by courts above it but its decisions are not binding.

Magistrates' and County courts

Magistrates try the vast majority of criminal cases (about 97%). When trying the least serious criminal cases they decide the facts, the law and the sentence. When hearing committal proceedings their role is to makes sure that there is sufficient evidence for a Crown Court trial. Magistrates' courts also have a very limited civil jurisdiction. County courts are at the bottom of the civil court ladder but process far more claims than any other civil court. They also deal with some family matters. As inferior courts, the magistrates' and county courts are bound by the superior courts.

Coroners' courts

The main function of coroners courts is to investigate unexplained deaths (such as those allegedly caused by medical negligence) and those where death was violent, unnatural or suspicious, e.g. suspected suicides. After a death has been reported a coroner may order a post-mortem examination to find out the cause of death. Depending on the outcome of this an inquest may be held. An inquest is not a trial but is held to establish how, where and when the deceased died. Sometimes a jury will be used at an inquest.

The European Court of Justice

This court's role is to ensure that European Union law is enforced and inter-preted uniformly throughout the EU. It sits in Luxembourg and hears cases against member states and proceedings against EU institutions.

Court of Human Rights

As a member of the European Convention of Human Rights it is possible for UK citizens who allege that a basic right of freedom has been violated to have their claim referred to the Court of Human Rights in Strasbourg. Access to the court may be restricted, however, once the Human Rights Act 1998 comes into force (due in October 2000).

Sources of law

English law derives from three main sources.

Legislation

This is now the main source of law. There are two types of legislation – primary and secondary. **Primary legislation** consists of Acts of Parliament (also called **statutes**). Before becoming law, Acts have to pass through several formal and, if they are controversial, fairly lengthy stages in both Houses of Parliament. All statutes start life as Bills. Their process through parliament consists of a First Reading and Second Reading in the House of Commons, during which time the proposals are debated, usually amended, and then voted on. The Committee Stage comes next, when the Bill is examined in detail by a parliamentary committee. Its report back to the House of Commons – when any proposed amendments are debated and voted upon – is called the Report Stage. The Third Reading follows, at which stage a vote is taken on whether to accept or reject the Bill. The next stage is for the Bill to go to the House of Lords. Here it also has three readings and will be returned to the House of Commons only if the House of Lords proposes changes. The House of Lords cannot, however, now block legislation that has been put forward by the House of Commons.

There are three types of Bill. **Public Bills** are initiated by the government of the day and reflect government policy. **Private members' Bills** are prepared by individual backbenchers but very few of this kind of Bill actually make the statute book because they depend on the government allocating parliamentary time – always in short supply – to debating them. They are nonetheless a useful way of drawing attention to controversial social or moral issues and do sometimes, as with the Abortion Act 1967, eventually become law. The third type of Bill is the **Private Bill**, which is usually introduced by a local authority or large public company.

Whatever its origins a Bill can only become law when it receives the Royal Assent. Even then the Act may not come into force immediately as it is not uncommon for several months, if not longer, to elapse before it is finally implemented.

New legislation can be influenced by many different factors. The work of law reform agencies such as the Law Commission and Royal Commissions are particularly persuasive, as are public enquiries, which are often set up following a major disaster. New legislation also typically follows a change of government. The internal market reforms introduced in the National Health Service and Community Care Act 1990 are a example of this type of party political legislation. It usually is preceded by a **Green Paper** (a consultation document), which will involve consultation with ministers, the civil service and other non-parliamentary bodies such as special interest pressure groups, charities, and so on. A **White Paper** may also then be issued, which sets out the government's intentions. An example is the proposals for the NHS set out in the 1997 White Paper *The New NHS: Modern, Dependable.*

Other Acts, especially those that deal with controversial moral or social issues, may be introduced as a swift response to a particular event or 'moral panic'. The Surrogacy Arrangements Act 1985, for example, was enacted very shortly after the 'Baby Cotton' case (in which an American couple commissioned an English woman to have their baby) hit the headlines, raising fears of 'baby selling' and 'womb leasing'. This kind of legislation is sometimes preceded by a committee of enquiry. One of the most well known of these was the Warnock Committee, which was set up to consider the implications of the reproductive technologies and advances that had been made in relation to conception and pregnancy. Its report in 1984 eventually led to the Human Fertilisation and Embryology Act 1990.

Much of the structure, organization and administrative framework of the health service is governed by legislation, e.g. the National Health Service Act 1977, the National Health Service and Community Care Act 1990 and the Health Act 1999. Legislation also governs the day-to-day work of nurses in the form of the Nurses, Midwives and Health Visitors Act 1997. Other Acts that regulate nursing practice include the Mental Health Act 1983, the Access to Health Records Act 1990 and the Data Protection Act 1998.

Delegated or **subordinate legislation** is the second type of legislation. It has the same legal force as primary legislation but is not subject to the same rigorous parliamentary scrutiny. Delegated legislation is passed by a wide variety of bodies ranging from government departments to local authorities and public corporations. There are several different types of delegated legislation but it typically consists of Statutory Instruments, usually in the form of Rules and Regulations. In its modern form this kind of legislation came into general use during the first half of the 19th century because the government was increasingly unable to deal with its ever-increasing legislative responsibilities. Reliance on this type of legislation has continued because many modern statutes are so complex that they can only be provide a broad framework and thus require much detailed and technical work before they can be implemented. Other reasons explaining the increase of subordinate legislation in recent years include speed and flexibility – it can be introduced very quickly and can be easily revoked if it turns out to be unworkable. Delegated legislation plays a major role in health service law – in fact its day-to day working depends on it (Miers and Page, 1990)

Common law

In the past, common law was the most important source of law. It dates from the 13th century but has roots going back even further, since it originates from local custom. Because it evolves over time as judges resolve particular disputes, the common law is also sometimes called **judge-made law** (or **case law**). Although statute law now far outstrips common law as a source of law, common law has significantly contributed to the development of health-care law, in particular the law of consent and negligence.

Common law develops through a system known as **precedent**, which requires courts to interpret similar cases – i.e. cases raising similar legal principles and involving similar facts and circumstances – in like manner. What this means is that in principle the courts are legally bound to follow earlier decisions. In other words, decided cases are binding authorities for the future. But not all the facts of a case are relevant to the decision that is eventually reached. Hence once the Gillick case (*Gillick* v. *West Norfolk and Wisbech AHA* [1986] AC 112 [1985] 3 All ER 402) established the legal principle that 'mature minors' could give consent to medical treatment and advice without their parents' knowledge or permission, subsequent cases had to apply that precedent irrespective of some of the 'facts' of subsequent disputes. Hence whether the minor is a boy or a girl, has red or brown hair or is 12 or 13, for example, is irrelevant. What counts is whether the minor is 'Gillick-competent', bearing in mind the nature of the treatment and all surrounding circumstances. Another famous example is *Donoghue* v. *Stevenson* [1932] AC 562, which laid the foundations for the law of negligence. The case involved a decomposing snail, a ginger-beer bottle and a woman who suffered shock and gastroenteritis as a result of drinking some of the ginger beer before the snail's remains floated out of the bottle. The precedent it established, the so-called 'neighbour principle', must be followed in subsequent cases that raise the same legal issues even though they may have nothing do with snails or ginger beer.

The system of binding precedent is based on the hierarchy of the courts. The hierarchical structure of the courts is in fact a distinctive feature of the English legal system. In general, the lower courts are bound to follow the decisions of the higher courts but appeals are usually possible. The system of judicial precedent is a complex process that has provoked much debate about the precise nature of the judges' role. Are judges neutral decision-makers who simply declare the law or do they have far more discretion and freedom to actually create new law? If so, what influences their decisions? For writers such as Griffith (1985) there is little doubt that judges' views of the 'public interest' are heavily influenced by their background and position in society. Others, for example Waldron (1989), concede that judges do exercise discretion and are influenced by political and ideological considerations, but claim that this is not necessarily a bad thing. In contrast, Dworkin (1977, 1986) asserts that judges have no real discretion in making case law. For him law is a 'seamless web of principles, which supply a right answer – and only one to every possible problem' (Elliott and Quinn, 1998, p. 11). Consideration of these questions is, however, outside the scope of this text. Nevertheless, it is clear that judges do have some choices. They can, for example, avoid 'inconvenient' precedents by resorting to various techniques such as 'distinguishing' the case in question from the precedent, i.e. showing that there are important factual differences between the two cases. Alternatively, if the precedent is obscure, or has been reversed or overruled, it can be ignored.

Although the common law is no longer a major source of law it has several advantages. These include certainty – as judges have to follow previous cases their decisions are more likely to be consistent. Furthermore, because the common law develops when 'real' cases come to court it can also be very flexible and respond quickly to changes in society and the needs of everyday life. But the common law does have disadvantages. One is that it can be a very lengthy process. It is not unknown, for example, for cases alleging professional malpractice to take 10 years to go through the various appeal stages in the courts. Moreover, some cases are so complex that it can be almost impossible to establish clear principles from them. Another major criticism is that it is too rigid a system, which can force judges to make illogical distinctions if they want to avoid a binding precedent. It can also develop far too slowly, if at all in some instances, since it depends on cases being brought before the courts (Geldart, 1995).

European law

As a member of the European Union the UK is subject to European law and treaties. European law can override both judge-made law and legislation as it takes precedence over national laws. There are four main types of European law:

- Treaties under which European law is established and operates are the highest source of EC law. They can create rights and obligations but require detailed legislation before they can be enforced.

- Regulations, which must be directly applied by all member states, closely resemble Acts of Parliament and become law as soon as they come into force.
- Directives set out broad objectives and so are much vaguer than Regulations. Nevertheless, they do have direct effect and so must be applied by member states.
- Decisions, which may apply to a state, a person or a company, are binding only on those to whom they are addressed.

Most of English law is unaffected by membership of the EU, which in legal terms deals mainly with economic activity. European law does nevertheless have an impact on nursing practice. In particular, it governs the mutual recognition of professional qualifications and regulates the pharmaceutical industry. Much of English health and safety legislation is also based on European Directives, as are equal-pay provisions of employment law. The European Court (which sits in Luxembourg) is responsible for ensuring that EU law is observed.

Other sources of law

In addition to the main sources of law noted above, law can also come into existence from other processes.

Equity

In simple legal terms, equity means fairness. It provides a body of rules that are distinct from the common law but just as binding. Many of these rules deal with a variety of discretionary remedies that may be available to a wronged party.

The European Convention of Human Rights

The Convention provisions have now been incorporated into UK law by the Human Rights Act 1998. Once the Act is in force individuals will be able to seek redress for breach of a human right without taking their case to the European Court of Human Rights. No specific health rights are granted by the Convention, although several have health-care implications, in particular the right to life and the right to marry and start a family.

'Non-legal' sources

Included in this final category are several very important non-legal 'rules'. While they cannot be described as 'law' in the strict sense of the word, i.e. they are not usually legally binding, they are nonetheless so influential in shaping nursing practice and setting the standards by which nurses will be judged that they arguably have the same status as law. This explains why they are often referred to as **quasi-law**. Montgomery (1997, p. 12), for example, describes their effect as follows: '[T]here may be no legal sanction against failure to obey such rules, but in most circumstances they will be followed, and therefore any survey of the norms which govern practice must take them into account.'

The primary source of quasi-law derives mainly from communications from the NHS Executive, which provide advice to health authorities, NHS trusts and individual practitioners. These can take several forms: Circulars (HCs); guidance (sometimes called health service guidelines, HSGs) and executive instructions (EIs). They can cover a variety of matters and, as they are designed to be accessible to the layperson, they are generally written in jargon-free language. When linked to a particular statute or case (the Gillick case, for example, was followed by HC(86)1), circulars are most likely to identify areas of change, explain underlying principles and discuss implications for policy and practice. Heath service guidelines are normally issued by the NHS Executive and give guidance on policy and operational matters. Executive letters are meant to give guidance about policy or legislative changes.

The other major type of quasi law is the code of practice and similar publications. A very important code for nurses is the UKCC *Code of Professional Conduct* (1992) and the more recent *Guidelines for Professional Practice* (1996). Note too other UKCC guidelines that are regularly issued on particular aspects of practice, for example the *Standards for the Administration of Medicines* (1992). Codes and professional guidelines are likely to be taken into account in disciplinary and complaints proceedings. Failure to comply with them could also be used in legal proceedings.

WHAT IS ETHICS?

Texts on nursing ethics are now almost commonplace. This is perhaps not surprising given that ethics has been described 'not only as at the heart of nursing, [but] as the heart of nursing' (Tschudin, 1996, p. 9). Yet, despite the widespread acceptance that the study of ethics is essential for nurses, the term is not an easy one to define. Why should this be so?

The main explanation is that when we talk about ethics several other terms typically come to mind, e.g. words such as 'rights', 'duties', 'obligations'. Often, too, the term is described in terms of 'morality' and so involves articulating certain moral principles and notions such as rightness and wrongness, guilt and shame, and so on (Routledge, 2000, p. 256). As a consequence, the terms 'ethics' and 'morals' have become almost synonymous, in the sense that an 'ethical' action is one that is morally acceptable, i.e. the right thing to do (Edwards, 1996, p. 3, see also Singer, 1979, p. 1; Johnstone, 1989, p. 28).

But even though both terms originally derived from the same roots and the general ideal of right and wrong – 'ethics' coming from the Greek and 'morals' from its Latin equivalent – morality is a distinct sphere within ethics and distinctions are sometimes drawn between them. Thus the word 'morals' (and 'morality') is more often used to describe the standards of behaviour actually held or followed by individuals and particular groups of people, whereas 'ethics' tends to refer to the science or study of morals, a much more academic approach, which has its own name – **moral philosophy** (Thompson *et al.*, 1994, p. 3).

How then should ethics be defined for the purposes of this book? A two-pronged approach will be taken. First, the convention of treating the terms 'ethics' and 'morals' interchangeably will be adopted. Secondly, ethics will be seen as concerning itself with what is right and wrong, good and bad in human actions. In other words 'with judging what we do and the consequences of what we do and considering the justifications that might be given for our moral positions' (Nuttall, 1993, p. 1).

ETHICAL THEORIES

According to Beauchamp and Childress (1994, p. 44), ethical theories: 'provide a framework within which agents can reflect on the acceptability of actions and can evaluate moral judgements and moral character'. Some knowledge of these theories is therefore indispensable if nurses are to deal with the ethical problems they often have to face. This is because the moral intuition that people ordinarily rely on in their everyday lives is of limited use in health-care settings. In hospitals, for example, where patients are in unfamiliar surroundings and may feel vulnerable, they may not act as they normally would. Medical technology, too, such as life-support procedures, is likely to involve nurses in very different situations from those they would have to deal with in normal circumstances (Edwards, 1996). There are many ethical theories but the two that have most influenced moral reasoning in modern times are **consequentialism** and **deontology**.

Consequentialism

Consequentialist theories are sometimes called **teleological** (from the Greek *telos*, meaning 'end'). For the consequentialist the rightness or wrongness of actions depends on their consequences. Put crudely, this means that the right (or moral) thing to do is that which produces the best possible outcome. But what is the best outcome? In health-care contexts this would include the prevention, elimination or control of disease, relief from unnecessary pain and suffering, amelioration of disabling conditions, the prolongation of life, promotion of health, and so on. More specifically, the best outcome will depend on the goal chosen by the particular teleological theory in question. There are many consequentialist theories but the best known is **utilitarianism**.

Utilitarianism

Put very simply utilitarians do not regard actions as inherently good or bad – they are valuable only in so far as they are a means to an end. A nurse who was a utilitarian would therefore make a decision about truth-telling on the basis of the consequence of her actions. She would have to decide what the consequences would be of telling the truth and not being truthful. The morally right approach for her would then be to act in the way that led to the desired consequence (Edwards, 1996). The most famous proponents of utilitarianism were two English philosophers: Jeremy Bentham (1748–1832) and John Stuart Mill (1806–73). Bentham wanted to provide a coherent and rational foundation for social and legal policy. To do so he adopted a 'scientific' approach to the study of law and morality that was based on his interpretation of human nature as developed through the concept of utility. In its most general sense, utility means simply 'useful'. But for Bentham it meant useful for promoting what he felt motivated human beings, namely to seek out pleasure and avoid pain. Accordingly, the morally right action was the one that produced the greatest net balance of pleasure over pain. Bentham's classic formulation has been immortalized in the famous slogan: 'the greatest happiness for the greatest number'. But his formula for measuring and classifying actions, in particular the 'felicific calculus' (the method he used to work out 'happiness sums'), was modified by Mill. The calculus involved working out how intense the happiness would be, how long it would last, how likely it was to occur, whether it had any unpleasant side-effects, and so on. But the calculation was based on a quantitative approach that treated all actions as equally good as long as they produced the same amount of pleasure. Mill rejected this approach. He believed that there were qualitative differences between different kinds of pleasure. He also wanted to ensure that individuals could think and behave as they wished as long as they did not interfere with the freedom of others (his famous 'harm principle'). Mill's conception of utility allowed him to grade activities into higher and lower ones. Scoring highest marks – because they were intrinsically more worthy – were the intellectual and aesthetic pleasures. The lowest scores were allocated to purely physical and sensual pleasures.

Bentham and Mill are both described as **hedonistic utilitarians** (from the Greek *hedone*, meaning 'pleasure') because they defined utility in terms of pleasure and happiness. Their versions of utilitarianism were certainly popular, not least because they reduced all moral judgements, however complex, to a straightforward calculation. In addition most people would support their overall aim of reducing suffering and maximizing happiness. Yet, many criticisms have been raised against them. Here are some:

- The felicific calculus is impractical because it assumes that such subjective concepts as pleasure, happiness and pain can be accurately measured and estimated (Thompson *et al.*, 1994; Gillon, 1985). It also assumes (wrongly) that the consequences of actions can always be reliably predicted.
- Because utilitarianism treats human beings as means rather than ends in themselves it is conceivable that the theory can lead to injustice, with individual rights being sacrificed for the sake of a greater quantity of happiness all round.
- Utilitarianism may treat individual persons equally, but only by effectively treating them as having no worth. This is because they are valued not as persons but as 'experiencers' of pleasure or happiness.
- The concept of utility is flawed, since it fails to identify or provide any satisfactory mechanism for deciding whose interests should be promoted. Should all members of a particular community, of whatever age, present or future generations, be included? What about all sentient creatures? As Harris

notes, unless the concept of utility can provide some kind of answer to these and similar questions, it is difficult to know where to draw the line (Harris, 1997).

• The utility principle is unworthy. Satisfying all human desires should not be the aim of morality, as some 'pleasures' are gross (e.g. torturing children) whereas some forms of suffering are ennobling (Harris, 1997).

In an attempt to respond to some of these criticisms different versions of utilitarianism have been proposed. 'Ideal utilitarians', such as G. E. Moore (1873–1958), claim that goodness cannot be defined in terms of pleasure and pain and regard values other than happiness as having intrinsic moral worth – values such as friendship, knowledge, love, beauty and health. Accordingly, the rightness of an action is judged in terms of how far it enables these values to be realized and enjoyed (Singer, 1993).

A distinction is also now recognized between **act utilitarianism** and **rule utilitarianism.** Act utilitarianism requires each and every action to be individually scrutinized. This means that whenever a decision has to be made the consequences have to be calculated and the option chosen that maximizes the benefits. Rule utilitarians, on the other hand, calculate the consequences of adopting a certain set of rules – such as 'Do not kill' or 'Do not lie'. It is these general rules that determine whether an act is right or wrong (Fletcher *et al.*, 1995). An act is right, therefore, if it falls under the right rule, because following the rule results in more happiness (or some other specified goal) than not following the rule. Accordingly, the rule should be adopted as a moral principle whatever the consequences of applying it in individual cases.

Deontology

The other major ethical theory that has dominated Western moral philosophy is *deontology* (from the Greek *deon* meaning 'duty' and *logos* meaning 'word'). Like utilitarianism, it is committed to promoting 'good' outcomes but unlike its rival (which regards motives as unimportant), deontology considers a person's intentions to be crucial in determining the moral worth of his or her actions. The deontologist believes that there are fundamental rules that must be followed whatever the consequences. In other words, there are certain sorts of act that are right or wrong in themselves because of the sort of act they are rather than what effect they have or may have. Deontological theories regard concepts such as duty and obligation as central. But as with utilitarianism there are several different versions.

Classic deontology, for example, has a religious basis according to which moral duties derive from 'divine command' as in the Ten Commandments (Johnstone, 1989). But the leading deontological theory is that of Immanuel Kant (1724–1804). The son of very pious parents of Scottish extraction, Kant was a brilliant German academic who studied and taught philosophy. Although he was a devout Christian he rejected a theological framework for his system of ethics and constructed instead a theory of morality independent of religion and irrespective of considerations about God's existence. Put very simply, Kant believed that morality was basically about complying with a set of compulsory rules and that it was through the use of reason rather than, for example, emotion, inclination or conscience that individuals – who were rational beings – could know what duties were expected of them and what was the right thing to do.

For Kant an action had moral worth only so far as it was done out of a sense of duty (Singer 1994). Acts motivated by self-interest, convenience or ambition were not therefore morally praiseworthy even if they involved or resulted in keeping a promise or, say, being kind and helpful to others. This is because Kant drew a moral distinction between an act done out of respect for duty – in which autonomy plays a central role – and one done out of inclination or coercion. The latter might well accord with moral duty but was not a moral action because it did not depend on 'the will' (the mind) being free to make moral decisions (Edwards, 1996).

To identify what the compulsory rules are and thus what actions could be considered moral, Kant devised a universal test called the 'categorical imperative' or more generally the Moral Law. He formulated his theory in *Groundwork of the Metaphysic of Morals* (1785). The best known version of the imperative (there are several versions) runs: 'Act only on that maxim through which you can at the same time will that it should become universal law'. This is the keystone of Kant's ethics, which establishes the standard by which all moral action was to be judged. It also coincides with the Judaeo-Christian golden rule: 'Do as you would be done by'. The essential features of Kant's ethical theory can be reduced to the following propositions:

1. If you wish to act morally, act as if your action in each circumstance is to become law for everyone, yourself included, in the future.
2. If you wish to act morally, always treat other human beings as 'ends in themselves' and never merely as 'means'. In other words, it is always wrong to treat people as objects, i.e. mere tools to be used to further your own ambitions and ends.
3. If you wish to act morally, always act as a member of a community where all the other members of that community are 'ends' just as you are (Seedhouse, 1988, pp. 97–98).

Overall, Kant's theory of morality amounts to the view that:

> *Moral beings are free, rational and capable of self-legislation. We call them 'persons' in order to distinguish them from the rest of nature, as the bearers of rights and duties. A person must always be treated as an end (he cannot be exploited, manipulated, abused, enslaved or trampled on). He is an equal member of an ideal community, and takes up his place in that community to the extent that he obeys the moral law. Towards the rational being I owe the same respect that I owe the moral law itself. This obligation is impartial and objective, and overrides all those arbitrary distinctions of race, creed and custom that divide the nations from each other.*   Scruton (1994, p. 286)

Kant's system of ethics is the best known and most influential secular moral theory, despite his own application of it, which led him to forbid lying, suicide, revolution against the existing political order, solitary sex and selling one's hair for wig-making. Yet it has been attacked on many fronts. Here are some of the main objections:

- It imposes rules that are too absolutist, rigid and insensitive and so cannot take account of differences between cases nor accommodate any exceptions to the compulsory moral rules it prescribes. As Seedhouse points out (1988, pp. 100–1), there may be situations in health-care contexts where it is justifiable to lie. He suggests, for example, that there is a duty not to tell a man badly injured in a car crash and fighting for his life that his wife and children have been killed. Only when the man's condition is no longer critical should that information be revealed.
- It provides no guidance on how choices should be made when duties conflict (e.g. between telling the truth and lying to protect someone). This is because 'trade-offs' between differing obligations are not part of the theory and so there is no routine procedure for dealing with conflict. What should a nurse do, for example, if she is asked by a terminally ill child patient not to tell his parents that he knows he is dying? Keeping that promise may mean that she has to lie to the child's parents. In this type of situation it seems that the nurse may not be able to keep her promise to the child and be truthful to his parents.
- It pays insufficient attention to consequences. Thus, while it is committed to the idea that patients should be autonomous and so have the right to decide and choose for themselves, it disregards considerations that may be no less important when determining the moral worth of an action. Thus in health-care contexts it may be equally important to consider other factors such as 'the probability of outcome and actual outcome' (Seedhouse, 1988, p. 103) irrespective of the treatment a patient may have requested.
- It seems to assume that people are saints rather than ordinary human beings. Hence it ignores the fact that we live in a complex world where life is messy and difficult to understand. In short, it is not always possible to act according to a universal code of conduct.

ETHICAL PRINCIPLES AND RULES

This brief account of the two most influential ethical theories is intended to provide an overarching justification for pursuing one course over another. However, the reason for reaching a particular decision or acting (or not acting) in a particular way will inevitably call upon some specific rule, which in turn will need to be justified by reference to a general principle. Ethical principles are fundamental moral rules that are used to justify actions (Fletcher *et al.*, 1995, p. 8). The relationship between ethical theories, principles and rules is well summed up by Melia (1989, pp 6–7):

First there are particular judgements that nurses make for individual cases.... At another level there are rules which state what ought and ought not to be done.... These rules are justified by more general principles.... Finally at the highest level of abstraction there are ethical theories....

So what are these principles? At a very general level they are basically about the kinds of values that health care can be said to be all about – in other words, compassion, desire to relieve pain and suffering, promote health, and so on. More specifically, the following are widely accepted as the most important: respect for autonomy, beneficence, non-maleficence and justice (Childress, 1997).

Autonomy

This cardinal principle means recognizing patients as persons who are entitled to such basic human rights as the right to know, the right to privacy and the right to receive care and treatment (Thompson *et al.*, 1994, p. 60). In relation to capable persons, it refers to an individual's ability to come to his or her own decisions and requires nurses to respect the choices patients make concerning their own lives. Respect for autonomy also means the protection of those incapable of autonomy because of illness, injury, mental disorder or age (see also Chapter 2).

Beneficence and non-maleficence

Often perceived as the overriding duty in health care, beneficence means the duty to do good and maximize good. It obliges nurses to help their patients and clients by promoting and safeguarding their health and welfare. As such it can require positive action by nurses, e.g. becoming an advocate for a patient or client who is vulnerable – through illness or age, for example. Non-maleficence is sometimes considered alongside the duty of beneficence but also sometimes distinguished from it. The principle of non-maleficence imposes a duty to do no harm or to minimize harm. Less onerous than beneficence in the sense that it generates fewer obligations to take positive actions, it nevertheless requires nurses to refrain from doing anything that could be detrimental to others (see also Chapter 3).

Justice

This principle is perhaps the most complex since it can be interpreted in several different (sometimes contradictory) ways. It is also the one that is most strongly associated with the law. In simple terms, justice requires equal treatment of equal cases and equitable distribution of benefits – in other words no discrimination on the basis of sex, race, religion, or because of youth, age, and so on. For health professionals its main impact is in relation to controlling and allocating health resources (see also Chapter 5).

The importance of principles in ethical reasoning is of course primarily acknowledged by those who adopt a principle-based approach to ethics. The most well-known proponents of this approach are Beauchamp and Childress (1994). They regard principles as indispensable not because they function as precise action-guides telling us what to do in every circumstance but because they are general guides providing substantive guidance for the development of more detailed rules. As such they describe the characteristics of actions that make them morally right or wrong and so provide an essential starting point for moral reasoning. Edwards, who also takes a 'four principles' approach to nursing ethics (1996, pp. 48–49), considers an understanding of the role of principles in nursing practice to be essential. They are, he asserts:

> *easily applicable to the vast majority of moral problems faced by nurses ... providing a structure for the moral intuitions that are typically brought to problems ... and allow one to develop a coherent, well-motivated strategy for solving dilemmas.*

In addition, they reflect specific obligations and responsibilities set out in the UKCC *Code of Conduct* (1992) and thus reinforce the standards nurses are expected to reach.

The principles approach has, however, come under criticism for being too superficial or too limited. But, as Cribb points out (1995, p. 30), those who take this approach are not arguing that all ethical thinking can be reduced to a few words, but rather that they provide a reminder of the key dimensions of ethical thinking and a common vocabulary and framework for individuals with different outlooks or philosophies.

Turning finally to the role played by rules, it would seem that, although derived from principles (and sometimes described as derivative principles), they are more specific than principles and more restricted in their scope (Beauchamp and Childress, 1994). Put simply, this means that they flesh out principles by adding substance to them in a way that makes them more practically useful. Yet despite their differences rules share with principles the overall aim of guiding behaviour by prescribing what we should or should not do. Examples of specific rules given by Beauchamp and Childress (1994, p. 39) are: veracity, which imposes a obligation to tell the truth and not to lie or deceive others; privacy and confidentiality, which together impose obligations to respect the 'personal space' of individuals and their right to decide how personal information about them should be used. The fourth rule is fidelity, which imposes obligations to keep promises.

LAW and *ETHICS* – a comparison

In this final section the role of law and ethics in health care will be compared. That there is a close association between the two was recognized over a century ago by Lord Chief Justice Coleridge when he asserted that: 'It would not be correct to say that every moral obligation involves a legal duty; but every legal duty is founded on a moral obligation' (*R v. Instan* [1893] 1 QB at 453). The moral dimension to law has also been acknowledged by Ronald Dworkin, a leading modern legal philosopher. In describing the nature of law he claims that a moral dimension is inevitable to an action in law because:

a judge must decide not just who shall have what, but who has behaved well, who has met the responsibilities of citizenship, and who by design or greed or insensitivity has ignored his own responsibilities to others or exaggerated their's to him. If this judgement is unfair, then the community has inflicted a moral injury on one of its members because it has stamped him in some degree or dimension an outlaw.   (Dworkin, 1986, p. 2)

To claim that professional practice develops within a moral framework – albeit one that is constantly being restructured by contemporary society (Mason and McCall Smith, 1999, p. 15) – is therefore unlikely to be contentious. There can be little doubt, for example, of the influence of both law and ethics on the formulation of Codes of Professional Conduct and the various other guidelines and circulars that guide and regulate professional practice. This is because law and ethics are not only both normative and so specify what ought to be done but also aim to distinguish between the acceptable and the unacceptable by reflecting public opinion. They can both, therefore, be described as forms of social control, using rules, principles and standards to prescribe behaviour and so determine what kinds of actions are prohibited, permitted or required (Farrar and Dugdale, 1990). Both also share a common vocabulary – in which terms such as rights, duties, responsibilities and obligations dominate, as do concepts such as justice, fairness and equity – and have common roots that can be traced back to Judaeo-Christian traditions.

The clearest example of the close relationship between law and ethics is, of course, the criminal law, especially its prohibition of violence, theft and sexual crimes – actions that are widely accepted as both illegal and immoral. Less immediately obvious but nevertheless still informed by moral values are civil areas such as tort law, in particular negligence – which is based on the moral idea that those who harm others may have to pay compensation for the injuries they have caused. As Lord Atkin noted in the famous snail case *Donoghue* v. *Stevenson* [1932] AC 562, the biblical principle of 'love thy neighbour' must include 'do not harm thy neighbour' (Elliott and Quinn, 1998, p. 445). Similarly, the law of consent reflects ethical considerations, namely autonomy and the obligations it generates to respect the choices that people make about their own lives. Moral values also underpin the law of contract, in particular the principle that people should keep their promises and perform their agreements (Atiyah, 1979). To the extent that contract law also attempts to counter inequality of bargaining power, e.g. between unwary patients who buy defective drugs and drug manufacturers who can hide behind their wealth and control of the market, it can also be said to be concerned with respecting autonomy by protecting the vulnerable.

But the close relationship between law and ethics is evident in more explicit ways. This is most easily seen in legislation such as the Surrogacy Arrangements Act 1985, the Human Fertilisation and Embryology Act 1990 and the Abortion Act 1990. Yet case law too is increasingly likely to be concerned with moral issues as the courts struggle to keep pace with rapidly advancing medical technology. That the law sometimes fails to move as quickly as medicine, public mores and the expectations of patients is perhaps not surprising, particularly when the 'big' moral issues such as euthanasia, embryo experimentation and reproductive technologies are at stake. Take, for example, the Bland case (*Airedale NHS Trust* v. *Bland*, [1993] AC 789, see Chapter 9), which concerned a young football fan who was crushed in the Hillsborough football stadium disaster. Tony Bland survived in a persistent (sometimes called permanent) vegetative state for almost 3 years, at which point the courts had to decide whether it was any longer in his 'best interests' to keep him alive. This required them to consider such morally loaded concepts as medical futility (see Chapter 9) and the scope of the right of self-determination.

Now too that it is possible for children born with severe disabilities to survive much longer than in the past it is not surprising that their treatment has also been adjudicated (in cases like *Re B*, [1981] 1 WLR 1421; *Re C* [1989] 2 All ER 782 and *Re J*, [1990] 3 All ER 930, discussed in Chapter 9). Again, this has taken the courts into new areas as they have had to develop the law to meet unfamiliar situations raised by the ability to sustain life artificially.

Other cases with obvious moral implications have tended to focus on the allocation of health resources. The most well known of these was *R* v. *Cambridge HA* ex p. *B* [1995] 2 All ER 129 (see also Chapter 5). It involved a 10-year-old girl with leukaemia who unsuccessfully challenged the health authority's decision not to fund life-saving treatment. The case prompted wide public debate about the role of law in regulating access to treatment. Particularly interesting, however, was that in refusing to overturn the health authority's decision one of the judges expressly applied utilitarian considerations and the public interest to justify his approach. While it is rare that judges so explicitly use philosophical arguments in their summing up there can be little doubt that ethical theories, principles and rules do influence their decisions, especially when they have to develop the law to meet new situations. In cases in which the rights of the fetus are at stake – the 'forced' caesarean cases, for example (Chapter 6), Mill's harm-to-others principle is especially relevant in deciding whether the fetus has a right to life. Mill considered that individuals should be free to choose their own conduct except when doing so harmed others. But who counts as another? Are fetuses included? Are they persons or potential persons? These questions are clearly at the heart of this kind of case as they are in legislation about abortion and experimentation on embryos (Lee, 1986).

It seems self evident, then, that law and ethics do overlap. Perhaps this is because, as Raphael (1994, p. 68) has observed, 'even though justice in law and justice in ethics are distinct but not separate concepts' they appear in both. This, he argues, is so despite the fact that the concept of justice is less pervasive in ethics – where it is one of the most basic of the social virtues – than in law (the whole of which can be said to be concerned with justice). Yet the relationship between law and ethics is a complex one. What this means is that, although what is ethical will usually be legal and *vice versa*, this is not always so. Thus certain ethical principles are too vague to be translated into law or the law may not be a suitable instrument to enforce a moral idea. Telling lies, for example, is widely condemned as immoral yet there are very few laws against it. It also explains why English law does not force people to be Good Samaritans. Nurses, therefore, have no legal obligation to provide first-aid or any other treatment in an emergency when they are 'off duty', irrespective of any moral obligation to do so. Another fundamental difference between law and ethics relates to their overall aims. Ethical standards – as set out, for example, in the UKCC code – are designed to encourage optimum standards. Thus an ethical decision is usually taken to mean one that results in the best possible outcome. As Stone and Matthews note (1996, p. 134), to behave ethically is to: 'behave rightly, to be morally conscionable, and to arrive at decisions after a careful weighing up of all the relevant facts, having considered rights and responsibilities, rather than as a result of thoughtless, arbitrary decision-making with no regard to consequences'.

In contrast, the law is concerned with deterring bad conduct and setting minimum standards below which practitioners must not fall. As such it accepts much lower thresholds of behaviour. Accordingly, the questions asked when legal decisions have to made are likely to be rather more instrumental, and include, for example, 'What can we get away with?; or 'Will we be punished if we pursue this course of action?' In practice, what this means is that a nurse may avoid legal liability, say in a negligence claim, because it is impossible to prove that his/her negligence caused (in a legal sense) the patient's injuries. Or a patient may have been unnecessarily exposed to risk but luckily escaped injury. In both these situations the nurse has acted in a morally dubious way even though s/he will not be sued. This is not to say, however, that s/he will be able to avoid all adverse consequences, since breaching ethical codes can result in proceedings for professional misconduct. Notwithstanding the heavy penalties (professional and social) that can follow the breach of professional rules it is nevertheless likely that failure to comply with legal duties is taken more seriously – no doubt because of the formal and official sanctions that back them up, which can result in loss of liberty or, in the case of professional malpractice, in the payment of large sums of money in compensation. In short, the UKCC can bar a nurse from practice but the courts can send her to jail (Fletcher *et al.*, 1995).

That there are fundamental differences between law and ethics raises another question, namely whether the law's intrusion into the care and treatment of patients always benefits them. Or does it, as some now claim, simply encourage litigation? Thus it is one thing to recognize that the law provides a framework within which professional practice can develop but quite another to say that medical decisions should always be subject to legal scrutiny and control. As Mason and McCall Smith (1999) point out, the crucial question is to determine the extent to which professional practice should be regulated by the law. There are, of course, two very different positions on this – one arguing that health professionals should be left to regulate themselves and the other that, even though the law may be imperfect and often inaccessible, it is the best way of controlling practice in the interests of the community as a whole. But perhaps the law's role and usefulness should be left to the reader to decide. Once, that is, subsequent chapters have clarified the relationship between professional practice, the law and ethics.

REFERENCES

Adams, J. N. and Brownsword, R. (1996) *Understanding Law*. Sweet & Maxwell, London.

Atiyah, P. S. (1979) *The Rise and Fall of Freedom of Contract*. Clarendon Press, Oxford.

Atiyah, P. S. (1995) *Law and Modern Society*. Oxford University Press, Oxford.

Beauchamp, T. L. and Childress, J. F. (1994) *Principles of Biomedical Ethics*, 4th edn, Oxford University Press, Oxford.

Childress, J. F. (1997) The normative principles of medical ethics. In: *Medical Ethics*, 2nd edn, (ed. R. M. Veatch). Jones & Bartlett, London.

Cribb, A. (1995) The ethical dimension. In: *Nursing Law and Ethics*, (eds J. Tingle and A. Cribb). Blackwell Science, Oxford.

Devlin, P. (1965) *The Enforcement of Morals*. Oxford University Press, Oxford.

Dworkin, R. (1977) *Taking Rights Seriously*. Duckworth, London.

Dworkin, R. (1986) *Law's Empire*. Fontana Press, London.

Edwards, S. D. (1996) *Nursing Ethics: A Principle-based Approach*. Macmillan, Basingstoke.

Elliott, C. and Quinn, F. (1998) *English Legal System*, 2nd edn, Addison Wesley Longman, Harlow.

Farrar, J. H. and Dugdale, A. M. (1990) *Introduction to Legal Method*, 3rd edn, Sweet & Maxwell, London.

Fletcher, N., Holt, J., Brazier, M. and Harris, J. (1995) *Ethics, Law and Nursing*. Manchester University Press, Manchester.

Geldart, W. (1995) *Introduction to English Law*, 11th edn, (prepared by Sir David Yardley). Oxford University Press, Oxford.

Gillon, R. (1985) *Philosophical Medical Ethics*. John Wiley, Chichester.

Griffith, J. A. G. (1985) *Politics of the Judiciary*, Fontana Press, London.

Harris, J. W. (1997) *Legal Philosophies*, 2nd edn, Butterworths, London.

Hart, H. L. A. (1968) *Law, Liberty and Morality*, Oxford University Press, Oxford.

Hart, H. L. A. (1994) *The Concept of Law*, 2nd edn, (eds P. A. Bullock and J. Raz), Clarendon Press, Oxford.

Johnstone, M. J. (1989) *Bioethics: A Nursing Perspective*, Baillière Tindall, London.

Kant, I. (1785) *Groundwork of the Metaphysic of Morals*. In: *The Moral Law*, (trans. H. J. Paton, 1948), Hutchinson, London.

Lee, S. (1986) *Law and Morals*. Oxford University Press, Oxford.

McLeod, I. (1996) *Legal Method*, 2nd edn, Macmillan, Basingstoke.

Mason, J. K. and McCall Smith, R. A. (1999) *Law and Medical Ethics*, 5th edn, Butterworths, London.

Melia, K. M. (1989) *Everyday Nursing Clinics*, MacMillan Education, Basingstoke.

Miers, D. R and Page, A. C. (1990) *Legislation*, 2nd edn, Butterworths, London.

Montgomery, J. (1997) *Health Care Law*. Oxford University Press, Oxford.

Nuttall, J. (1993) *Moral Questions: An Introduction to Ethics*. Polity Press, Cambridge.

Raphael, D. D. (1994) *Moral Philosophy*, 2nd edn, Oxford University Press, Oxford.

Routledge (2000) *Routledge Encyclopedia of Philosophy*, Routledge, London.

Scruton, R. (1994) *Modern Philosophy*, Mandarin, London.

Seedhouse, D. (1988) *Ethics – the Heart of Health Care*, John Wiley, Chichester.

Simpson, A. W. B. (1988) *An Invitation to Law*, Blackwell, Oxford.

Singer, P. (1979) *Practical Ethics*, Cambridge University Press, Cambridge.

Singer, P. (1993) *Practical Ethics*, 2nd edn, Cambridge University Press, Cambridge.

Singer, P. (ed.) (1994) *Ethics*, Oxford University Press, Oxford.

Stone, J. and Matthews, J. (1996) *Complementary Medicine and the Law*, Oxford University Press, Oxford.

Thompson, I. E., Melia, K. M. and Boyd, K. M. (1994) *Nursing Ethics*, 3rd edn, Churchill Livingstone, Edinburgh.

Tschudin, V. (1996) *Ethics: Nurses and Patients*, Baillière Tindall, London.

Twining, W. and Miers, D. (1991) *How to Do Things With Rules*, 3rd edn, Weidenfeld & Nicolson, London.

UKCC (1992) *Code of Professional Conduct*. United Kingdom Combined Council, London.

UKCC (1996) *Guidelines for Professional Practice*. United Kingdom Combined Council, London.

Waldron, J. (1989) *The Law*, Routledge, London.

White, R. C. A. (1999) *The English Legal System in Action*, 3rd edn, Oxford University Press, Oxford.

Wolfenden Committee (1957) Report of the Committee on Homosexual Offences and Prostitution, *Cmnd 247*, HMSO, London.

FURTHER READING

Elliot, C. and Quinn, F. (2000) *English Legal System*, 3rd edn, Addison Wesley Longman, Harlow.

Fletcher, L. and Buka, P. (1999) *An Introduction to Law and Ethics in Health Care*, Macmillan, London.

2 AUTONOMY AND CONSENT

INTRODUCTION

Respect for a person's autonomy and the right to consent to or refuse treatment are now widely accepted as central values in health care. This was acknowledged in 1991 in the Patient's Charter, which gave people the right to have any proposed treatment, including any risks involved in that treatment and any alternatives, clearly explained to them before they decided whether to agree to it or not. Yet in spite of the era of consumerism and partnership with patients that the Charter seemed to usher in there is still some resistance to providing information to patients (Hogg, 1999). Nor, as we shall see, has English law yet fully embraced the concept of 'informed consent'. Nevertheless, the phrase is now part of the lore of medical ethics (Mason and McCall Smith, 1999) and is commonly used in non-legal texts even though there is no single concept of informed consent. This is because its meaning varies depending on the context in which it is used (Skegg, 1999). It is unsurprising, therefore, that very few judges (or others) have provided a definition of the term. Yet the fact that 'informed consent' is now in common usage is in itself significant as it reflects the importance of autonomy as an ethical imperative even if in practice it is only recognized to a limited degree. Perhaps this is inevitable, however, as it is one thing for philosophers to enjoy the luxury of propounding abstract theory but quite another to accept responsibility for the actual outcome of applying such theory, especially when that outcome can have so profound an impact on a person's life (Brazier and Bridge, 1996). This chapter looks at the principle of autonomy and what happens when autonomy is limited. It also outlines the law of consent. But, as in other chapters, it begins with some hypothetical case studies the answers to which will be given at the end.

CASE STUDY 2.1 BELLA'S TREATMENT

Bella is in her early thirties and has two young children. Recently, breast cancer – from which her mother and eldest sister both died – was diagnosed but Bella has refused all treatment even though she knows that she will die very soon without it. Carla, a nurse, is very upset by Bella's decision, believing that treatment is her only hope, if not of a cure then at least of several more years of life. She wonders whether Bella can be forced to have treatment against her will or if there is any reason to ignore her wishes.

CASE STUDY 2.2 JOHN'S CONSENT

John is in his late fifties and has suffered for many years from a chronic condition. Until a few weeks ago he was cared for by his partner, James, but following his death his condition has deteriorated very quickly. John is particularly worried about the tests his GP has recommended, especially some blood tests. Once in hospital few details of the tests are explained to John other than in very broad terms. This is because Alison, the doctor, is very busy but also because John has said several times that he wants to leave all the decisions to the 'professionals'. Eileen, a nurse in whom John has confided, realizes that John is confused about the tests and is convinced that he has only reluctantly agreed to them for fear of upsetting Alison. She also thinks that part of his anxiety stems from his assumption that he is going to be tested for AIDS.

Is John's consent 'real'? Does respecting his autonomy mean respecting his choice not to participate? Has he been given enough information about the tests or has it been justifiably withheld?

CASE STUDY 2.3   HELEN'S AUTONOMY

Helen, a 15-year-old girl was perfectly fit and well until about 3 months ago. Then she suddenly developed heart failure and has only 1 week, or thereabouts, to live. Her parents have consented for her to have a heart transplant but, on learning that her only chance of survival is the operation, Helen has refused her consent. Her reasoning appears to be logical in that she has told those treating her that she knows death is final and that she cannot change her mind. However, she is insistent that she would rather die than have the transplant and someone else's heart. As she poignantly says: 'I would rather die with 15 years of my own heart.' All the adults involved want Helen to have the opportunity to live by undergoing the heart transplant except Miriam, a nurse, who thinks Helen's autonomy should be respected.

Should Helen's wishes prevail?

AUTONOMY

There are many conceptions of autonomy, a word that comes from the Greek: *autos* ('self') and *nomos* ('rule' or 'law') (Dworkin, 1988, p. 12). In the literature it is a term that is usually associated with several ideas such as self-determination, self-government, self-mastery, voluntariness and choosing one's own moral position (Beauchamp, 1997, p. 195). Broadly, it can be defined as 'the capacity to think, decide, and act on the basis of such thought and decision freely and independently and without let or hindrance' (Gillon, 1985). To be an autonomous person therefore means being able to runs one's own life according to a set of self-chosen rules and values. Such a 'life plan', i.e. whatever it is that a person broadly wants to do with his/her life (Young, 1986, p. 78), requires not just a sense of self but also awareness of options and knowledge of the implications and consequences of choosing a particular course of action. In health-care ethics, however, it is the principle of respect for autonomy to which writers most often refer (see, for example, Beauchamp and Childress, 1994; Gillon, 1985). Although treated by many as the most fundamental of moral principles (Downie and Calman, 1994, Edwards, 1996), respect for autonomy can, at least in relation to complex medical decision-making, be fraught with difficulty. Nevertheless to say that we should respect a person's autonomy means that we should ensure that people are able to make informed decisions and be as self-determining as possible (Rowson, 1996, p. 37). Basically, as we shall see below, what this involves is discussing proposed treatment or care with patients, allowing them to make decisions and, if they are competent, accepting their choices.

Respect for autonomy is a value that has long been acknowledged in Western society, whether it is seen as a good in itself or as a component of well-being. But its prominence in health care is more recent – dating from the late 1950s. Although justified by numerous ethical theories (both religious and secular), the two classic notions of autonomy that have most influenced modern thinking are those of Mill and Kant.

Kant assumed that people were essentially rational, although desires might at times blind them. Decisions that were made as a result of such desires he called 'heteronomous'. They were not truly the desires of the self because they were caused by the non-rational aspects of human nature (Randall and Downie, 1996). Kant's approach to autonomy was based on his dominant thesis that every person is an end in himself and deserves to be treated as such. Respect for autonomy is in fact a universal law and is supported both by the categorical imperative (see Chapter 1) and the concept of respect for persons. However, he argued that respect for the autonomy of any one individual had to be seen within the context of respect for the autonomy of all. Note that Kant was concerned with what is called the autonomy of will. To will was to decide on a particular course of action. But this course of action was only morally good where the reason for taking it was not only to act in accordance with duty, but for the sake of duty (Devereux, 1997). What this basically means is that people can be held morally responsible for their actions if they (1) are free to decide how to act and (2) do so not through ambition, fear, vanity or some other motive but purely out of respect for duty. To be autonomous in a Kantian sense is therefore to act morally (O'Neill, 1993, p. 179).

In contrast, Mill's support for the principle of autonomy derived from his concern with liberty, which he expressed in his famous 'harm principle', i.e. that we have the right to do whatever we want unless it can be shown that we are harming others. He justified this principle by appealing to the concept of utility (Chapter 1). In other words, allowing every person the freedom to act autonomously and pursue their own goals made them happier and thus increased the sum total of happiness in society. Note also that for Mill autonomy was a 'vital interest' (i.e. one that must be satisfied in order to flourish) not just because it was usually a means to other ingredients of happiness but also because it was a constituent of happiness itself.

Practical implications of respect for autonomy

In health-care contexts it is now taken for granted that one of the main ways patients exercise autonomy is through the concept of consent (or informed consent as it is often called). As Ian Kennedy has stated:

> *Consent in the context of modern medicine is an ethical doctrine about respect for persons and about power. It seeks to transfer some power to the patient in areas affecting her self-determination, so as to create the optimal relationship between doctor and patient ... namely a shared endeavour in pursuit of the clients' interests. (Kennedy, 1991, p. 178)*

But what does respecting autonomy mean in practice? In particular, what obligations does it impose on nurses and other health professionals?

Although there is no general agreement as to the essential elements of consent it would seem to include the following (Beauchamp and Childress, 1994, Chapter 3 and Kohner, 1996):

Communication

Communication with patients is now recognized as an essential part of good practice. It is not only important as a means of discovering or conveying information but it is also acknowledged as the single and most important way of securing cooperation and compliance (Thompson *et al.*, 1994, p. 113). Furthermore, if it is accepted that nurses have a moral obligation to tell the truth (see below) then it must be part of that obligation that nurses communicate as effectively as possible (Rowson, 1996, p. 54). Communication is, however, a two-way collaborative process. Note too that it involves listening to patients and talking to them in a language that is familiar to them, is jargon-free and that they can understand (Rumbold, 1999).

Giving information

The importance of information disclosure cannot be overstated. Without accurate information patients cannot make rational choices and so cannot act autonomously. In practice, of course, giving and receiving information can be seen as a continuum from patient education to individual autonomy (Hogg, 1999). According to the 1996 UKCC *Guidelines for Professional Practice*, patients must be given adequate information so that they can make a meaningful decision (clause 28). Yet despite wide acceptance that patients have a moral right to information there is little detailed guidance in the literature on exactly what the information should comprise, i.e. precisely what a nurse should disclose when obtaining consent. Nevertheless, Beauchamp and Childress (1994, p. 147) state that the core information should include:

- those facts or descriptions that patients or subjects usually consider material in deciding whether to refuse or consent to the proposed intervention or research;

- information the professional believes to be material;
- the professionals' recommendations; and
- the purpose of seeking consent.

Note also Department of Health guidance: *A Guide to Consent for Examination or Treatment* (HC(90)22), which gives fairly detailed guidelines on information disclosure. The combined effect of this guidance and the UKCC guidelines suggest that the following should be disclosed:

- the nature of the patient's condition and what would happen if no treatment was provided;
- treatment options and their respective benefits;
- substantial or usual inherent risks and side-effects associated with each option;
- any 'dangers' that may be special in kind or magnitude or special to a particular patient.

Of these the most controversial is the question of risk disclosure. Should every risk, however remote or inconsequential, be disclosed? If not, where should the line be drawn? As we shall see below, this aspect of consent has long troubled the courts. But as a moral matter – and certainly if consent is to truly 'informed' – it has been suggested that health professionals should disclose whatever information a reasonable person would want to know, plus whatever else the actual person wants to know (Brock, 1993, p. 50). Finally, it is worth noting the General Medical Council's latest guidance to doctors on obtaining consent and information disclosure. It is very detailed and specific reflecting the growing demands for greater openness and accountability (Jones, 1999).

Truthfulness

At its very simplest the obligation to tell the truth (or 'the duty of veracity' as it is sometimes called) means that nurses should not lie to or deceive patients. Indeed, some have argued that if a nurse is directly questioned about, for example, rare side-effects or adverse outcome, then it is morally indefensible to withhold information from that patient (Fletcher *et al.*, 1995, p. 43). Truth-telling is an obligation that the UKCC guidelines acknowledge: '[P]atients who want information are entitled to *honest* answers' (clause 24). However, not all patients want to be involved in decision-making and some may not want to know the truth about their health or treatment at all. If so, their 'right not to know' should be respected. The UKCC guidelines confirm this when they state: 'If patients and clients do not want to know the truth it should not be forced on them' (clause 25).

Voluntariness

For consent to be free it must not be obtained by fraud, coercion, duress or manipulation. The nature of voluntariness has been examined in detail by Beauchamp and Childress (1994). They adopt a fairly narrow definition of the term and suggest that a person acts voluntarily 'to the degree he or she wills the action without being under the control of another influence' (p. 163). Voluntariness can, however, also be diminished or voided by conditions such as debilitating disease, psychiatric disorders or drug addiction. Although this definition may be uncontroversial in practice it may be very difficult to distinguish acceptable forms of influence – which may include persuasion but only in so far as it fosters understanding, discussion and rational decision-making – and objectionable forms of influence such as 'informational' manipulation (Kennedy and Grubb, 1994).

Competence

To give consent to treatment a person has to be mentally competent to make that decision. Yet most texts on nursing ethics do not distinguish between competence and autonomy (e.g. Benjamin and Curtis, 1992, Seedhouse, 1988). Edwards, however, argues that while the two concepts are related they are distinct (1996, p. 57). Hence autonomy refers to a general capacity of an individual whereas competence refers to an ability to perform specific tasks. What then is meant by the term 'competency'? Given the many competing theories about its nature (Beauchamp and Childress, 1994, p. 80) there is no one definition that is widely accepted. Nevertheless, it is clear that being competent to make a decision requires several types of ability. These include the ability to understand facts; to grasp causal connections between alternative treatments and their effects; to think logically; to imagine situations and feelings; and to relate all these to the making of the decision (Rowson, 1996, p. 58). Competence is therefore a fairly sophisticated concept that can operate on many different levels. The degree of competence required will also vary according to the complexity and seriousness of the proposed medical procedure.

Accepting patients' preferences

If patients' autonomy is to be respected the choices they make must be accepted whatever the outcome. This is made quite explicit in the UKCC guidelines, which state: 'respect for patients' and clients' autonomy means that you should respect the choices they make concerning their own lives' (clause 20). In other clauses (e.g. clause 31) the guidelines also make it clear that a competent adult patient's decision to refuse consent must be respected even if the refusal will shorten his or her life.

Is respect for autonomy an absolute principle?

As many have observed, fully autonomous choice is largely an ideal and none of us is wholly autonomous all of the time (Brazier and Lobjoit, 1999, p. 186). Indeed, there are many things that can in practice undermine the individual's capacity for choice (Harris, 1985, p. 195). Clearly, for example, a newborn baby is incapable of acting autonomously. Older children too may be unable to exercise autonomy because of immaturity or the complexity of proposed treatment. Similarly, adults may, for a variety of reasons, such as family commitments, not be able to make decisions that are fully autonomous. This is why it is common to describe autonomy as something we all possess but only to some degree (Bird and White, 1995, p. 120). Yet even though the extent to which someone can act autonomously is in practice affected by many factors there are some patients whose level of understanding or reasoning is so limited that others must act on their behalf.

So what kind of things can undermine or limit a person's autonomy? Harris (1985, pp. 195–200) identifies several different kinds of 'defect' that may do this, namely defects in control, reasoning and information. For convenience these will be grouped into the broad categories of mental impairment and information impairment.

Mental impairment

This is a very loose term (and it incorporates Harris's defects in control and reasoning). It covers all those situations that might impair a person's ability to make or communicate his/her decision. These can be temporary reasons such as sedative medicine or long-term ones such as illness (physical or mental), drug addiction or unconsciousness. If a decision has been based on a false belief or is influenced by, say, pain, fear or anger, then a person's ability to act autonomously is also in question. 'Mental impairment' can of course affect adults as well as children. Nevertheless children may be more susceptible to pressures than adults and can also sometimes be more impetuous (Brazier and Bridge, 1996, p. 92).

Information impairment

Just as mental impairment can affect autonomy, so too can lack of information. As Lindley notes (1986, p. 50), autonomy requires not just that people rationally pursue their not-irrational goals as best they can, but that they actually not be deluded about the nature of their goals and the consequences of their actions. If patients are 'deluded' – because they have been given misleading or inaccurate information – their ability to make decisions is inevitably affected. In other words, a choice based on false or incomplete information is not a true choice. Similarly, the way in which information is presented and choices are formulated can be significant not least because it may affect a patient's understanding – of the risks or available options, for example (Rumbold 1999).

Practical implications of limited autonomy – paternalism

If autonomy is impaired or diminished patients are either not involved at all (or only minimally) in the decision-making process or alternatively their choices are overridden or disregarded. The ethical justification for dispensing with consent derives from two ethical principles: beneficence, the duty to do good, and non-maleficence, the duty to do no harm (both of which are discussed in more detail in Chapter 3). When health professionals apply these principles and make decisions about a patient's nursing care or treatment irrespective of their wishes or judgements or without consulting them they are usually described as acting paternalistically.

Paternalism – which traditionally has been applied far more assiduously in the care of women and children – is a complex concept (Rumbold, 1999). It can be demonstrated in several ways, e.g. in attitudes, language, and treatment decisions (Beauchamp and Childress, 1994; Benjamin and Curtis, 1992). Briefly, however, in whatever way it is described it basically involves overriding someone's autonomy for what is considered to be their own good (Chadwick and Tadd, 1992, p. 188).

Yet even though it can be said that paternalism degrades the adult patient and risks achieving a result where the disease not the patient is treated (Brazier and Lobjoit, 1999, p. 180), some paternalistic interventions are appropriate. Thus in cases involving patients who are unable to exercise autonomy – if, for example, they are unconscious or very young and so not capable of making any decision at all or even of expressing their wishes – it is not difficult to justify making treatment decisions on their behalf without consulting them. More controversial, however, are those treatment decisions made by competent patients that are considered harmful by their carers – for example a patient refusing life-saving surgery. Here the temptation to act paternalistically may be overwhelming but is morally dubious just as it is in relation to those patients whose competence is uncertain, typically children, adolescents, elderly people and those who are mentally ill. That is, of course, unless a proper assessment of their competence has been made. Much would ultimately depend on the circumstances of each particular case and whether the reasons that have traditionally be given for acting paternalistically are valid. According to Benjamin and Curtis (1992) these are that:

- patients may lack the professional skills and expertise of health professionals and thus be unable to understand the complexities of medical terminology and treatments, risks, side-effects, and so forth – as a consequence they are too ignorant to make a informed choice;
- capacity for rational reflection may be significantly impaired;
- patients are likely to be significantly harmed unless interfered with;
- at a later time it can be assumed that the patient will ratify the decision to interfere by consenting to it.

All the justifications have been much debated (see, for example, Gillon, 1985; Edwards, 1996) but limited space prevents any further discussion here. What is nevertheless beyond doubt is that paternalistic interventions are much more likely to be questioned now than in the past. Some writers have in fact rejected paternalism altogether, claiming that it cannot fit in with the 'new ethic' of nursing (Rumbold, 1999). Whether or not this is widely accepted, a belief that one is acting in a person's best interests is unlikely now to be a sufficient reason for overriding autonomy, and a much more cogent justification will be necessary.

Children and autonomy

As Fortin notes (1998, p. 20), claims that children have a right to autonomy are derived from liberal political philosophies that emphasize the need to promote as fully as possible an individual's freedom to make rational autonomous decisions. These claims are based on the fundamental moral principle that respect for persons is not only owed to Kantian persons (i.e. fully rational beings) but also to children as developing persons (because of their potential to become such persons – Ross Friedman, 1998). And certainly few would disagree with the general principle of respect for autonomy given the benefits it is said to confer. These include increasing personal well-being by enabling people to lead happier, more fulfilling lives, and never treating people simply as means to ends but as ends in themselves, thereby preventing coercion, exploitation and oppression (Hendrick, 1998). However, when applied to children and young people these benefits are commonly questioned, even though it is often accepted that mature children are able to take on much more responsibility than adults give them credit for. This denial of children's capacity to make autonomous decisions is due largely to the many myths and assumptions about the nature of childhood and misconceptions about children's needs and desires for autonomy. Even John Stuart Mill, who attached enormous importance to autonomy (most notably articulated through his famous 'harm principle', Chapter 1) seemed to consider it self-evident that children were too immature to be autonomous:

> *It is perhaps hardly necessary to say that this doctrine is meant to apply only to human beings in the maturity of their facilities. We are not speaking of children, or of young persons below the age which the law may fix as that of manhood or womanhood. Those who are still in a state to require being taken care of by others, must be protected against their own actions as well as against external injury.* (1972, p. 73)

But, as Wieczorek and Natopoff (1981) point out, the length, essential nature and meaning of childhood are culturally determined and so vary from country to country. Childhood is also a concept that changes over time. Thus, while in Victorian times the idea that children should be seen and not heard might have been acceptable, today such an attitude would not suit society, given its need for more sophisticated children (Fortin, 1998, p. 12). Yet despite the widely held view that children should now be given greater opportunities to develop their decision-making capacities it is still commonly claimed that they lack the developed sense of self that an autonomous person requires or that they lack the ability to make rational choices or the experience to make wise ones. As such, they do not have a will of their own but must rely on others to make decisions for them. Denying children the right to participate fully in decision-making, far from being inconsistent with their autonomy, therefore, actually enhances it by enabling them to develop their potential as adults. To do otherwise, i.e. to burden them with the choices that they are incapable of making, is to deprive them of the chance of becoming full human beings. In other words, children should be allowed to be 'children' and should be protected from being forced into adulthood before they are sufficiently mature (Campbell, 1992).

Notwithstanding these claims, Alderson and Montgomery (1996) assert that if children are to exercise autonomy they must be given the opportunity and the permission to do so. They cite studies, such as Solberg's (1990), that suggest that children's competence and independence follow adults' expectations and that they increase with mutual respect and trust. This does not mean that all children should be forced to make decisions against their will or always have the final say, since respect for autonomy is not an absolute principle (Harris, 1985). Thus, if treatment is complex and carries serious risks, respecting autonomy may involve no more than letting a child express his/her wishes freely. It may even be appropriate to refer the decision to someone else. However, if the treatment is relatively minor a child's wishes could be determinative despite opposition (parental or otherwise).

THE LAW OF CONSENT

The legal principles that underpin the law of consent – now the most significant legal expression of the principle of respect for autonomy – were first recognized in a famous 1914 American case (*Schloendorff* v. *Society of New York Hospital* 105 NE 92 (NY, 1914), when the judge said: 'Every human being of adult years and sound mind has a right to determine what shall be done with his body'). More recently, the right to bodily integrity has been acknowledged in Department of Health guidance (HC(90)22) and guidelines from the NHS Executive (Department of Health, 1999), and likewise the Patient's Charter. It is a right that the law takes very seriously, not least because it is based on the strong moral conviction that everyone has the right of self-determination (Mason and McCall Smith, 1999). The modern practical significance of the law of consent has been summed up by Lord Donaldson (in *Re T* [1992] 4 All ER 649). He described it as serving two distinct functions. One is the clinical function, which is designed to foster patients' trust, cooperation and confidence. The other, legal, function is to protect practitioners from criminal charges and civil claims when they treat and care for patients. Consent law has been developed almost entirely through the courts rather than legislation and even though most have involved doctors the precedents set apply to all health professionals. Nurses, therefore, are bound by them.

Nurses have two roles in the consent process. In respect of treatment for which they are directly responsible – say, taking a blood sample or giving an injection – then they have prime responsibility for obtaining consent. Similarly, when responsibility for treatment has been delegated to them – even if this involves treatment that has been traditionally undertaken by doctors – again nurses have the primary responsibility for obtaining consent. Nursing care, too, such as washing, dressing and feeding patients, requires consent. In other situations nurses may not be the primary carers but their advocacy role may require them to take an active part in the consent process (Rumbold, 1999); for example, advising patients who are uncertain or confused or helping to determine the competency of those whose capacity is in question.

An understanding of the law of consent is thus essential for nursing practice. However, it is a vast area of law only a brief outline of which can be provided here. A good starting point is the most recent important case to reach the Court of Appeal, in which some fundamental legal principles were outlined. This was *Re MB* [1997] 2 FLR 426. It concerned a woman who was 40 weeks' pregnant. Initially she agreed to have a caesarean (and signed a consent form) as her unborn child was in breech position. But after she went into labour the operation was cancelled twice because she refused to consent to anaesthesia because of a phobia about needle pricks. The hospital sought and won a court order authorizing treatment necessary for the purposes of labour including a caesarean, the insertion of needles, and for reasonable force to be used in the course of such treatment. MB appealed immediately to the Court of Appeal but it turned down her appeal, claiming that her fear of needles rendered her incapable of making a decision about medical treatment. As a consequence, and given the emergency, doctors were free to administer the anaesthetic since to do so was in her best interests. The Court of Appeal stressed the following:

1. Subject to (3) below, it is an assault to perform physically invasive treatment, however minimal, without the patient's consent.
2. A mentally competent patient has an absolute right to refuse to consent to medical treatment for any reason, rational or irrational, or for no reason at all, even where that decision may lead to death.
3. Medical treatment may be undertaken in an emergency even if, through a lack of capacity, no consent has been competently given, provided the treatment is necessary and the minimum required in the patient's best interests.

This summary of the law is a good starting point but it needs to be supplemented by the other basic criteria that must be satisfied for consent to be legally valid. These are as follows.

Consent must be effectively obtained and voluntary

In a few situations, such as in mental health settings, abortion and assisted conception, the law prescribes what form consent should take. In all other cases the law is silent, although it is now standard practice for written consent forms to be signed for any treatment or other invasive procedure received under the NHS (Brazier, 1992). While not a legal requirement, written consent provides the best evidence that consent was actually given, although it is not always full-proof. A patient who signs a form without understanding its implications is thus not giving valid consent. Furthermore, even though written consent has been given it can be withdrawn at any time, in which case a fresh consent has to be obtained before treatment can be given or reinstated. Other forms of consent include express oral consent – typically used for routine procedures – and implied consent. Implied consent, which is the weakest, is based on the patient's actions or behaviour (rather than words), say a nod of the head or rolling up a sleeve for an injection.

Consent (or its refusal) is not legally valid unless it is freely given, i.e. obtained without force, manipulation, coercion or undue pressure (Kennedy and Grubb, 1994). Although the law on this is very clear, it is, of course, quite another matter to actually pinpoint what amounts to a free or voluntary consent and what does not, despite guidance given in *Re T* [1992] 4 All ER 649. This case concerned a 20-year-old woman injured in a car accident when she was 34 weeks' pregnant. She was rushed to hospital where, following an emergency caesarean, her baby was stillborn. Shortly afterwards her condition deteriorated as she developed an abscess on her lungs – treatment for which she refused on religious grounds. The hospital sought a court order overriding her refusal. The central issue was a difficult one – just how 'free' her refusal was, bearing in mind that she was an ex-Jehovah's Witness who, while retaining some beliefs, was by no means as committed as her mother (a 'fervent and devout' Jehovah's Witness). The major problem was to try and determine just how much influence her mother had exerted in the time she had spent alone with her daughter soon after she was admitted. As the court put it:

> [T]he real question in each case is: Does the patient really mean what he says or is he merely saying it for a quiet life or to satisfy someone else or because the advice and persuasion to which he has been subjected is such that he can no longer think and decide for himself? In other words: Is it a decision expressed in form only, not in reality?

The answer will, of course, turn on several factors, in particular the personalities of the individuals concerned, the institutional setting, the effect of pain, tiredness, drugs, and so on. The relationship of the 'persuader' to the patient may also be of crucial importance.

In answering its own question the Court of Appeal decided that it could ignore T's refusal because 'her will had been overborne' by her mother. Furthermore, as a result of the various drugs she had taken she was in any event in no fit state to take a decision. Accordingly, treatment that was in her best interests could be carried out. But, as the court pointed out, deciding what is a 'free' and 'real' consent will also largely depend on the information a patient receives. It is to this we now turn.

What information must patients be given?

As was discussed above, for patients to exercise autonomy they need accurate information. The legal control of information is therefore very important since it not only determines the balance of power between health professionals and patients but, more importantly, at least in this context, shows just how committed the law is in practice to the principle of respect for autonomy. Not surprisingly, case law in recent years has focused primarily on the provision of information, especially the disclosure of risks.

Broadly, two different approaches can be taken. One is the 'patient' standard, which is based on what an average 'reasonable' patient (with that particular illness or condition) would expect and want to know. In its most extreme form this approach requires disclosure to a rational patient of all the relevant facts. This approach has not found favour in English courts, even though it has become more common in Australia (see, for example, *Rogers* v. *Whittaker* [1992]

109 ALR 625), and Canada (McHale *et al.*, 1997; Skegg, 1999). The other approach to information disclosure is the 'professional' standard. As the name suggests, it allows nurses and other health professionals to set their own standards of disclosure and decide what patients should know and be told. In other words the Bolam test is applied. This test was endorsed in the seminal Sidaway case (see below) and states that providing health professionals comply with accepted practice they will not be liable for negligence (for further details of *Bolam* see Chapter 3).

The choice between the patient standard and the professional standard is a difficult one, not least because there are persuasive arguments in favour of each and whatever standpoint is taken there will be a case somewhere that endorses it (Mason and McCall Smith, 1999). In English law, however, it is the professional standard that has traditionally been adopted, as the courts have not adopted the concept of informed consent but have talked instead of 'real' consent (Jones, 1999; Skegg, 1999). Yet there are signs that this conventional stance might possibly be changing. Recently, for example, the courts have been more willing to modify the Bolam test, albeit only when there is no rational basis for the professional standard. In *Smith* v. *Tunbridge Wells HA* [1994] 5 Med LR 334, for example, a consultant surgeon was found negligent for failing to inform a 28-year-old man of the potential for impotence and bladder dysfunction following an operation to treat rectal prolapse, despite medical support for his decision. The court held that the only reasonable course of action was to disclose the risk (see also *McAllister* v. *Lewisham and North Southwark HA* [1994] 5 Med LR 343; *Bolitho* v. *City and Hackney HA* [1998] AC 232; *Lybert* v. *Warrington HA* [1996] 7 Med LR 71 for a similar approach).

But despite these few exceptional cases it is clear that the amount of information that nurses and other health professionals have to disclose is still largely governed by *Sidaway* v. *Board of Governors of Bethlem Royal Hospital* [1985] AC 871. Thus the answer to the question 'What does English law require health professionals to disclose?' is basically 'that which no reasonably prudent health professional would fail to disclose'. Yet, even though Sidaway remains the leading case on information disclosure, because some of the Law Lords made contradictory speeches it is very difficult to state with any certainty precisely what the law requires to be disclosed in all situations. That said, the duty of disclosure required under Sidaway may be somewhat cryptic but is not fixed. Thus, as expectations of patients change about their involvement in their treatment, so do the levels of disclosure required of practitioners also change – imposing obligations on them to reveal more they would have done in the past (McHale, 1998, p. 74). Some commentators suggest that there are signs that this is happening already and that the two approaches, i.e. the professional and patient standard, are approximating *de facto* even if not *de jure* (Mason and McCall Smith, 1999, p. 287).

Mrs Sidaway suffered severe disability and partial paralysis following an operation on her spine some 10 years earlier to cure persistent pain. One of the recognized risks of the operation was damage to a nerve root, assessed as between 1% and 2%. Another more serious risk – to the spinal cord – was said to be less than 1% likely. Mrs Sidaway was told of the first risk but not the second, which regrettably occurred even though the operation was performed properly. She sued in negligence on the basis that she would not have had the surgery had she been told of that risk. The case took 9 years to reach the House of Lords, by which time the surgeon who had performed the operation had died. Nevertheless the court held that he had acted reasonably (and so was not negligent) in failing to reveal the risk to the spinal cord because in 1974 it was accepted medical practice not to do so. At the time the Sidaway judgement generated considerable debate, much of it critical of the almost unanimous acceptance by the Law Lords of the professional standard of disclosure (Montgomery, 1997). It is also worth noting that a failure to provide adequate information can result in a claim in either battery or negligence.

Battery (trespass to the person)

This kind of claim can be made if consent is obtained by fraud, such as when no information is provided at all or the nature of the treatment is so misrepresented that a patient accepts treatment that s/he would otherwise refuse (Hendrick, 1997). A similar claim could be made if the wrong operation was performed on the wrong patient. Note that actions for battery cannot be brought once the patient has been informed 'in broad terms' of the nature of the treatment (*Chatterton* v. *Gerson* [1981] QB 432). This requires only the most basic of information, i.e. the nature and effect of treatment and its likely risks.

Negligence

A negligence claim alleges that although consent is valid it is inherently flawed. The 'flaw' here is that crucial information was withheld. What this amounts to is that to avoid being sued for negligence nurses must give 'adequate' or 'sufficient' information, i.e. they must tell patients in broad terms about the nature of the procedure but also those risks that are so obviously necessary to an informed choice 'that no prudent medical man would fail to make them' (Lord Bridge in Sidaway). As a general rule this means that the more serious the risk of harm the more likely it is that it should be disclosed (even if in percentage terms its likelihood is very remote). So patients should always be told of 'substantial' risks (note that in *Pearce* v. *United Bristol Healthcare NHS Trust* [1999] PIQR reference was made to the need to disclose 'significant' risks that would effect the judgement of a reasonable patient). It seems, however, that there is no obligation to inform patients about everyday risks associated with surgery, such as bleeding, pain, scars from incision and so on (Jones, 1999). As to alternative forms of treatment, these too should be disclosed. This is made clear in Department of Health guidance HC(90)22 and HSG(92)32, which add that patients should also be told 'of dangers which may be special in kind or magnitude or special to that particular patient'. But even supposing a patient can prove that what was disclosed was insufficient, to win a negligence claim another hurdle has to be overcome, namely convincing the court that the patient would not have agreed to the treatment had the relevant information been given.

There is one situation, however, when the law allows information to be withheld. It is known as the doctrine of 'therapeutic privilege' and was confirmed in Sidaway as appropriate in those cases where revealing certain facts would harm a patient, i.e. damage his or her health or cause psychological distress. Note too that Sidaway also confirms there is no duty to disclose information where patients indicate that they do not want to know.

Sidaway was concerned with therapeutic treatment. It was therefore conceivable that the law would take a more pro-patient attitude in other situations such as when contraceptive advice and treatment is sought or where patients seek more detailed information and ask direct questions. But case law suggests otherwise: if anything, the courts have adopted a very conservative interpretation of Sidaway on these specific issues. In *Gold* v. *Haringey HA* [1987] 2 All ER 888, a woman agreed to be sterilized after the birth of her third child but sued because she was not warned either of the risk of the sterilization reversing itself or of alternatives (i.e. her husband having a vasectomy). The Court of Appeal rejected Mrs Gold's claim because, even though some gynaecologists did warn of the risk of failure, others did not (at least not in 1979, when the sterilization was carried out). Accordingly there was no negligence since the level of disclosure conformed to acceptable medical practice.

In another controversial case, *Blyth* v. *Bloomsbury HA* [1993] 4 Med LR 151, the scope of the duty to answer questions was considered. In this case a nurse asked her doctor about the side-effects of the long-term contraceptive Depo-Provera. When she suffered menstrual irregularity and bleeding she sued, claiming that she should have been told of all the risks inherent in the drug, which were known to the hospital at that time. She won her claim in the High Court (a decision which was very 'pro-patient') and was awarded £3,500, but the Court of Appeal reversed the decision. It held that the standard that applied when specific questions were asked was the same as when information was volunteered. In short, it was the 'professional' standard – i.e. the 'proper' answer is determined in accordance with 'responsible medical opinion and practice'. The decision in Blyth has been described as 'frankly astounding', one that appears to take paternalism to Draconian levels (Davies, 1998, 174) and one that appears to show that English law does little more than pay lip-service to autonomy. Note finally that, in common with other negligence, claims the plaintiff has to prove that had appropriate information been given s/he would have refused treatment, thereby avoiding the risk that had materialized (Jones, 1999).

Competency

To give consent patients must be mentally competent (note that the words 'capacity' and 'competence' are commonly used interchangeably). Although the law presumes that, in the absence of evidence to the contrary, adult patients are able to consent to or refuse treatment, the term has yet to be defined by statute. This means, at least until the recommendations on the assessment and definition of capacity made by the Law Commission (1995) are adopted (in late 1999 the Government indicated that these are expected to be incorporated into new legislation when parliamentary time allows), judges are responsible for establishing legal guidelines on competence. The Law Commission proposed a functional approach to determining capacity, which focuses on whether the individual is able, at the time when a particular decision has to be made, to understand the nature and effect of the decision. But for the moment the leading case law is *Re C* [1994] 1 All ER 819. Here a 68-year-old Broadmoor patient with paranoid schizophrenia and a gangrenous foot – which doctors were convinced he must have amputated – refused his consent, saying he wanted to die with two feet rather than live with one. He therefore applied to court for an injunction preventing surgery without his consent. Notwithstanding his mental illness and his delusions, which were both persecutory and grandiose – he believed he had an international medical practice – the High Court held C to be legally competent.

The 'new' test for capacity it laid down was a three-stage one:

- was the patient able to comprehend and retain information;
- did he or she believe it; and
- could the patient weigh up the information?

Re C was welcomed by many as evidence of a more enlightened judicial attitude towards the mentally ill. It also seemed to reaffirm the law's commitment to the value of patient autonomy – at least at an intuitive level (Stauch, 1997). Yet some commentators took a different line and expressed scepticism as to the true extent of judicial support for autonomy, not least because all the elements in the *Re C* test are vague and open to interpretation. But despite the uncertainties of the test it was applied in *Re MB* (p. 39). In that case the Court of Appeal also outlined the considerations that should be borne in mind when assessing competence. These are that:

- panic, indecisiveness and irrationality do not as such amount to incompetence, but they may be symptoms or evidence thereof – note that 'irrationality' is used here to connote a decision that is so outrageous in its defiance of logic or of accepted moral standards that no sensible person who had applied his mind to the question could have arrived at it;
- the greater the consequence of a decision, the commensurately greater the level of competence that is required to take it;
- temporary factors such as confusion, shock, pain, or drugs may completely erode capacity but those concerned must be satisfied that such factors are operating to such a degree that the ability to decide is absent;
- equally, fear may paralyse the will and so destroy capacity – but, again, careful scrutiny of the evidence is necessary because fear of an operation may be a rational reason for refusal to undergo it.

Exceptions to the principle of consent

In this section an outline of certain special scenarios will be covered, with the exception of the care and treatment of the mentally ill (see Chapter 7).

Unconscious and incompetent adult patients – proxy consent?

When faced with an emergency situation – typically an unconscious patient arriving in the A&E department – nurses may have to make on-the-spot decisions as to how to treat them. The question which then obviously comes to mind is whether anyone can consent to medical treatment on behalf of an incompetent adult. In other words, is proxy consent in respect of adults lawful? The answer is an unequivocal no. English law does not recognize any general doctrine whereby a spouse or near relative is empowered to give a legally effective consent to medical procedures to be carried out on an adult. This statement of the law was most recently confirmed by Lord Donaldson in *Re T* [1992] when he said:

> *There seems to be a view in the medical profession that in emergency circumstances the next of kin should be asked to consent on behalf of the patient and that, if possible, treatment should be postponed until that consent has been obtained. This is a misconception because the next of kin has no legal right either to consent or to refuse to consent.*

That said, however, if the patient is accompanied by relatives it may be appropriate to involve them in the decision-making process – but only so far as they can shed light on what the patient would have wanted. What then is the legal justification for treatment of an adult patient without consent? The answer lies in the doctrine of necessity (Mason and McCall Smith, 1999, p. 246). This means that (subject to any evidence to the contrary such as a valid 'living will' – see Chapter 9) such emergency treatment can be carried out as is necessary to save the patient's life and health. Note that a health professional cannot use this doctrine 'to take advantage of unconsciousness' so as to perform procedures that are not essential for the patient's survival (*Marshall* v. *Curry* [1933] 3 DLR 260; *Murray* v. *McMurchy* [1949] 2 DLR 442).

As to other incompetent patients, i.e. those who are not unconscious but do not have the capacity to make a decision about treatment, it is now clear that treatment that is in the patient's 'best interests' can be carried out. This includes routine procedures as well as major surgery (*Re F* [1990] 2 AC 1). The patient's best interests are determined by the Bolam test and thus must accord with practice accepted by a responsible body of relevant medical opinion. Whether this profession-oriented approach necessarily always benefits patients or indeed supports them is of course another matter (Mason and McCall Smith, 1999), which will be explored further in Chapter 7.

Children

16- and 17-year-olds

Giving consent

Children generally achieve adult status at 18 but in relation to medical treatment young people reach maturity at a younger age by virtue of the Family Law Reform Act 1969. This Act gives 16- and 17-year-olds the same rights to consent to medical treatment as adults, providing they are competent (as defined above). The effect of the Act is that the consent of competent 16- and 17-year-olds cannot be overridden by their parents (or others with parental responsibility for them) but can be overridden by a court. If a young person in this age group is incompetent, consent can be given by a proxy – almost always in practice someone with parental responsibility.

Refusing consent

Competent 16- and 17-year-olds were once thought to have the same rights to refuse treatment as adults but this assumption was not accepted by the courts in one of the most poignant cases to reach the courts on the autonomy of young people. This was *Re W* [1992] 4 All ER 627. It concerned W, a 16-year-old anorexic with whom, as one of the judges said, fate had dealt very harshly. Orphaned at 8, she had been fostered (unsuccessfully) several times. In one home she had been bullied and in another collapsed because her foster mother had surgery for breast cancer. Her grandfather, to whom she was greatly attached, died when she was almost 14 and a psychologist who had been treating her left the area soon after. Recently, another psychiatrist who had been caring for her had suffered a heart attack. The last straw was that her current foster parents had indicated that if W was discharged they could not continue to offer her a home. Before the case came to court W had been fed (with her consent) by a nasogastric tube. But by the time the case was heard by the Court of Appeal she was refusing this 'treatment' and apart from drinking 12 cups of tea a day had refused all food for the previous 9 days. As a result her weight had dropped to 35 kg, which for a girl of 1.7 m was considered dangerously low. Medical opinion was unanimous that, if she continued to refuse food, within a week her capacity to have children would be seriously at risk and a little later her life might be in danger. Given these circumstances and the fact that the court believed that anorexia was capable of destroying her ability to make an informed choice, it concluded that her refusal could be overridden. This was despite Lord Balcombe conceding that 'in logic there is no difference between an ability to consent to treatment and an ability to refuse treatment'.

The judgement in *Re W* was controversial not least because of the potential long-term and damaging consequences of coercion (Hogg, 1999). But even more controversial were the general principles the court laid down about how future cases involving refusal of treatment by any young person under 18 should be resolved. Briefly these are that, even if they were competent, their refusal could be overridden not just by a court but also by parents or by anyone else with parental responsibility. For many, this judicial paternalism and the wide discretion it gave judges to ignore young people's wishes was unacceptable, not least because of the judges' failure to take sufficient notice of the developing autonomy of adolescents. However, as Fortin notes (1998, p. 75), the U-turn from the law's apparent commitment to adolescent autonomy enshrined in the landmark 1986 Gillick case (see below) was probably predictable if society was to retain a means of exercising a form of benevolent paternalism to prevent adolescents risking their own lives.

Under-16-year-olds – Gillick-competent

Giving consent

The law in relation to giving consent for this age group was established in *Gillick* v. *West Norfolk and Wisbech AHA* [1986] AC 112. At the time the decision – that 'Gillick-competent' young people under 16 had the independent legal right to consent to treatment – appeared to usher in a new era of respect for children's rights in health-care contexts, not least because within a short time the concept was applied to all medical treatment, not just contraceptive care. But the Gillick test sets an evidential standard of competence, which means that children must understand what is to be done to them, why it is proposed to treat them in this manner and, in general terms, what consequences follow from agreeing to or refusing treatment. It is therefore a fairly stringent test and arguably a higher one than is required of adults and 16- and 17-year-olds. This is because the latter group of people are presumed to be competent in the absence of evidence to the contrary. In relation to children, however, the onus of proof is reversed in that health professionals must satisfy themselves that they do in fact enjoy the necessary intelligence and understanding to be deemed Gillick-competent (Brazier and Bridge, 1996).

Furthermore, the concept of Gillick competence suffers from an inherent weakness, notably uncertainty. As Fortin acknowledges (1998, p. 73), the fact that an adolescent's legal capacity hinges on notions as debatable as under-standing and maturity fundamentally hampers its effectiveness as a means of settling family conflicts. Note finally that a court, but not a person with parental responsibility, can override a Gillick-competent child's consent.

Refusing consent

As to the right of under-16-year-olds to refuse consent, there is no doubt, following *Re W*, that just like 16- and-17-year-olds their informed refusal can also be overridden both by a court and by anyone with parental responsibility, providing of course the treatment is in the child's best interests. It is therefore not surprising that the courts have done just this in several controversial cases. In *Re E* [1993] 1 FLR 386, for example, a Jehovah's Witness teenager who was nearly 16 refused (as did his parents) a life-saving blood transfusion urgently needed to treat his leukaemia. The court nevertheless ordered the treatment to proceed. At the time the judge was no doubt faced with a very difficult decision but with hindsight it may be that his decision was wrong, since it is now known that once E reached 18 he refused further treatment and subsequently died.

Despite this eventual outcome the court took a similar approach in *Re L* [1998] 2 FLR 810. Here the court authorized a blood transfusion that a 14-year-old – very badly burnt after accidentally falling into a bath of scalding hot water – had refused on religious grounds (she was a Jehovah's Witness). The decisions in *Re E* and *Re L* were predictable given that there are no reported cases in England and Wales in which the court has allowed a Jehovah's Witness child to refuse a blood transfusion (nor have their parents been allowed to do so on their behalf). But in both cases the young people concerned were denied very crucial information, in particular that their deaths would be prolonged and painful. In the absence of such information (which the court sanctioned), questions can at least be raised as to whether they were ever given a real opportunity to make an informed decision. Indeed it can be argued that in both cases the court and health professionals made it impossible for the teenagers to give or withhold consent.

Under-16-year-olds – not Gillick-competent

Children under 16 who are not 'Gillick-competent' cannot give consent and permission has to come from someone else. Again this 'proxy' will typically be a parent or other person with parental responsibility. The guiding principle is that treatment must be in the child's best interests. In the vast majority of cases this is not problematic – despite the uncertainty of the meaning of 'best interests' in relation to children (Hendrick, 1993). In cases of dispute when, for example, health professionals are keen to provide treatment that parents reject the courts will resolve the issue by deciding what will be best for the child. If they accept that this involves treatment they will authorize it despite parental objection.

This is what occurred in *Re S* [1993] 1 FLR 376, when the parents of a 4-year-old child with T-cell leukaemia had refused consent for a blood transfusion on religious grounds. *Re S* makes it clear that, even when children are too young to make their own decisions, parents cannot veto treatment that is thought to be medically essential (see also *Re C* [1999] 2 FLR 1004, in which the Court of Appeal authorized an HIV test for a 6-month-old baby despite her mother's opposition). And, as the case of *Re C* [1998] 1 FLR 384 shows, they cannot demand treatment either. In *Re C* the court refused to respect the wishes of parents to continue treatment of their 16-month old daughter, who was suffering from spinal muscular atrophy.

Refusal of consent

The kind of situation that poses one of the most acute dilemmas for nurses is when patients refuse life-saving treatment or treatment without which their health will be irreparably damaged. In some cases refusal of treatment may lead to death. And if the patient is pregnant the dilemma is more acute (see Chapter

6 for further discussion of so-called 'forced caesarean' cases). But whatever the probable outcome the law is now well-settled. Providing patients are competent they have the legal right to refuse treatment. This issue was dealt with by the courts in *R* v. *Blaue* [1975] 1 WLR 1411, when it was decided that a doctor was not justified in overriding the refusal to consent to a blood transfusion by a Jehovah's Witness even though it was necessary to save her life.

The difficulty with this absolute legal principle in practice, of course, is that, according to cases like *Re MB* [1997], it applies to all competent adults even if their decision is an irrational one. Thus, although it might be thought that irrationality sits uneasily with competence the law states clearly that irrationality in itself does not amount to incompetence. Whether or not irrationality is a symptom or evidence of incompetence is, however, another matter. Perhaps the best approach to take when a patient's refusal of treatment seems irrational is that recommended by Kennedy (1991): that an 'irrational' decision should be respected where it derives from long-held beliefs and values on the basis of which a patient has run his or her life but not if it is the result of a temporary delusion. In practice, of course, distinguishing between different 'irrational' decisions may be an almost impossible task.

CASE STUDY 2.1   BELLA'S TREATMENT – A DISCUSSION

(Refer to the scenario presented on page 29.)

If Bella's decision to refuse treatment is to be respected it must be a decision she is capable of reaching of her own free will. In other words, she must be capable of acting autonomously. Bella's capacity is clearly therefore a central issue. In the absence of any obvious physical or psychological factors – she does not appear to be suffering from any long-term mental illness or other incapacitating factor such as drugs or pain – the assumption must be that Bella is competent. It would seem too that her refusal is not based on a false belief. However, given the seriousness of Bella's decision it is at least arguable that she would have to satisfy the most stringent of competency 'tests'. For Edwards (1996, p. 66), this would mean that she must be able to reach a reasonable decision (as judged, by example, by a 'reasonable person' standard).

Another limitation on Bella's autonomy could arise because crucial information has been withheld from her. But again, this does not appear to be the case as Bella knows that without treatment she has no chance of surviving (for argument's sake it will be presumed that no alternative treatment is possible). Ethically, therefore, there is no justification for acting paternalistically and so Bella's refusal must be accepted.

But what does this mean for Carla, who wants to do all she can to prolong – if not save – Bella's life? It means basically that Carla is faced with a conflict of principles. Her wish to do the best she can for Bella, the principle of beneficence, is difficult to reconcile with her moral obligation to respect Bella's autonomy. Yet in the absence of any reason for acting paternalistically Carla has little choice but to go along with Bella's decision. As the UKCC guidelines state: 'you must respect the patient's refusal just as much you would their consent' (clause 31).

Let us turn now to the law, which also focuses on Bella's competence and the issue of information disclosure. In so far as the case study assumes that she has been informed as to the nature of her illness, treatment options, their respective risks and her prognosis without treatment, it would seem that at the very least the 'professional' standard of disclosure has been met, as is required by the Sidaway case. It is also arguable that the higher patient standard of disclosure has also been met, since Bella seems to have been fully informed. But is Bella legally competent, bearing in mind that in law every adult is presumed to have the capacity to consent or refuse medical treatment? The test laid down for capacity in *Re C* [1994] (which was recently confirmed in *Re MB* [1997]), i.e. that Bella is able to comprehend and retain information, believes it and can use it so as to weigh it in the balance, appears to be satisfied. In legal terms, then, Bella's refusal of treatment must be respected whatever the consequences. Note that, as far as the law is concerned, even if Bella's refusal of treatment was considered irrational this in itself would not be a good enough reason to ignore her wishes. As the Court of Appeal said in *Re MB*: 'a competent woman may, for reasons, rational or irrational, choose not to have medical intervention even though the consequence may be her own death'.

CASE STUDY 2.2   JOHN'S CONSENT – A DISCUSSION

(Refer to the scenario presented on page 29.)

John has apparently consented to several procedures, but is his consent valid? It seems that he has voluntarily decided to waive his right to be informed, i.e. he has delegated decision-making to Alison. Patient waiver is widely accepted as a justification for not obtaining consent (Beauchamp, 1997). It is, in other words, an exception to the informed consent requirement, assuming, of course, that the waiver has not been obtained by coercion or manipulation. In short, John is exercising his right not to be informed. But the facts of the case study suggest that John's deference to the 'professionals' can be questioned.

And this is where Eileen comes in. As patient advocate she can play a very important role in safeguarding John against abuse and violation of his rights (Rumbold, 1999). As the 1996 UKCC guidelines assert: 'the nurse may often [be] best placed to know about the emotions, concerns and views of the patient or client and may be best able to judge what information is needed so that it is understood' (clause 29). Eileen should therefore take steps to let her concerns be known, namely that John has not been fully informed about the various tests. It may even be appropriate for her to discuss details of the tests with him. She must take care, however, to make sure that if his waiver of consent is genuine it is respected.

The HIV test, however, is especially problematic. Recognising the potentially enormous impact of a positive result, advice from the UKCC in 1994 recommends that non-consensual testing should only be carried out in 'rare and exceptional circumstances where this was necessary in the patient's interests'. It is arguable that, given John's current frame of mind and general anxiety, he fits into this category. But with little detailed guidance on what amounts to 'rare and exceptional circumstances' it is not possible to be certain that this is the case. A way to resolve the ethical dilemma posed by testing for HIV may be that proposed by Brazier and Lobjoit (1999). They suggest that the best response is to recognize that patients and professionals form a partnership (in which both partners have responsibilities and rights) and that the therapeutic alliance is best represented by developing the concept of the fiduciary relationship (one that calls for frankness by both parties).

In legal terms the main issue is whether the legal standard of information disclosure has been met. Assuming that John is competent his consent should be obtained, otherwise his consent is legally invalid. Note, however, that the information that has been given – although just about sufficient to avoid a claim in battery – would not satisfy the professional standard, i.e. accepted medical practice. This latter standard would require more detailed information to be given about the tests. As a result, Alison could face a negligence claim unless she could justify withholding information on the basis of therapeutic privilege. In practice, this is a very broad doctrine which is rarely questioned and thus, given John's anxiety, could well be defended since information, especially about a potentially fatal illness, could be detrimental to his health.

Also worth noting is the recent legal emphasis on the importance of how information is communicated. In short, it is not now good enough simply to tell patients about risks without making any attempt to see that the patient has understood the information (Smith v. Tunbridge Wells HA [1994] 5 Med LR 334).

The HIV test is, however, another matter on which there are divergent opinions but no decided case. As Brazier and Lobjoit wryly observe (1999, p. 181), if you gather two or three lawyers together to debate screening for HIV you are likely to gather four or five different opinions as to whether testing for HIV without express consent constitutes an assault. Thus some legal commentators claim that patients must specifically consent to an HIV test. Others disagree, claiming that as long as general consent has been given to a blood sample and diagnostic testing then any additional tests, including HIV, will be lawful because they will have been tacitly consented to as well (Mason and McCall Smith, 1999). The essential question seems to be whether the HIV test is of such a nature as to remove it from the scope of those tests to which the patient may be said to consent implicitly. Until this question is finally resolved by the courts – when the legality of non-disclosure would probably be measured in Bolam terms – withholding information about an HIV test may be legally justified on the basis of therapeutic privilege. It is on this basis that it would arguably be lawful not to tell John about it, given the uncertain state of the law.

CASE STUDY 2.3   HELEN'S AUTONOMY – A DISCUSSION

(Refer to the scenario presented on page 30.)

The issue at the heart of this case is whether Helen's right to autonomy should be respected. It is the kind of situation that requires parents and carers to exercise great sensitivity and foresight. It is also the kind of case that inevitably causes controversy. Thus those, like Miriam, who think that the wishes of young people, however misguided, should be respected even in life-and-death situations will strongly oppose Helen being forced to undergo the heart transplant. In contrast others, including Helen's parents, would support such an outcome believing that she should have the opportunity to live.

The main question, however, is to determine whether Helen is competent. According to Rumbold (1999, p. 233), in order to make decisions children must have three attributes. These are:

- possession of a set of values and goals;
- the ability to communicate and understand information; and
- the ability to reason and deliberate about their choice.

They are attributes that, Rumbold believes, do not suddenly develop at any fixed age, since moral development, as with all other aspects of development (physical, mental, social and emotional), varies from one individual to another. It may well be, therefore, that even though Helen is 15 she may have developed these attributes to a sufficient degree at least to be able to participate in decision-making.

Indeed, not involving Helen in the decision-making process would be unthinkable, given the model of parent–child relations that Rumbold argues is now the most preferable in health-care contexts, namely the partnership model. Within the model the parent–child relationship is viewed as one of almost equality, in which parents and children negotiate and agree actions. It is also one that he argues is the 'most morally acceptable one' for the nurse to adopt (1999, p. 232). Furthermore, it recognizes children as 'full human beings who are due respect for their feelings, interests, and desires in relation to their own health care' (Bandman and Bandman, 1990).

Does that mean, then, that Helen's refusal of treatment should be accepted? If we are to treat young people in the same way as adults then, providing Helen can demonstrate the three attributes, it would seem ethically dubious to deny her the same rights as she would be afforded as an adult, in particular the right to refuse treatment. Nevertheless, given the seriousness of the decision it could be argued that Helen would have to reach a very high level of competency.

In legal terms, the main point that needs to be decided is again whether Helen is Gillick-competent. But how is this to be assessed? And what role should Miriam have in the assessment process? Guidance to lawyers and doctors issued in 1995 jointly by the Law Society and the British Medical Association states that, among other things, assessment of capacity should include consideration of a young person's ability to understand that there is a choice and that choices have consequences. It also includes assessing whether they understand the nature and purpose of the proposed procedure as well as risks and side-effects. Although these guidelines were issued to doctors, there is no reason why Miriam should not be involved in assessing Helen's capacity, as she is a member of the health-care team. She should also, as Helen's advocate, make known her views, especially if she is a lone voice, i.e. the only person who thinks that Helen's wishes should prevail.

Assessing Gillick competence is a complex process. Nevertheless, the concept is flexible, enabling the courts to demand capacity commensurate with the gravity of the consequences of the decision in question (Diduck and Kaganas, 1999). Note too that competence, according to *Re R* [1991] 4 All ER 177 is a developmental concept that must be assessed on a broad, long-term basis, taking into account a child's whole medical history, background and mental state. This means that a child is not Gillick-competent if his/her capacity to understand fluctuates on a day-to-day or week-to-week basis.

Yet even though the Gillick decision was once interpreted as giving the competent child the right to make mistakes (Eekelaar, 1994), judges in subsequent cases have been very reluctant to recognize this right and have interpreted it very restrictively (see, for example, *Re E* [1993] 1 FLR 386 and *Re L* [1998] 2 FLR 810). They have also now made it very clear that, even if a child is Gillick-competent, his/her wishes can be overridden, in particular her refusal of treatment. In other words, Gillick establishes only that competent children can give valid consent; it does not give them a right of veto (*Re W* [1992]).

The courts, therefore, have very wide powers and can impose whatever decision they choose, providing is in the child's best interests. Whether health professionals would be willing to carry out intrusive treatment against the wishes of an articulate and intelligent teenager is, of course, another matter (Downie, 1997, p. 500). In conclusion, then, and following *Re M* [1999] (unreported), the facts of which are identical to this case study, it is most unlikely that the courts would respect Helen's wishes. In short, they would, albeit very reluctantly, sanction the surgery.

LAW and *ETHICS* – a comparison

What do these case studies and the discussion of autonomy and the law of consent that preceded them tell us about the relationship between law and ethics? That they overlap in several ways is self-evident, not least at a theoretical level in that both Mill and Kant support the principle of respect for autonomy, albeit from different perspectives. More specifically, both law and ethics are concerned with protecting patients' 'rights' – to make autonomous choices, to self-determination and bodily integrity. Both too are committed to preventing coercion, manipulation and duress and to ensuring that patients give their consent freely. The same basic elements, in particular truthfulness and volun- tariness are also central components of each, as is the concept of competency.

Indeed, as Beauchamp and Childress (1994) have pointed out, even though autonomy and competence are different in meaning the criteria of the autonomous person and of the competent person are strikingly similar. So much so in fact that they assert that an autonomous person is necessarily a competent person for making decisions, and that judgements of whether a person is competent to authorize or refuse treatment should be based on whether the person is autonomous (1994, p. 135).

In law too, the concept of competence is a central one in that there is no question of consent being legally valid unless it is given by someone whom the law deems capable (as established in *Re C* [1994]). How the ethical and legal test of competence compare is, however, difficult to assess. Arguably there is little difference in practice between the law and ethics on this except that case law has provided rather more detail of those factors that are specifically relevant in assessing competence.

Notable too are the similar mechanisms law and ethics adopt to provide ways of making decisions for patients when they cannot do so for themselves. The law does this by the 'best interests' test, which for all its vagueness is arguably better than any alternative. Paternalistic intervention is also justified ethically when patients' autonomy is limited. Similar paternalistic principles justify the legal doctrine of therapeutic privilege in which information is withheld from patients in certain circumstances.

But despite the many similarities between law and ethics there are differences. Perhaps the greatest distinction is that the moral approach to information-giving is more 'informed' than the law's. As we have seen, English law does not have a concept of informed consent except in a very limited form (see *Chatterton* v. *Gerson* [1981] Q.B 432). And, although the courts now seem more sympathetic to the idea of autonomy, the basic structure of the law in this context remains strongly paternalistic (Jones, 1999). What this effectively means is that to conform to an ethical standard of information disclosure – e.g. the standard set by the 1996 UKCC guidelines (see also guidance from the Senate of Surgery of Great Britain and Ireland) – more detailed information should be disclosed than the law currently requires. It seems therefore that the ethical standard of disclosure is more patient-oriented.

Yet not all legal commentators condemn the law's stance. Skegg (1999), for example, while conceding that the current law has no less than ten significant weaknesses, nevertheless argues that at least it has not imposed unrealistic or counterproductive standards of disclosure, i.e. those that would require health professionals to thrust unwanted information on patients or require them to spend so much time discussing risks and alternatives with some patients that others cannot be assisted.

It is also worth noting that, although both law and ethics are concerned with competence and patients' ability to be self-governing, their different perspectives have resulted in different conceptions of the role played by rationality. Hence the law has always insisted – most recently in *Re MB* [1997] – that as far as the law is concerned autonomy includes the right to make irrational decisions and that as a consequence a mentally competent patient has an absolute right to refuse to consent to medical treatment for any reason whatsoever, however irrational. In practice, of course, the courts have not been unwilling to challenge irrational choices as they have found it too tempting to construe irrationality as a symptom of incompetence, especially if the patient has unusual beliefs or attitudes. Rationality is also an important aspect of the moral approach to consent – at least in the sense that the inability to give a rational reason is a test (albeit a very demanding one that only needs to be satisfied for the most weighty of decisions) that many adopt as a criterion for determining competence (see, for example, Edwards, 1996, pp 60–68 and Beauchamp and Childress, 1994, pp 136 – 142).

Finally let's look briefly at the obligation to tell the truth – an important ethical principle that nurses are forcibly reminded of in the UKCC guidelines. The law also endorses this principle in theory but its commitment to it can be described as weaker – at least in the context of answering patients' questions. This is because, even though it is unlawful to misinform patients, the law currently only requires a 'proper' answer to be given, i.e. one that accords with acceptable practice. This does not of course mean that the law sanctions dishonesty but rather that its concern for candour and openness is arguably more symbolic than real.

REFERENCES

Alderson, P. and Montgomery, J. (1996) *Health Care Choices: Making Decisions with Children*, Institute for Public Policy Research, London.

Bandman, E. L. and Bandman, B. (1990) *Nursing Ethics through the Life Span*, 2nd edn, Prentice-Hall, Englewood Cliffs, NJ.

Beauchamp, T. L. (1997) Informed consent. In: *Medical Ethics*, 2nd edn, (ed. R. M. Veatch), Jones & Bartlett, London.

Beauchamp, T. L. and Childress, J. F. (1994) *Principles of Biomedical Ethics*, 4th edn, Oxford University Press, Oxford.

Benjamin, M and Curtis, J. (1992) *Ethics in Nursing*, 3rd edn, Oxford University Press, Oxford.

Bird, A. and White, J. (1995) An ethical perspective – patient autonomy. In: *Nursing Law and Ethics*, (eds J. Tingle and A. Cribb), Blackwell Science, Oxford.

Brazier, M. (1992) *Medicine, Patients and the Law*, 2nd edn, Penguin Books, Harmondsworth.

Brazier, M. and Bridge, C. (1996) Coercion or caring: analysing adolescent autonomy. *Legal Studies*, 16(1), 84–109.

Brazier, M. and Lobjoit, M. (1999) Fiduciary relationship: an ethical approach and a legal concept? In: *HIV and AIDS: Testing, Screening, and Confidentiality*, (eds R. Bennet and C. A. Erin), Oxford University Press, Oxford.

Brock, D. W. (1993) *Life and Death: Philosophical Essays in Biomedical Ethics*, Cambridge University Press, New York.

Campbell, T. (1992) The rights of the minor. In: *Children, Rights and the Law*, (eds P. Alston, S. Parker and J. Seymour), Clarendon Press, Oxford.

Chadwick, R. and Tadd, W. (1992) *Ethics and Nursing Practice: A Case Study Approach*, Macmillan, Basingstoke.

Davies, M. (1998) *Textbook on Medical Law*, 2nd edn, Blackstone Press, London.

Department of Health (1990) *Patient Consent to Examination and Treatment, HC(90)22*, HMSO, London.

Department of Health (1992) *HSG(92)32*, HMSO, London.

Department of Health (1999) *Consent to Treatment, HSC 1999/031*, HMSO, London.

Devereux, J. (1997) *Medical Law: Text, Cases and Materials*, Cavendish Publishing, Sydney.

Diduck, A. and Kaganas, F. (1999) *Family Law, Gender and the State*, Hart Publishing, Oxford.

Downie, A. (1997) The doctor and the teenager – questions of consent. *Family Law*, 499.

Downie, R. S. and Calman, K. C. (1994) *Healthy Respect*, 2nd edn, Oxford University Press, Oxford.

Dworkin, G (1988), *The Theory and Practice of Autonomy*, Cambridge University Press, Cambridge.

Edwards, S.D. (1996) *Nursing Ethics, A principle-based approach*, Macmillan, London.

Eekelaar, J. (1994), The interests of the child and the child's wishes: the role of dynamic self-determinism. *International Journal of Law and the Family*, 8, 42.

Fletcher, N., Holt, J., Brazier, M. and Harris, J. (1995) *Ethics, Law and Nursing*, Manchester University Press, Manchester.

Fortin J. (1998) *Children's Rights and the Developing Law*, Butterworths, London.

Gillon, R (1985) *Philosophical Medical Ethics*, John Wiley, Chichester.

Harris, J. (1985) *The Value of Life*, Routledge, London.

Hendrick, J. (1993) *Child Care Law for Health Professionals*, Radcliffe Medical, Oxford.

Hendrick, J. (1997) *Legal Aspects of Child Health Care*, Chapman & Hall, London.

Hendrick, J. (1998) Legal and ethical issues. In: *Textbook of Children's Nursing*, Stanley Thornes, Cheltenham.

Hogg, C. (1999) *Patients, Power and Politics: From Patients to Citizens*, Sage, London.

Jones, M. (1999) Informed consent and other fairy stories. *Medical Law Review*, 7(2), 103–134.

Kennedy, I. (1991) Consent to treatment. In: *Doctors, Patients and the Law*, (ed. C. Dyer), Blackwell Scientific, Oxford.

Kennedy, I. and Grubb, A. (1994) *Medical Law: Text and Materials*, 2nd edn, Butterworths, London.

Kohner, N. (1996) *The Moral Maze of Practice*, King's Fund, London.

Law Commission (1995) *Mental Incapacity*, Report No. 231, HMSO, London.

Lindley, R. (1986) *Autonomy*, Macmillan, London.

McHale, J. (1998) Consent to treatment: general principles. In: *Law and Nursing*, (eds J. McHale, J. Tingle and J. Peysner), Butterworth Heinemann, Oxford.

McHale, J. and Fox, M., with Murphy, J. (1997) *Health Care Law: Text and Materials*, Sweet & Maxwell, London.

Mason, J. K. and McCall Smith, R. A. (1999) *Law and Medical Ethics*, 5th edn, Butterworths, London.

Mill, J. S. (1859) In: *Utilitarianism, On Liberty and Considerations on Representative Government* (1972), J. M. Dent, London.

Montgomery, J. (1997) *Health Care Law*, Oxford University Press, Oxford.

O'Neill, O. (1993) Kantian ethics. In: *A Companion Guide to Ethics*, (ed. P. Singer), Blackwell, Oxford.

Randall, F. and Downie, R. S. (1996) *Palliative Care Ethics*, Oxford Medical Publications, Oxford.

Ross Friedman, L. (1998) *Children, Families and Health Care Decision Making*, Clarendon Press, Oxford.

Rowson, R. (1996) Informed consent. In: *Ethics: Nurses and Patients*, (ed. V. Tschudin), Baillière Tindall, London.

Rumbold, G. (1999) *Ethics in Nursing Practice*, 3rd edn, Baillière Tindall, London.

Seedhouse, D. (1988) *Ethics – the Heart of Health Care*, John Wiley, Chichester.

Skegg, P. D. G. (1999) English medical law and 'informed consent'. *Medical Law Review*, 7(2), 135–165.

Solberg, A. (1990) Negotiating childhood; changing constructions of age for Norwegian children. In: *Constructing and Reconstructing Childhood*, (eds A. James and A. Prout), Falmer Press, Basingstoke.

Stauch, M. (1997) *Re MB* (an adult: medical treatment). *Nottingham Law Journal*, 6, 74–86.

Thompson, I. E., Melia, K. M. and Boyd, K. M. (1994) *Nursing Ethics*, 3rd edn, Churchill Livingstone, Edinburgh.

UKCC (1992) *Code of Professional Conduct*, United Kingdom Central Council, London.

UKCC (1994) *Acquired Immune Deficiency Syndrome and Human Immune Deficiency Virus Infection (AIDS and HIV Infection)*, United Kingdom Central Council, London.

UKCC (1996) *Guidelines for Professional Practice*, United Kingdom Central Council, London.

Wieczorek, R. R. and Natopoff, J. N. (1981) *A Conceptual Approach to the Nursing of Children*, J. B. Lippincott, Philadelphia, PA.

Young, R. 1986 *Personal Autonomy: Beyond Negative and Positive Liberty*, Croom Helm, London.

FURTHER READING

Alderson, P. (1990) *Choosing for Children*, Oxford University Press, Oxford.

Skegg, P. D. G. (1984) *Law, Ethics and Medicine*, Clarendon Press, Oxford.

3 RESPONSIBILITY, ACCOUNTABILITY AND NEGLIGENCE

INTRODUCTION

This chapter begins with a discussion of the ethical principles of beneficence and non-maleficence, both of which have very significant implications for nurses. Indeed, in so far as health is a moral endeavour that involves working to promote a good, namely that of restoring health, it can be said that the moral foundation of health care involves the principle of beneficence (Edwards, 1996, p. 161). Non-maleficence too is of central importance in that nurses are, at the very least, expected not to harm their patients. But, as was noted in Chapter 1, ethical principles can only provide a moral framework for practice or, to put it another way, 'rules of thumb' (Cribb, 1995). They thus provide little guidance on the day-to-day practice of nursing or on the specific duties that nurses owe and the standards of care they are expected to provide. This is why this chapter also focuses on the concepts of responsibility and accountability. As we shall see, an analysis of the scope and limits of the notion of responsibility tells us more about the specific roles nurses have and the tasks they can be expected to perform. And when mistakes are made and 'things go wrong' the concept of accountability enables us to ask why a person acted in a particular way, what were their reasons and whether they can justify their actions. In so far as the law of negligence is concerned with attributing responsibility and, in some instances, blame, its place in this chapter is arguably self-evident, especially because the fault principle, on which it is based, clearly has a moral dimension (Phillips, 1997).

CASE STUDY 3.1   HOW RESPONSIBLE IS LISA FOR PAUL'S ACCIDENT?

Paul, a 65-year-old patient, has one leg in a sling and the other on a pillow. It is mid-morning and the staff nurse, Lisa, rushes in. She is in a hurry because the ward is short-staffed. She quickly gives Paul a cup of tea without giving him any time to say anything nor checking that he can manage. As Paul tries to drink the tea it spills and burns one of his hands badly.

What is Lisa's responsibility for this accident, bearing in mind that when the ward was adequately staffed more time would have been spent ensuring that Paul could cope safely with drinking the tea?

CASE STUDY 3.2   SHOULD AYEESHA QUESTION PAT'S DECISION?

Staff nurse Ayeesha is concerned about the drug dosage written on the medicine chart. She is sure the dosage is too high but, mindful that Pat, the doctor who prescribed the drug, has a formidable temper and is known to make life very difficult for anyone who challenges her, is uncertain what to do.

Should Ayeesha obey Pat's instructions? What if she does and the patient is harmed?

CASE STUDY 3.3 WHO IS ACCOUNTABLE – ANNE OR PATSY?

Anne, a recently qualified nurse, has been asked by Patsy, the sister, to do an intravenous injection. Patsy did not check whether Anne had the necessary skills. She simply assumed that she was capable. But Anne, who is new to the ward, is well aware that she is not qualified to do the infusion. She is reluctant to admit it, however, for fear of being thought incompetent. So she goes ahead. Patsy does not check what Anne has done and Sanjay, the patient, suffers as a result.

Who is responsible for Sanjay's injuries? Should Patsy have delegated the task to Anne? Should Anne have carried out the infusion?

BENEFICENCE AND NON-MALEFICENCE

In health-care contexts beneficence initially appears to be a relatively straight-forward term. It is commonly seen as a moral injunction always to do good (Rumbold, 1999, p. 217) and has long been a cornerstone of nursing ethics (Tschudin, 1996, p. 52). In a very general sense, beneficence requires nurses to benefit others and is enshrined in clause 1 of the UKCC Code of Conduct (1992a, hereafter referred to as 'the Code'), which states that registered nurses must 'act always in such a manner as to safeguard and promote the interests and well-being of patients and clients'. As Edwards notes (1996, p. 42), the similarity between this clause and the principle of beneficence is significant. This is because the clause makes clear that beneficence is a major part of a nurse's professional duty, one that generates moral obligations to act in ways that promote the well-being of others. In practice, however, working out precisely what obligations it imposes on nurses in everyday contexts is a much more difficult task. What, for example, counts as a benefit? And who decides what is in the patient's or client's interests? Far from clear, too, is to whom nurses owe moral obligations, i.e. who they have to benefit.

Although these are fairly basic questions, the Code itself provides no clear answers. This is not surprising, however, given that it is only intended to provide very general statements of the ethical principles that underpin practice rather than detailed guidance on the different situations nurses face (Singleton and McLaren, 1995). More specific guidance is nevertheless provided in the UKCC Guidelines for professional practice (1996, hereinafter called 'the Guidelines') in a section called 'Duty of Care'. Here there is more detailed advice on the practical implications of beneficence and what nurses should do in certain circumstances – i.e. if they are walking along the street and come across a person injured in a road traffic accident. The Guidelines make it clear that, although the nurse does not have a legal duty to stop and provide care, 'she does have a professional duty' that operates at all times. The scope of this duty is, however, limited, in that in this situation it is reasonable to expect a nurse 'to do no more than comfort and support the injured person' (clause 14). Other advice given in the Guidelines tells nurses what to when they find a women giving birth alone in a hospital corridor. Here all that they can be reasonably be expected to do is to call a midwife or obstetrician and stay with the woman until appropriate help arrives.

Also worth noting in this context is that the standard adopted by the Guidelines for determining whether a nurse has acted reasonably (in accordance with a professional duty of care), is the case of *Bolam* v. *Friern Hospital Management Committee* [1957] 1 WLR 582, which, as we shall discuss below, is one of the most important cases in the law of negligence.

But, even supposing it is possible to establish how nurses are required to act in the kinds of scenario mentioned in the Guidelines, there are other difficulties with the concept of beneficence. What, for example, do the words 'benefit', 'well-being' and 'interests' mean? These all constitute the 'good' that nurses are expected to promote and as such include both physical and psychological benefits and are broadly to have a positive value (Edwards, 1996). Thus they include the prevention of disease, the restoration of health and the reduction of pain and suffering (Davis and Aroskar, 1991). Yet all these are subjective terms that depend on an individual's evaluation of the situation. In other words, what counts as a benefit and how it is assessed cannot be objectively determined because people can have very varied attitudes to illness, disease, pain and disability (Singleton and McLaren, 1995). So, for example, a young, 'sporty' patient is likely to regard the amputation of a limb in a very different way from an elderly patient whose mobility has been severely restricted for many years. As a consequence their respective views on the benefits of treatment, risks, and so forth, are also likely to be very different. A related question is whether health benefits (likewise 'well-being' and 'interests') should be very broadly interpreted so as to include psychological, social, economic and religious benefits (Veatch and Fry, 1987).

Finally, there is the crucial question: Who must nurses benefit? That nurses have a primary duty towards their patients and clients is widely accepted. What this means is that they have more weighty obligations towards patients on their own wards, i.e. their own case load. Nevertheless, nurses arguably also have obligations, albeit less onerous ones, towards patients on neighbouring wards. As Edwards (1996) suggests, if a nurse is aware of, say, gross malpractice on a neighbouring ward, then presumably, her obligations of beneficence would extend to those suffering as a result of that malpractice (p. 70). Note too that the Code seems to impose professional obligations not just towards patients but also to other nurses and health professionals, patients' and clients' relatives, and the general public. That nurses also have obligations to themselves, their dependants and their employers is also recognized by some (e.g. Edwards, 1996).

In summary it seems therefore that the principle of beneficence is potentially very broad in that it can be said to generate significant obligations towards all those who may be affected, directly or indirectly, by a nurse's conduct.

Let us turn now to the principle of non-maleficence. Put simply, this means that nurses have a duty not to harm patients or subject them to risk of harm (Rumbold, 1999; Beauchamp and Childress, 1994). Although it is a well-estab-lished, almost sacred principle, its origins are somewhat obscure (Gillon, 1985). It is enshrined in clause 2 of the Code, which states that nurses 'must ensure that no action or omission on their part or within their sphere of responsibility is detrimental to the interests, condition or safety of patients and clients' (Edwards, 1996). Similarly, it is plausible to suggest that it also underlies clause 9.2 of the UKCC document *The Scope of Professional Practice* (1992b). This tells nurses that they 'must honestly acknowledge any limit of personal knowledge and skill and take steps to remedy any relevant deficits in order effectively and appropri-ately to meet the needs of patients and clients'.

Non-maleficence is commonly described as less morally demanding than beneficence because it generates fewer obligations (Henry, 1996). Or, to put it another way, it does not demand positive action. This means that it imposes no obligation on us to act as Good Samaritans, i.e. to help strangers in distress. Rather, it simply requires us not to harm them. Nevertheless, the moral requirement not to harm or injure others can be problematic in practice. This is because it presupposes that terms such as 'harm' and 'injury' are neutral and value-free and so can be defined objectively. But, like the concept of benefit, they too are evaluative terms and depend very much on how the individual assesses the situation. In short, what counts as a harm to one person may not be a harm at all to another person, because of their different outlooks on life. 'Harm' can be physical and so include pain, disability, discomfort and death. But it can also be psychological and thus include mental stress, and so forth. Beauchamp and Childress (1994) adopt a fairly broad definition of harm: 'thwarting, defeating or setting back the interests of one party by causes that include self-harming conditions as well as the (intentional or unintentional) actions of another party' (p. 193). Note too that this definition is broad enough to include the harm caused by intimidation, undue influence or pressure. Similarly misleading and misinforming patients so that they accept treatment that they would otherwise reject can be a form of harm. Finally, as Beauchamp and Childress's definition indicates, the causes of harm can be very varied, ranging from the intentional (resulting from, say, abuse, assault or exploitation) to the unintentional, deriving from careless or negligent care and treatment.

Having looked briefly at the principles of beneficence and non-maleficence the final issue to consider is the relationship between them. That they are closely connected is widely accepted, given that the moral objectives of medicine are both beneficence – to help those who are sick and suffering – and non-malefi-cence – to prevent harm in terms of both preventing deterioration of existing illness, damage, and disease (Gillon, 1985). Indeed some philosophers join them together as a single principle, claiming that non-maleficence is merely an aspect of beneficence (Frankena, 1973). But even those who treat them as separate principles (such as Beauchamp and Childress, 1994) acknowledge that they are intertwined. This is because almost every nursing or medical intervention that aims to benefit a patient may at the same time result in harm. As Rumbold observes (1999, p. 222), sometimes the harm will be unavoidable, even intentional. But at other times it can be unintentional and unexpected. For example, an operation may restore health but it can also carry risks. Similarly, drugs may cure but can have side-effects (Tschudin, 1994). So a patient with bone cancer may have to lose a leg to have a chance of surviving.

It seems clear, therefore, that beneficence and non-maleficence usually have to be considered and weighed together. In other words, benefits and harms need always to be balanced against each other (Singleton and McLaren, 1995). From this balancing exercise – the outcome of which will depend on each individual's own evaluation of what is harmful and good for them – will emerge what is the morally justified course of action, in other words that which causes the least harm and the most good. Note that this balancing exercise should also reveal that neither beneficence or non-maleficence are absolute principles and that sometimes they come into conflict. This then raises the question as to which one should have priority.

For Gillon the claim that non-maleficence should normally override beneficence is untenable (1985, p. 81). Of course, in some situations this may well be the case. Thus if the risks associated with a particular procedure are very high and serious then it will almost certainly be morally indefensible to carry out the procedure if the potential benefit is very small. But in others, however, non-maleficence can be overridden. An example commonly given here is the case of immunization programmes. If non-maleficence were to be prioritized it would mean that nobody could be immunized – because of the risk the procedure poses to a minority of people who may suffer side-effects. Such a conclusion is illogical, according to Rumbold (1999, p. 221), because the benefit of immunization programmes to the wider community carries more moral weight.

More controversially, it has been argued that it is justifiable to override non-maleficence in mental health contexts. In other words, it is justifiable to harm someone – by compulsorily detaining them – so as to protect society at large (Edwards, 1996).

RESPONSIBILITY AND ACCOUNTABILITY – MORAL AND PROFESSIONAL ASPECTS

The principles of beneficence and non-maleficence may provide the moral foundation for the various obligations set out in the Code and the Guidelines but they tell us little about the day-to-day activities of nurses or what happens when 'things go wrong'. For more practical guidance on the duties and standards of care that are expected of nurses we have, therefore, to look elsewhere, in particular at the concepts of responsibility and accountability. As we shall see, although these concepts are closely connected they are not the same and should not be used synonymously (Marks-Maran, 1996). Nevertheless, as Tschudin notes (1996, p. 94), the two concepts do overlap and depend on each other.

Responsibility

Scruton (1994) describes responsibility as of the greatest importance in human life because without it would be impossible 'to manage or adjudicate the web of human relations' and because it allows us to 'reward the good and punish the delinquent' (p. 231). Whether or not the concept is as fundamental as Scruton suggests, it is certainly true that there is now renewed and widespread discussion of the nature of responsibility (Giddens, 1999). Yet as it is used today, 'responsibility' is a multilayered term that can be understood or conceived of in different ways.

The notion of legal responsibility, for example, is reflected in the law of negligence (see below). According to Beauchamp and Childress (1994), this legal model of responsibility provides a general framework that can be adapted to express the idea of moral responsibility. For Hunt (1991), moral responsibility means 'accepting and carrying the burden of judgement and decision in matters of right and wrong'. It is based on the person's free will and freedom to use that judgement. This means that when they cannot – for whatever reason – exercise that freedom then they have less than full moral responsibility. Note too that responsibility, in both its legal and moral forms, can be personal or institutional. Thus a nurse's personal responsibility is to herself, patients and clients, colleagues, the profession and society at large (Rumbold, 1999). In contrast, an institution's responsibility is to its employees. As such, it must provide equipment, beds, a safe system of work and so on (Tschudin, 1996). In this context, however, the two aspects of responsibility that need to be emphasized are as follows.

Causal responsibility

Being responsible for something in this sense means that a person has caused something to happen (or produced something). It generally refers to consequences, results and outcome and includes actions or omissions (Hart, 1968). A nurse, therefore, who neglects to give a patient pain relief can be said to have caused that patient harm. In some cases, however, it might not be so easy to link a nurse's actions or omissions with the harm that a patient has suffered. The nurse may have been working as part of a team, for example, another member of which may also have been negligent. So there may have been several causes for a patient's injuries. Or the procedure may have been very complex and technical, making it difficult to establish exactly what went wrong. As we shall see below, proving negligence (i.e. that the nurse is legally responsible) in this kind of case can be very difficult, if not impossible. Yet morally the nurse is clearly responsible. Note too that it is not only human beings who can cause something to happen, since conditions (e.g. staff shortages, poor equipment, inadequate resources, and so forth) may also cause accidents or result in a patient being injured.

In professional terms a nurse will be responsible for causing a patient harm when s/he has fallen below the standard of care that s/he is expected to reach. But what is the required standard? The Code may well provide nurses with a valuable reminder of the special responsibilities they have but given their very general nature they are really no more than statements of belief, i.e. about the nature of the profession of nursing (Benjamin and Curtis, 1992). More guidance is given in the Guidelines, most notably in the section that deals with the nurse's duty of care. In explaining generally what this means, the Guidelines draw heavily on negligence law. The guiding principle, however, in deciding whether nurses have taken proper care, is whether they acted 'reasonably' in all the circumstances.

Note that the concept of reasonableness, again, is determined very much by the legal standard of care. This strongly suggests that professional and legal standards are very similar if not identical. Yet, as the guidelines point out, sometimes the legal and professional approaches to responsibility are different. Thus, although in law the courts can only find a nurse negligent if a person suffers harm because s/he has failed to care for them properly, the UKCC's Professional Conduct Committee can find nurses guilty of misconduct and remove them from the register if they failed to care properly for a client, even though the client suffered no harm. Take the following example. A nurse makes an avoidable and careless mistake when administering a drug – he is in a hurry to finish his shift so that he can go home and get ready for a party. If the patient is unaffected by the mistake, i.e. suffers no ill-effects and is unharmed, in law the nurse will escape liability (because the third element in a negligence claim, namely causing harm, is missing). But professionally, should the nurse admit his mistake (which he may or may not decide to do – see Fletcher *et al.* (1995), pp. 110–111), he could face disciplinary action.

Role responsibility

A person is responsible for something in this sense if it is his/her job or task to deal with it (Downie and Calman, 1994, p. 80). The focus here is the nurse's role. Role responsibility, according to Hart (1968, p. 212), arises whenever people occupy a distinctive place or office in a society to which specific duties are attached. In such cases they can then be said to be responsible for doing what is necessary to fulfil them.

Role responsibility can be either legal or moral. A nurse's shift – the nurse's legal (i.e. contractual) responsibility may, for example, finish at lunchtime, at which time she can go home. But supposing she has promised a particularly anxious young patient that she will stay with her until her mother comes to visit her. It can at least be argued that she has a moral responsibility to keep her promise.

Note also that different roles bring with them different responsibilities. Thus while all nurses have a fundamental responsibility to promote health, prevent illness, restore health and alleviate suffering (ICN, 1973), the way they carry it out varies according to the setting in which they practise. Thus, the responsibilities of a nurse working on a hospital ward will include administering medicines, maintaining records and perhaps teaching students. In contrast, the duties of a practice nurse based in a health centre will include advising on health promotion and giving vaccinations (Fletcher *et al.*, 1995, p. 106).

A nurse's role therefore should be defined in terms of the rights and obligations accorded to the particular position the nurse occupies (Rumbold, 1999, p. 187). This means that specialist nurses – e.g. those working in paediatrics or palliative care – will have different responsibilities from those traditionally taken on by nurses. Similarly, nurses whose role has been expanded and who perform tasks previously carried out by doctors will have wider responsibilities than in the past. Nurses now, for example, undertake tasks such as carrying out ECGs, performing defibrillation after a heart attack, verification of death, taking blood samples, performing male catheterization. There are also nurse-led minor injury units where nurses carry out a variety of tasks such as suturing, X-ray (Tingle, 1998a).

Although role expansion has generally been welcomed it has nevertheless been controversial. One major concern is the issues it raises about the boundaries of practice, in particular where ultimate responsibility should lie. Thus it is one thing for a nurse to take on additional responsibility as an independent practitioner because she feels she has the necessary skills, but it is quite another for her to have a task delegated to her inappropriately. It is important to note, too, that a nurse's role is not just about performing particular tasks but also about issues such as competence and maintaining appropriate standards of care. This is confirmed in the Code, which states that nurses must 'maintain and improve [their] professional knowledge and competence'. Similarly, the UKCC document *The Scope of Professional Practice* states that nurses 'must endeavour always to achieve, maintain, and develop knowledge, skill and competence and respond to the needs and interests [of patients and clients]'. Note also the UKCC Post-Registration Education and Practice Project (PREP), which encourages personal updating (Tingle, 1998c, p. 23). In addition, as Rumbold observes (1999, p. 81), nurses have a responsibility not just to ensure that their knowledge and skills are constantly being improved but also to contribute to the development of knowledge and skills within the profession as a whole.

Accountability

Like responsibility, the concept of accountability can be understood and conceived of in several different ways. Before looking at its various meanings, however, it is important to distinguish it from the concept of responsibility, with which it is often mistakenly confused. Thus you can be responsible for something – in the sense that you caused it to happen – without being accountable. A student nurse, for example, who makes a mistake and harms a patient would almost certainly not have to account for her actions if responsibility had been inappropriately delegated to her. Instead, accountability would rest with the trained nurse who should have supervised her. Put very simply, accountability is about justifying actions, explaining why something was (or was not) done. The purpose of calling people to account for their actions is therefore to establish whether they had good enough reasons for acting in the way they did. It is a process that the Guidelines state involves 'weighing up the interests of patients and clients in complex situations, using professional knowledge, judgement and skills to make a decision (UKCC, 1996). Echoing this, Marks-Maran (1996) states that an accountable person is one who: 'examines a situation, explores the various options available, demonstrates a knowledgeable understanding of the possible consequences of options and makes a decision for action which can be justified from a knowledge basis' (p. 123).

In recent years, accountability has become a very pervasive term in health-care contexts whose importance is constantly emphasized, even though, as Hunt (1994) notes, demanding accountability does not in itself say anything about whom one is accountable to, what things one is or ought to be accountable for, and according to what criteria.

It is possible too to distinguish several types of accountability. Hence, as we shall see below, **legal accountability** can be defined as the extent to which nurses can be held in law to be liable for their actions (Dimond, 1995). **Moral accountability** is very similar but it does not necessarily overlap with the legal model. Indeed, they can conflict, as in the following example. A patient's prescription for pain relief is too low and the patient is in severe pain. If the nurse ignores the prescription and tops it up she will have to account for her actions legally, since she has overstepped the prescription. Morally, however, she may feel she has done the right thing in relieving the patient's pain. Another kind of accountability is **professional accountability**. The Code identifies 16 guidelines for standards of professional practice. As was noted above, the Code is not designed to provide comprehensive answers to all the situations a nurse will encounter but nevertheless does establish principles to aid decision-making and so enable members to exercise accountability (Singleton and McLaren, 1995).

But complying with the Code, i.e. acting in the professionally 'right' way, does not necessarily mean that a nurse's actions are always morally right too. In other words, professional and moral accountability do not in practice neces-sarily coincide. Supposing, for example, a nurse allows a young child, whose prognosis is hopeless, to die in his arms without taking any steps to resuscitate her. If he later faces disciplinary action – for ignoring resuscitation policy – and so fails to justify his actions to his employers – he could nevertheless probably justify his actions in his own personal moral terms and according to his own value system. In other words, by allowing the child to die peacefully he has acted in a caring way that he thought was morally 'right' (Hunt, 1994, pp 134–142). Similarly, a nurse who is off duty and comes across an accident victim to whom she only provides 'comfort and support' (as the Guidelines stipulate) could almost certainly justify her action in professional terms. Morally, however, she might be expected to do more and so can be said to have to account morally for her failure to give any further assistance.

LEGAL RESPONSIBILITY AND ACCOUNTABILITY

As we have seen above, nurses may perform a variety or roles. That they have a moral and professional obligation to carry them out diligently and with due care is self-evident. What we will consider in this section is the legal consequences of their failure to do so. In other words, in what circumstances can those who hold positions of responsibility be held accountable in law for their conduct?

There are several channels of accountability. But the main focus will be on the tort system, notably the law of negligence, which is the most common action in health-care contexts for NHS patients seeking compensation. For the private patient, i.e. a person who is being treated privately, the law of contract exists as an additional alternative to this tort liability but it will also not be considered further here. Note too that, because it is only very exceptionally that nurses face criminal prosecutions, the role of the criminal law will not be considered here (see Mason and McCall Smith, 1999, pp. 240–243). Similarly, limited space prevents a discussion of alternative processes by which standards are controlled, notably complaints and UKCC disciplinary procedures (on which see Tingle, 1998b, ch. 3; Pyne, 1995, ch. 3).

NEGLIGENCE

Liability for medical negligence has a long history – the first significant malpractice case in English law dates back to the 14th century (*Stratton* v. *Swanland* (1374)). But until fairly recently it was very rare for patients to sue health professionals. Indeed, conventionally such an action was considered almost a presumptuous thing to do (Teff, 1994). But reluctance to sue is now a relic of the past, since there can be little doubt that since the early 1980s the number of claims against all health professionals have dramatically increased. In 1989–90, for example, the NHS spent approximately £45 million on malpractice cases. By 1996–97 the figure had risen to £300 million – the vast majority of which concerned hospital patients (Mason and McCall Smith, 1999, p. 215).

How can this increase be explained? The most widely accepted explanation is the nature of modern medicine. Not only is it very intrusive but advances in medical technology, new forms of treatment and transplant surgery, 'miracle' drugs and so forth all increase the opportunities for things to go wrong as procedures become more complex and risky and the skills required ever more intricate (Teff, 1994; Phillips, 1997). Changing patterns of consultation and attitudes to illness and health also now encourage patients not just to seek treatment for conditions once seen as untreatable but also to expect cures. When these are not met it is hardly surprising that in the current culture of consumerism – fuelled by the language of commerce and the market that pervades patients' and citizens' charters and Department of Health publications – aggrieved patients will want to blame someone or something. As Mason and McCall Smith note; 'there are no longer any accidents – somebody, somewhere must be made to answer for what happened' (1999, p. 215).

The media's role, too, has been significant. Keen to disclose malpractice and report successful claims it has certainly contributed to both the public's increasing consciousness of health-related issues and its intolerance of medical mistakes. A better-educated public is also much less inclined to accept assurances about medical care and to challenge practitioners when accidents occur (Teff, 1994).

Although it is currently not possible to identify the number of accidents that occur each year or the number that result from negligence – such information is not systematically collected (Jones, 1996) – it is clear that the negligence action is a popular one and will almost certainly remain so, given the implementation of new procedural rules in 1999. These were introduced to produce just outcomes in civil cases and reduce the delays, inequalities in access to justice and uncertainties that had plagued the old system.

What then is the purpose of negligence law? Obtaining compensation is perhaps the most obvious function (McHale *et al.*, 1997, p. 145). It seeks to minimize the effect that negligence can have on a victim's life. Thus, injured patients may lose all or most of their earning capacity and require long-term nursing care, especially if they are harmed at birth or as children. Others, less seriously injured, may nevertheless find their income significantly reduced. Damages awarded are thus expected to compensate them for their lost earning potential and higher living expenses. But the problems with a negligence action as a method of providing compensation are well documented. They include: delay; the cost of bringing an action (which is notoriously high); problems of proof (which make the outcome of proceedings unpredictable); and the complexity of modern medicine, which makes proving fault and causation extremely difficult, if not impossible (Jones, 1996, p. 8).

The other main function of negligence law is the deterrent one. Legal action and its impact on professional reputations is thought to be a very effective in promoting good practice and maintaining high standards. In other words, the fear of a lawsuit is believed to make practitioners more careful and so reduce the number and seriousness of accidents. But this idea too can be undermined. First, as we shall see below, negligence may exist but be impossible to establish, and even where established can fail because of the causation hurdle. Secondly, the use of insurance and the fact that in most cases it is employers who actually pay damages mean that individual responsibility is, if not extinguished, then at least diluted (Phillips, 1997).

However, despite the known shortcomings of the tort system, which have prompted various proposals to replace the tort action altogether – such as no-fault compensation schemes, where victims of medical accidents get compensation without having to establish fault (see Phillips, 1997, pp. 176–183) – the negligence action is likely to remain the main method of dealing with malpractice for the foreseeable future. This is so despite the fact the vast majority of claims never actually come to trial (but fail or are settled before then). Its continuing popularity may be that litigation may be the only way to prompt an investigation and, ultimately, an apology. Indeed, evidence from organizations representing patients' interests suggests that information and accountability are just as important to victims of medical accidents as compensation, not least because of the satisfaction it may provide that the error will not be repeated (Jones, 1996).

Basic elements in negligence

To succeed in a negligence claim, patients or clients have to establish the following elements, which they must prove on the 'balance of probabilities' (Montgomery, 1995). These are that:

- the nurse (the defendant) owed a duty of care to the plaintiff;
- the defendant breached that duty;
- damage (that the law recognizes) was caused by the breach.

Duty of care

It is for the law to determine whether a duty of care exists, depending on the particular facts of each situation. In essence, this means deciding whether a practitioner has assumed responsibility for the patient, i.e. has undertaken to use his/her skills for that patient (Davies, 1998). In most professional contexts this is fairly easy to establish – at least in relation to existing patients and clients – and is rarely a matter of dispute (Brazier, 1992). Hence nurses clearly owe a duty to patients on their wards as they do to those they are caring for and treating in other health-care settings, e.g. in outpatients departments, in the community or when they are attached to specialist clinics such as family planning clinics. In some situations, however, the existence of a duty of care is less obvious. Is one owed, for example, to accident victims nurses come across while off-duty? As the Guidelines (clause 14) make clear, nurses do not have a legal duty to stop and care in this situation. Note that if a nurse does decide to treat the victim then a duty of care arises (Hendrick, 1997, p. 24).

Another not uncommon question concerns the duty owed to clients arriving for treatment at a hospital without an accident and emergency department. As Tingle notes (1998c, p. 18), the answer to this question will depend on the circumstances of each case. In general, however, establishing whether duties are owed in these and similar situations turns on applying the 'neighbour test'. This test was established in the famous case of *Donoghue* v. *Stevenson* [1932] AC 562 (Chapter 1). It states that a duty is owed **to anyone who is reasonably likely to be affected by their acts or omissions**. The neighbour test is an objective one and involves asking a hypothetical question about what a 'reasonable' person would have done in the circumstances. Furthermore, it is not only owed to patients but extends to all those who may be affected by a nurse's actions or omissions, as well as patients' relatives and visitors. Although this approach might suggest that nurses could find themselves responsible for the welfare of a large number of people, the law does set limits. One way in which it does this is to say that the relationship between the nurse and the patient or victim is not close enough to be legally significant. This explains why English law does not require nurses (or other health professionals) to be Good Samaritans rescuing strangers whenever they happen to be on hand. Another way is to claim that on public policy grounds a duty of care should not be recognized since otherwise it would make the law too impractical, costly and unwieldy (Nelson-Jones and Burton, 1995).

So far we have looked at the personal responsibility of nurses. In some situations, however, a duty of care may be owed by hospitals to patients. This **direct** or **primary liability** was first signalled in *Cassidy* v. *Ministry of Health* [1951] 2 KB 343, where Lord Denning said that: 'when a patient puts himself in the hands of a hospital he expects there to be sufficiently qualified people and adequate facilities to look after him properly and hopefully make him better; if that fails to materialize then it is fitting that the health authority should be made liable'.

Claims based on this type of duty typically allege that a reasonable regimen of care has not been provided – because of, for example, defective equipment, inadequate facilities or too few suitably qualified and competent staff. In the past this kind of claim has been controversial and difficult to win. Yet in *Bull* v. *Devon AHA* [1993] 4 Med LR 117, the Court of Appeal found the hospital authority liable for organizing its maternity services in such a way that Mrs Bull's son's birth was delayed for 68 minutes – as a result of which he suffered asphyxia. In so doing it rejected the hospital's defence that given available resources it had provided the best care possible. Whether claims against hospital authorities will be more successful in the future remains to be seen. But many commentators predict that they will be, given the growing dissatisfaction of hospital staff with conditions under which they are now expected to practise (see, for example, Davies, 1998).

Note too the doctrine of **vicarious liability**. Although nurses are personally liable for their own negligence it is rare that they will be able to bear the cost of claims against them or will have to (because of the NHS Indemnity Scheme). This explains why in the vast majority of cases their employers – the hospital, health authority NHS trust – are sued instead. Under the doctrine of vicarious liability employers are indirectly liable for the negligent acts or omissions of their employees (whether clinical or non-clinical), providing the negligence occurred in the course of their employment. Employers can, of course – at least in theory – recover the amount paid out on an negligent employee's behalf, although in practice they rarely do this, not least because NHS guidance advises against it (UKCC, 1996). Usually there is little difficulty in determining whether or not a hospital is vicariously liable but the position is less certain when a nursing agency supplies a nurse. The supplying agency is unlikely to be liable for the torts of the nurse during the course of her work. But ultimately liability would turn on the contractual terms, the representation made by the agency and the steps taken by the agency to provide a competent nurse (Nelson-Jones and Burton, 1995, p. 137).

The duty of care owed by nurses has been described as a single indivisible duty (Khan and Robson, 1997), yet it has many different aspects. Thus, although it means that they must take reasonable care for the well-being of their patients throughout all stages of advice and treatment (Phillips, 1997), it consists of various specific duties, of which the following are particularly relevant to nurses.

Duty to keep up to date

Nursing journals, research articles, technical papers, practice guidelines, circulars, and so on can vary considerably in both their frequency and status. How can busy nurses read them all? Do they have to? As far as the law is concerned it is now well established that practitioners are expected to keep reasonably up to date and must know of all major developments in their particular field. The duty to do so is nonetheless a reasonable one (*Crawford* v. *Charing Cross Hospital* (1953) *The Times* 8 December). So nurses do not have to read every single article or research paper but they should be aware of mainstream literature and be familiar with mainstream changes in diagnosis, treatment and practice in their field and new techniques that have been widely adopted (*Gascoine* v. *Ian Sheridan & Co.* [1994] 5 Med LR 437). In addition, they should be familiar with relevant guidance and instruction from the NHS Executive and senior nurse management. As Tingle notes (1998a, p. 55), clinical guidelines (which may be evidence-based) and protocols are an increasingly important aspect of nursing, setting out the procedure to be followed in, for example, advanced practice situations. A nurse practising in a context where such guidelines have been issued would almost certainly, therefore be expected to be familiar with those which have been widely followed (see further Tingle, 1998a, Chapter 4).

Duty of candour

Here the main issue is whether there is a general duty to inform patients that something has gone wrong. Several cases in the past have strongly suggested that there is such a duty. In *Gerber* v. *Pines* (1935) 79 Sol J 13, for example, the court held that when a foreign substance was left in a body the doctor had a duty to inform patients of that fact even if there had been no negligence. In that particular instance a patient was having injections for rheumatism but a muscle spasm caused a needle to break, which could only be removed by an operation. While there have been few cases directly on this point and there is still some doubt about its legal basis (Jones, 1996, p. 565), the principle of truthfulness seems to have been affirmed in *Naylor* v. *Preston AHA* [1987] 1 WLR 958, when Lord Donaldson not only stated that: 'in medical negligence cases there is a duty of candour resting upon the professional man', but also that: 'doctors have a duty to tell patients that they have a right to sue'.

Exceptionally, however, this duty of candour may not apply – such as when the effect was very minor or could be easily rectified. However, given the increasing legal emphasis on patient autonomy, even these exceptions could now be questioned (Davies, 1998, p. 81). Note too that, although these cases concerned doctors, there is no reason to suppose that the law would except any lesser degree of honesty from nurses. Indeed, Dimond (1995, p. 106) asserts that if a nurse makes a mistake her duty to the patient means that she must ensure that the mistake is made known and must also take steps to prevent the error recurring.

Duty in emergencies

Nurses who work in accident and emergency departments – where the workload can be erratic and staff can suddenly find themselves under a lot of pressure – may sometimes fail to exercise the skill and professional judgement they would normally hope to provide. How does the law react? In other words, does the law demand the same duty of care in emergencies as it does in other health-care settings? Take another example, that of a nurse who stops to help an accident victim. Will the law take account of the fact that she is acting in an emergency situation without the usual medical backup and so forth?

There have been few cases directly on this point but, as Lord Mustill said in *Wilsher* v. *Essex AHA* [1986] 3 All ER 801, 'an emergency may overburden the available resources, and if an individual is forced by circumstances to do too many things at once, the fact that he does one of them incorrectly should not lightly be taken as negligence'. It is likely that the law would probably recognize that in emergencies practitioners are more likely to make mistakes. While this does not mean that the courts would overlook a practitioner giving substandard treatment, they would nevertheless judge the practitioner according to the standard expected of other reasonably competent nurses acting in an emergency. In this way, any special 'emergency' circumstances would be taken into account.

Duty to be extra vigilant

Over the years there have been a steady stream of cases – several of which have involved nurses – that suggest that there are certain categories of patients who are especially vulnerable, such as children and those suffering from mental illness, in respect of whom the law expects extra precautions to be taken. Although the scope of the duty to such patients is uncertain, it is clear from case law that a duty to care for patients 'at risk' of harming themselves and others is established (Davies, 1998, p. 78). This does not mean that a constant watch has to be kept on them but rather that a stricter regime of supervision might have to be put in place.

Thus in *Selfe* v. *Ilford & District Management Committee* (1970) 4 *British Medical Journal* 754 the hospital authority was found liable for failing to provide adequate supervision in respect of a 17-year-old with suicidal tendencies. He took an overdose and was put on the ground floor, with an unlocked window behind him. There were 27 patients on the ward and he was grouped with three other suicide risks at one end. Three nurses were allocated to the ward (all of whom knew that the young man was a suicide risk) but all disappeared at the same time without telling the others – one to the kitchen, one to the lavatory and one to attend to another patient. In their absence the patient climbed through the window and eventually threw himself from a roof. As a result of the fall he became a paraplegic. The basis of the court's decision was that the degree of care required was proportionate to the degree of risk, and that in this case there had been a breakdown in proper nursing supervision, which had caused the accident (see also *Mahmood* v. *Siggins* [1996] 7 Med LR 76).

Breach of duty

Once a duty of care has been established the prospective claimant has to prove that the duty has been breached. The law expects nurses, like all other health professionals, to exercise reasonable care and skill in all the tasks they undertake – although they will not inevitably be liable if an accident occurs, since not all mistakes and errors will amount to negligence. Nevertheless, even though the borderline between a negligent and non-negligent mistake can be difficult to draw, case law suggests that there are particular areas of nursing practice that are most likely to result in claims. Typical actions involving nurses concern allegations that they have not properly supervised patients (see the Selfe case, above and *Newham and Another* v. *Rochester and Chatham Joint Hospital Board* (1936) *The Times*, 28 February).

Many others focus on substandard treatment or aftercare. Thus in one case three nurses on duty in the post-anaesthetic recovery rooms went for a coffee break, leaving only two nurses to observe seven patients. Because of their absence no-one noticed that a young patient, who had had plastic surgery for over-prominent ears, had suffered respiratory failure followed by cardiac arrest. He died a few years later without having regained consciousness (*Krujelis* v. *Esdale et al.* (1971) 25 DLR 557). The hospital authority was held vicariously liable for the negligence of the three nurses, i.e. their inadequate observation. In another case a nurse was found negligent for passing a rigid catheter vaginally, causing a bladder perforation (*Powell* v. *Streatham Nursing Home* [1935] AC 243). So too was a midwife who injected pethidine into the inside of the plaintiff's right thigh (*Walker* v. *South West Surrey DHA*, 1982, unreported). Negligence was also proved against a matron who failed to notice a developing infection under a plaster cast that she had put on, as a result of which the child patient became severely disabled (*Baylis* v. *Blagg* (1954) 1 *British Medical Journal* 709).

A wrong diagnosis can also lead to a claim. Thus in *Sutton* v. *Population Services Family Planning Ltd* (1981) *The Times*, 7 November a nurse failed to follow prescribed procedure for referring a patient with a lump in her breast. As a consequence, the tumour was detected and removed much later than it should have been.

Errors in the dispensing of prescribed drugs have also led to successful claims, as in the case of *Strangeways-Lesmere* v. *Clayton* [1936] 2 KB 11, which concerned two nurses who administered a fatal dose of 6 ounces of paraldehyde instead of 6 drachms – one poured out the dose, the other checked it but neither of them read the bed card. And in another case (*Smith* v. *Brighton and Lewes Hospital Management Committee* (1958) *The Times*, 2 May) a ward sister was held responsible for a patient who suffered permanent loss of balance when she received 34 streptomycin injections instead of 30. The sister was negligent because, even though she did not administer the drugs herself, she had failed to make an appropriate record on the notes.

In several cases too nurses have been held responsible for accidents arising out of routine quasi-domestic aspects of their jobs (see, for example, *Trew* v. *Middlesex Hospital* (1953) 2 *The Lancet* 343 and Nelson-Jones and Burton, 1995, pp. 137–139).

From this brief account of the kinds of claim that have involved nurses it should be clear that they can cover a wide range of tasks. And as nurses take on more responsibility and extend their role so the chances of incurring liability increase, whether it is in respect of diagnosis, nursing care, treatment, counselling (e.g. giving information and disclosing risks) or communicating with other health professionals (for a detailed discussion of the legal aspects of a nurse's expanded role, see Tingle, 1998a, chapter 4). But whatever the mistake or error and in whatever context it occurs, the legal test for liability is the same, namely whether the nurse's performance fell below the legally recognized standard of care. What then is that standard and secondly, who sets the standard?

Legal standard of care

In determining what is the legal standard of care advice would have to be sought from other nurses practising in the same area. Should the case go to trial, the judge would hear expert evidence and then draw conclusions as to the appropriate standard of care (Tingle, 1998c, p. 19). The guiding principles, however, would derive from case law, most notably the landmark case of *Bolam* v. *Friern Hospital Management Committee* [1957] 1 WLR 582. This case and the standard of care it established – popularly known as the Bolam test – has been applied in all cases of negligence law for the last 40 years (Mason and McCall Smith, 1999, p. 224). It has been endorsed time and time again in the courts – even though it has been the subject of sustained criticism, especially in the last decade (see, for example, Sheldon and Thompson, 1998; Kennedy and Grubb, 1994).

According to Bolam the required standard is that of:

the ordinary skilled [person] exercising and professing to have that special skill. A [person] need not possess the highest skill. It is well-established law that it is sufficient if he exercises the ordinary skill of an ordinary competent [person] exercising that particular art.

In other words a nurse's conduct is judged according to what an ordinary skilled nurse practising in the same speciality would have done in the circumstances. Points worth noting about the Bolam test are as follows.

- Even though the case concerned a doctor, the principles it established applies to all health professionals.
- The test is an objective one. This means that practitioners are judged by their peers, i.e. by those who do the same kind of work. So a sister is judged by the standards of other sisters, a specialist nurse (e.g. a neonatal nurse) according to the standards expected of other neonatal nurses. A nurse whose role is

expanded and who has more independence – e.g. in diagnosis and treatment – would thus be judged according to the standards that would be expected of other reasonably competent nurses who had taken on those additional responsibilities.

- Nurses do not have to have the highest level of skills; rather they must show that they have reached the same standard as the ordinary competent nurse.

Having established the relevant standard of care the next issue is to determine how the courts actually ascertain it in individual cases. The answer again comes from the Bolam case. It states that doctors (likewise nurses and all other health professionals) will not be liable in negligence if they have: 'acted in accordance with a practice accepted as proper by a responsible body of medical men skilled in that particular art'.

Points to note here are as follows:

- The 'accepted practice' test has been applied in several areas, including treatment, diagnosis, counselling, prognosis and more recently consent and information disclosure.
- It sets a minimum standard below which practitioners must not fall.
- Because of the courts' traditional deference to the medical profession (which means that they have almost never seriously challenged professional judgement), compliance with accepted practice has almost always been conclusive proof that the health professional was not negligent. As a consequence, standards of care have, until now, in practice been set, controlled and monitored unilaterally by health professionals themselves.
- In the future the courts may be more willing than in the past if not to reject professional opinion then at least to question its reasonableness. This is because of the important case of *Bolitho* v. *Hackney Health Authority* [1997] 3 WLR 1151, in which five Law Lords unanimously held that judges must not simply accept the word of experts who give evidence for doctors that a particular course of action is acceptable. Rather, they would have to be satisfied that experts had 'weighed up the risks and benefits and reached a defensible conclusion'. Although regarded by many commentators as a development that represents a 'significant nail in the Bolam coffin' (Mason and McCall Smith, 1999, p. 225), it is unlikely that this approach will be adopted very enthusiastically by the courts. This is because, as Lord Brown Wilkinson himself conceded, 'in the vast majority of cases the fact that distinguished experts in the field are of a particular opinion will demonstrate the reasonableness of that opinion'.

Other important questions that typically arise in settling standards of nursing competence are the following.

What if there are differences of opinion?

This was in fact one of the central issues in the Bolam case. It is an important question because often there are several different approaches and techniques which can be adopted. How then is the law to decide what is a responsible professional practice? In such cases the answer is clear. The judges will not choose between competing views and practices. In other words, they will not decide which they think is the best (*Maynard* v. *West Midlands RHA* [1985] 1 All ER 635). So the fact that some nurses would have done things differently is not in itself evidence of negligence. This means that a nurse would almost certainly avoid liability if s/he could show that at least some other reasonably competent nurses would have acted in a similar way. It is of course always open to the courts to reject the particular approach taken (see *Bolitho* v. *City and Hackney HA*, above). Note too that, according to *De Freitas* v. *O'Brien* [1995] 6 Med LR 108, the courts will not require the responsible body of opinion to be large. What this means is that in theory a body of two practitioners could outweigh the views of a much larger group – a precedent that could, rather worryingly, legalize the practice of a small fringe group of practitioners using experimental techniques that are contrary to the norm (Khan and Robson, 1997).

When is accepted practice judged?

Often, several years can have passed between the time of the alleged negligence and a trial. During that time professional practice might have significantly changed. But for legal purposes the crucial time for determining whether or not there has been a breach of duty is the date of the accident and not the trial date. The classic illustration of this approach is the case of *Roe* v. *Minister of Health* [1954] 2 QB 66 (see also now *HIV Haemophiliac Litigation* (1990) 140 NLJ 1349). *Roe* v. *Minister of Health* concerned a patient who became permanently paralysed below the waist after being injected with a spinal anaesthetic in 1947. This was caused by phenol leaking through invisible cracks in the glass ampoules containing the anaesthetic. However, the dangers of phenol leakage were unknown at the time of the operation, being first written about and published in 1951. The patient sued the anaesthetist but lost his claim. This was, according to Lord Denning because: 'We must not look at the 1947 accident with 1954 spectacles'.

Can a nurse deviate from accepted practice?

Suppose, for example, that a nurse decided to use a new and different technique rather than the orthodox one. If something went wrong would the nurse automatically be found liable? The answer would depend on whether departing from the conventional practice could be justified, bearing in mind all the circumstances. These would include the seriousness of the patient's condition, the patient's previous or likely response to the usual treatment, evidence of previous trials, the implications of changing practice and appraisal of new research (*Clarke* v. *MacLennan* [1983] 1 All ER 416).

The intention behind this approach is that new innovative techniques should not be discouraged but neither should the patient be exposed to reckless experiments. Thus in *Hepworth* v. *Kerr* [1995] 6 Med LR 139 an anaesthetist was found to be negligent for reducing a patient's blood pressure to a lower level than the accepted norm. He had done this previously with 1500 patients but this was not enough to show that his approach was valid, not least because he had failed to follow any of them up and there was no expert support or endorsement of his work.

Does the law take inexperience into account?
The law does not except a defence of inexperience, lack of ability or lack of knowledge. The leading case on this is *Wilsher* v. *Essex AHA* [1988] 2 WLR 557. Martin Wilsher was born 3 months prematurely. He needed extra oxygen to survive, which was administered by an inexperienced junior doctor who mistakenly inserted a catheter into a vein rather than an artery. The error was not spotted by the senior registrar (whose advice the junior doctor sought) and when replacing the catheter the registrar did exactly the same thing himself. The registrar was found liable (because he should have known better), but not the junior doctor (because he had consulted the registrar). Several general principles about the liability of trainee or inexperienced staff were laid down in this case. In brief these are:

- Junior staff 'learning on the job' and thus attempting specialist skills who make a mistake (which a more experienced professional would not make) satisfy the required standard of care if they seek the advice and help of a superior when necessary.
- Inexperienced professionals occupying a post in a unit providing specialist care must exercise the skill and expertise that patients would normally expect from a reasonably competent person occupying such a post and holding themselves out as having the necessary skills.
- The standard of care must be set according to the post occupied rather than according to the actual postholder and his/her personal ability.
- There is no such thing as team liability, since this would require each member to reach the high standard that the team as a whole could provide (i.e. a primary nurse would be expected to provide the same care as a consultant). Nevertheless, each team member is responsible for his/her own conduct.
- Nurses who take on delegated tasks they are not qualified to carry out remain personally liable.

Are some cases easier to prove than others?
To succeed, the plaintiff must prove breach of the standard of care. In medical negligence cases this is no easy task but there are some cases when plaintiffs have an inbuilt advantage because the acts or omissions that caused them injury give rise to the presumption of negligence, which the defendant then has to rebut. In other words, negligence can be presumed from the mere fact that an accident happened. This is basically a rule of evidence and is generally known by its Latin name of *res ipsa loquitur* ('the thing speaks for itself'). How the rule works was explained by Lord Denning in *Cassidy* v. *Ministry of Health* [1951] 1 All ER 574 when he said: 'I went into hospital to be cured of two stiff fingers. I have come

out with four stiff fingers, and my hand is useless. That should not have happened if due care had been used. Explain it, if you can.'

Causation

The third element in a negligence claim is the causation one. In practice this is one of the biggest hurdles for potential claimants, even though at first glance the burden of proof this imposes does not seem very heavy. First, all the parties are competing on fairly equal terms as plaintiffs only have to prove that, on the balance of probabilities, their injuries were caused (or were materially contributed to) by the nurse's acts or omissions. In other words, the court has to be convinced that their version of the truth was 50% likely. Second, in some cases the so-called 'but for' test works well, in that patients may easily be able to show that if it were not for the nurse's conduct they would not have been injured. For example, the nurse gave the wrong drug, administered an overdose or left a patient unattended. But in many cases proving causation is far harder. One particular problem is the lengthy delays in negligence cases, which typically take several years to reach the courts, during which time memories may have faded, important facts may have been forgotten and records may have been mislaid.

The case of *Whitehouse* v. *Jordan* [1981] 1 All ER 267 is a good example of the causation hurdle. It concerned a claim by a baby that the severe brain damage he suffered at birth was due to the doctor's negligence. His mother was small (just under 4 ft 11 in – 61.5 cm) and was unable or refused to have an internal examination or lateral X-ray. Initially 'trial by forceps' was undertaken but after five or six attempts the baby was delivered by caesarean. Mrs White-house claimed that the obstetrician, Mr Jordan, pulled too hard or continued traction too long, actions that caused the baby's head to become wedged. The case took 9 years to reach the House of Lords. Mrs Whitehouse's evidence consisted of what she remembered, notably being lifted up off the delivery bed by the pulling. In contrast, two expert witnesses (retired obstetricians) gave evidence based on reading the hospital notes that she had in fact been pulled down off the bed. Mr Jordan could not remember the facts in any detail but on the basis of his notes and usual practice was certain he could not have pulled too hard. Two midwives who were present – who could have been very reliable and useful neutral witnesses – could not be traced so could not give evidence. Other witnesses included four consultant obstetricians, who based their evidence on hospital notes and concluded that Mr Jordan had not been negligent. Faced with this conflicting and incomplete evidence it is perhaps not surprising that the plaintiff lost his case.

One other point raised by this case and worth noting here is the importance of maintaining accurate and comprehensive records of patients' care and treatment (guidance on standards for records and record-keeping was issued by the UKCC in 1993). Although not proof of the truth, medical and nursing records may well be used in evidence should a dispute arise.

Other major problems that commonly arise in relation to causation include the difficulty of proving that it was the nurse's negligence – rather than the natural progression of the patient's illness or underlying condition (or perhaps even a natural, albeit rare, accident) – that made the patient's ill health worse. Sometimes too cases collapse because a patient's injuries could have been caused by several factors unrelated to and irrespective of negligence. In this kind of situation it may be impossible to establish which factor was legally significant because the plaintiff cannot prove that on the balance of probabilities the negligence caused or materially contributed to the injuries. It was just this 'multiple cause' problem that hindered Martin Wilsher's claim (although an out-of-court settlement was finally reached). Although in that case it was clear that too much oxygen had been negligently administered – which was well known to cause blindness – there were at least five other possible causes of blindness in premature babies. With so many potential causes competing, the scientific evidence linking the negligence with the blindness was at best ambivalent and at worse inconclusive.

Nor are cases much easier to win if there are only two possible causes of the plaintiff's injuries, because here too there are problems. So in *Kay v. Ayrshire and Arran HB* [1987] 2 All ER 417, a 2-year-old boy with meningitis was given a massive overdose of penicillin (300 000 units instead of 10 000), which quickly produced toxic effects. Although the mistake was rectified and he recovered, he became profoundly deaf – which he claimed was due to the overdose. Negligence was admitted, yet the boy's claim failed because his expert evidence was unable to show that a penicillin overdose had ever caused deafness, whereas meningitis commonly did.

Other claims likely to fail are the so-called 'lost opportunity' cases in which the claim is essentially that the defendant's negligence lost the patient a chance of a full recovery or at the very least a 'better medical result'. In *Hotson* v. *East Berkshire HA* [1987] 2 All ER 909, a boy fell out of a tree, injuring his hip. The hospital did not notice the fracture and sent him home. He returned 5 days later, when his injury was correctly diagnosed and treated, but by then it was too late to prevent permanent disability. The boy conceded that even if the fracture and been diagnosed straight-away he would still have had only a 25% chance of being cured. But the House of Lords rejected his claim on the grounds that to succeed he had to prove that treatment would have cured him. This he could not do because there was a 75% chance that he would have suffered from avascular necrosis even if he had been properly treated.

Finally it is important to note that before any compensation can be claimed patients must show that the injuries they suffered were 'reasonably foreseeable', i.e. they were not too remote (in law compensation is known as 'damages' and is designed to cover any loss of earnings and other financial losses, as well as compensation for pain and suffering and loss of amenities). In the vast majority of malpractice claims this foreseeability test is easy to establish in that usually the victim can show that his original illness or condition has not been cured or a new injury has been inflicted. But rarely a consequence may be too remote and so not the responsibility of the defendant – perhaps because the chain of causation has been broken by some intervening event or because the courts have refused to recognize a certain type of injury. It was this reluctance which, until fairly recently, prevented plaintiffs who 'witnessed' medical accidents from getting compensation for 'nervous shock'. This is now recoverable, however, and is likely to generate an increasing number of claims from parents following the neonatal death of their children as a result of negligence – see *Krali* v. *McGrath* [1986] 1 All ER 54, in which, following what was described as 'a particularly horrendous piece of mismanagement' one of the plaintiff's twins died 8 weeks after birth.

DISPUTE SETTLEMENT OUTSIDE THE COURTROOM – COMPLAINTS AND DISCIPLINARY PROCEEDINGS

In this last section we will look very briefly at various ways in which nurses may be held accountable that do not involve the courts (for a more detailed account see Montgomery, 1997, Chapters 5 and 6). There are several options, the one chosen by aggrieved patients usually depending on what they hope to achieve.

Complaints

Patients can have many different reasons for complaining. Alleged negligence is one, lack of information another. Some may want an apology or just an explanation of what has taken place, while others will want to ensure that policies or practice change so that the same incident does not recur. In more serious cases, the purpose of the complaint might be to ensure that the 'guilty' health professional is appropriately punished. It is clear that, just as negligence claims have increased in recent years, so too have the number of complaints. In the past, complaint procedures were very complex and largely ineffective but major reforms introduced in 1996 have streamlined the system, making it (at least in theory) simpler, fairer, more responsive, accessible, accountable and open.

Complaints relating to care and treatment in NHS hospitals are governed by the Hospital Complaints Procedure Act 1985. Complaints about family health services are dealt with by health authorities. Both categories are dealt with under the same structure, however, which operates basically on two levels, local resolution and independent review, and includes clinical and non-clinical complaints. Note that under the Clinical Negligence Protocol it is possible that mediation will be seen as an essential part of the process of complaints handling. Finally there is the Health Service Commissioner. Operating as the final complaints forum the Commissioner is only intended to be involved after all other avenues of complaint have been exhausted. The Commissioner's powers are extensive, covering allegations of maladministration as well as failures in the provision of health services.

Disciplinary proceedings

There are two types of disciplinary proceeding that nurses may face. Nurses are accountable to their professional body, the UKCC, which has a statutory obligation to investigate allegations of misconduct. If a nurse is found to be guilty of professional misconduct – defined as 'conduct unworthy of a registered nurse, midwife, or health visitor as the case may be and includes registration by fraud' – there are several possible sanctions, including formal cautions and suspension and removal from the register. In addition, nurses may be disciplined by their employers for poor performance. The ultimate sanction is dismissal but in less serious cases the nurse might receive a warning, oral or written, demotion or suspension.

CASE STUDY 3.1   LISA'S RESPONSIBILITY – A DISCUSSION

(Refer to the scenario presented on page 58.)

The main issue in this case study is the effect of staff shortages. Although it focuses on fairly routine quasi-domestic aspects of Lisa's job, the ethical and legal issues it raises are identical to those that would apply whatever the nature of the task she was performing. The relevant ethical principles here are beneficence and non-maleficence. Together they impose a duty on Lisa to safeguard and promote Paul's well-being and to do him no harm. In practical terms, this means that she has at the very least a professional responsibility to ensure that he can cope with drinking his tea safely before she rushes off. But the crucial question then is whether Lisa is personally accountable for Paul's burn. Has she, in other words, failed to reach a professional standard of care, bearing in mind the pressures under which she was working?

When lack of resources jeopardize the provision of safe and appropriate care, procedures recommended by the UKCC should be followed. According to clause 38 of the Guidelines, if the environment of care is inadequate with the result that a nurse finds herself 'unable to provide good care' she will 'need to report her concerns (verbally and/or in writing) to the appropriate person or authority'. Similar advice is given in clauses 11, 12 and 13 of the UKCC Code (1992a). Together they are said to constitute 'the minimum action to be taken' (1996, clause 44).

Lisa may, of course have already reported her concerns – perhaps finding it easier to do so now than in the past because of the Public Interest (Disclosure) Act 1998, which was passed to help whistleblowers pass on information about poor practices in the NHS. However, other factors are relevant here. Was the ward so short-staffed, for example, that even when priorities were set it would have been impossible for another member of staff to help Lisa? Was such an accident reasonably foreseeable, so that additional precautions should have been taken, or was it an inevitable accident and therefore unavoidable? Perhaps it would have been safer to postpone giving Paul his tea? According to Dimond (1995, p 53), these are the kinds of question that should be asked.

And if the conclusion is that the accident was avoidable and that another nurse should have been assigned to help Lisa, then this will not automatically relieve

Lisa of her responsibility, especially if she was in charge of the ward. If so, then unless it was the first time that staff shortages had compromised standards of care, it would be important to know whether Lisa, in addition to reporting her concerns, had suggested some kind of remedial action, such as employing agency nurses. As Dimond notes (1995), failure to take such action – if Lisa had a management role – would mean that she would have to share some responsibility for Paul's burn.

Lisa's legal liability turns on similar issues to those that were raised above, in particular whether she had informed senior management of staffing shortages and whether appropriate priorities had been set. Legally too it would be significant to know if another nurse or anyone else could have helped Lisa and if she had a managerial role. If so, what did it normally involve? Note that, while these are important questions, it is nevertheless necessary to remember that, in the absence of any specific legislation on minimum staffing levels, ultimately Lisa's liability (and that of the hospital) would depend on the general issue of whether sufficient resources had been provided to ensure that patients being cared for were provided with the approved accepted standard of care (Dimond, 1995). In assessing this, evidence would be sought from relevant experts, who would be expected to advise on the minimum level consistent with good practice, bearing in mind available resources. In a case that was similar to the facts of this case, *Trew v. Middlesex Hospital* (1953) 1 *Lancet* 343, a nurse was held to be negligent when she 'breezed into a room, put down a tray and went out', giving the patient – who was sitting in bed with one leg in a sling and another on a pillow – some tea. She placed a tray on his lap but it tilted and hot water from the jug spilt on the plaintiff.

Let us assume, though, that appropriate priorities had been set and Lisa had made her concerns known but no new extra staff had been employed or allocated. What then? Is it a defence to say to Paul: 'Sorry you spilled the tea but I was very busy yesterday because we were so short-staffed that I did not have time to check that you could cope'. The answer is no. Patients are entitled to the approved standard of care (Dimond, 1995). Or, to put it another way, it is no defence to plead lack of resources as a defence (Lee, 1995). Thus in *Bull* v. *Devon AHA* (p. 70) the hospital authority was found liable for organizational failures in the delivery of its maternity services even though it argued that it was the best it could provide given available resources. It is possible then that the hospital could be liable to Paul for his injuries in failing to provide a safe system of institutional treatment and aftercare. Lisa too, however, might have to share responsibility if it was decided that in the circumstances she had failed to reach the legal standard of care. Her legal duty was towards Paul and she has to act in his best interests without reference to the interests of other patients or even potential patients (Jones, 1996, p. 220). Thus, in *Jones* v. *Manchester Corporation* [1952] 2 QB 852 a hospital was held responsible for 80% of the damages and the doctor 20% in respect of an anaesthetic accident caused primarily by the inadequacy of support and supervision provided for a junior doctor.

CASE STUDY 3.2   Ayeesha's Dosage Dilemma – a Discussion

(Refer to the scenario presented on page 58.)

The core issue here is obeying instructions. The principle of non-maleficence imposes an obligation on nurses not to harm patients. In this situation it must at the very least mean that Ayeesha should not just blindly follow orders but should act as an autonomous practitioner. To do otherwise, i.e. not to seek some kind of confirmation that the drug is the correct one, would constitute a breach of the UKCC document *Standards for Administration of Medicines* (1992c). This states that, as a matter of basic principle, the practitioner will be satisfied 'that she is able to justify any actions taken and is prepared to be accountable for[that] action' (clause 9).

This means that practitioners are expected not just to scrutinize carefully the prescription and the dosage but also to question the doctor as appropriate and, where necessary, to refuse to administer it. Ayeesha therefore has a professional obligation to question Pat. Note too that she should make sure that she keeps an accurate record of the problems that have arisen (in accordance with UKCC Guidance: *Standards for Records and Record Keeping*, 1993). This is very important, since any document that records any aspect of the care of a patient can be required as evidence before a court of law (or in disciplinary proceedings). Note, finally, that Ayeesha also has a moral responsibility not to administer a drug about which she has such grave doubts, given its potential harmful effects (Fletcher *et al.*, 1995). If Ayeesha fails to take these measures, gives the drugs and the patient is harmed there is little doubt that she is morally and professionally accountable for her actions.

Turning now to the law. Although several cases have established that as a general rule nurses can avoid liability if they follow a doctor's instructions – even if the directions turn out to be wrong – certain provisos apply (Montgomery, 1995 and see *Gold* v. *Essex County Council* [1942] 2 KB 293). Thus as the judge said in Gold, if a doctor ordered an 'obviously incorrect and dangerous dosage of a drug a nurse who administered it without obtaining confirmation from a doctor or higher authority might well be found negligent'. It seems then that when administering any drug it is the nurse's personal responsibility to ensure that it is the right drug, at the right time, in the right place, at the right dosage and in the right way, to the right patient (Dimond, 1995, p. 49). This means that nurses should challenge any order which seems to be wrong.

So whatever concerns Ayeesha has should be dealt with first by taking appropriate action. Otherwise she would be liable in negligence for failing to follow the reasonable standard of care expected of a nurse. Finally, it is worth repeating that, even after confirmation has been sought and has been obtained, nurses should still refuse to administer any order that is 'manifestly wrong' (*Junor* v. *McNicol* (1959) *The Times*, 26 March).

CASE STUDY 3.3   ANNE'S ACCOUNTABILITY – A DISCUSSION

(Refer to the scenario presented on page 59.)

The central issues in this case study are competency, supervision and delegation. Let's deal first with Anne, the junior nurse, who, despite not having the necessary skills, has been asked to administer an intravenous drug. The UKCC Code (1992a) and *Guidelines for Professional Practice* (1996) make it very clear that nurses should 'acknowledge their limitations and decline any duties or responsibilities unless able to perform them in a safe and skilled manner'. Similarly, the UKCC *Standards for Administration of Medicines* (1992c) states that administering intravenous drugs is acceptable provided that 'the practitioner is satisfied with her competence and mindful of her personal accountability'. But even without these reminders there can be little doubt that the principles of beneficence and non-maleficence impose a duty on nurses not to undertake tasks that they are not qualified to carry out. Anne should therefore tell Patsy that she has not developed the skills, competence and knowledge to undertake that task. And if she does attempt it she should at least ask Patsy to check that she has carried it out correctly. She should do this irrespective of the consequences to her reputation and whether (or not) the task is one that other reasonably competent nurses in her position would be able to carry out.

If, however, Anne keeps silent and goes ahead with the infusion, thereby harming Sanjay, she would be professionally accountable for her actions and would probably face disciplinary action. She would also be morally accountable, not only because she is clearly aware of her own limitations but also because her motives for failing to reveal her incompetence are self-interested. In other words she is putting her own interests above those of her patients.

But Patsy too has acted inappropriately in delegating a task to Anne that she has failed to ensure is carried out according to a reasonably competent standard. As such, she remains accountable for the delegation of the work and for ensuring that the person who does the work is able to do it (UKCC, 1996). According to Young (1994, p. 58), three checks should be made if a task is to be delegated. These are:

- the extent of the nurse's knowledge;
- how skilful the nurse is in the task delegated – a verbal check may be sufficient; and
- supervision while the task is carried out.

It seems that Patsy has done none of these and so has failed to comply with the standard of acceptable professional practice.

Legally, Sanjay has a right to a reasonable standard of care (Dimond, 1993). The fact that he was treated by an inexperienced nurse is no defence in law for Anne, who should, at the very least, have called for assistance. Then, even if she had made a mistake, the very fact that she had called for help would have been a responsible thing to do and would normally provide a defence (Montgomery, 1995). In other words, the law allows inexperienced staff to 'learn on the job' but only if they rely on supervision and guidance from a superior when tackling new or unfamiliar tasks (*Wilsher* v. *Essex AHA* [1988] above).

Patsy's liability for Sanjay's injuries will turn on whether or not in delegating the task to Anne she knew (or ought to have known) that Anne was incapable of undertaking it competently (*Bolam* v. *Friern Hospital Management Committee* [1957]). Had she checked that Anne had been trained? Had she supervised her before? If the answer to these questions is no, then Patsy would share liability with Anne for the harm Sanjay has suffered (although in practice their employers would be sued under the doctrine of vicarious liability).

LAW and ETHICS – a comparison

What do these case studies and the concepts of responsibility and accountability tell us about the ethical and legal expectation that nurses should avoid harm and do good? That there are many similarities is self-evident.

Indeed, as Stanton has argued (1994), no-one who has read *Donoghue* v. *Stevenson* [1932] AC. 562, could doubt, first, that the principle of fault liability that underpins the law of negligence is a form of ethical response to the problem created by accidents and the damage they cause, and second, that Lord Atkins's 'neighbour' principle, which that case established, is a limited legal response to the commandment to love one's neighbour. We have seen too how the legal and ethical concepts of responsibility and accountability do not only share a common vocabulary – of fault (which in ordinary linguistic terms connotes some degree of moral blameworthiness), duty of care and reasonableness – but also have a common function, most notably, setting acceptable standards of care. Similarly, both attempt to provide mechanisms by which those who fail to reach or maintain acceptable standards can be deterred from so 'failing' in future. Thus nurses can be disciplined (and removed from the register) if they are found professionally accountable and sued if they are found liable in negligence.

Yet despite the obvious overlap in the legal and ethical response to regulating conduct and allocating blame the wide assumption that the fault principle incorporates a moral dimension (Jones, 1996) can be questioned. Indeed, one commentator has suggested (Cane, 1993) that the fault principle is not a moral principle at all because a defendant may be negligent without being morally culpable and *vice versa*. That this is so was highlighted in the example given above, i.e. when a nurse makes an avoidable mistake when administering a drug but no harm is caused. Here she is morally to blame but will not be liable in negligence (because her action did not result in any injury).

It is also important to note other ways in which law and ethics differ in this context. Apart from deterrence, for example, the main purpose behind a negligence action is to win compensation for the injuries victims have suffered. In contrast, the principal function of professional codes (and the ethical principles they enshrine) is to set, maintain and improve standards of care. This explains why the legal standard of care is lower than the ethical standard, which aims if not for the highest level of care then at least for the 'best possible level' circumstances will allow. Or, to put it another way, the law is more concerned with setting a minimum level of competence below which practitioners must not fall. As such it does not require them to reach the highest standards (Rumbold and Lesser, 1995).

The ethical concept of duty of care is also wider than the legal duty of care. For example, nurses may have a professional and moral duty to help strangers in certain situations. In contrast, the 'neighbour test' (derived from the case of *Donoghue* v. *Stevenson* [1932]) is more limited (in the sense that it generally requires much less positive action to be taken in respect of strangers and other 'non-patients'). Note too that ethical principles and guidance are typically expressed in much more general and vague terms than legal principles – which specify (not surprisingly perhaps) precisely when, for example, a duty is owed, in what circumstances it can be breached and how the causation link must be established.

It is this causation link that highlights the final difference between law and ethics. If causation is not proved there can be no legal liability (even if the patient has been harmed). As we have seen above, this means that the nurse may well have breached the duty of care but, because of the need to prove fault (on the balance of probabilities) and all the technical and procedural difficulties this may entail, it might not be possible to link – in legal terms – the breach with the harm. But a different approach is taken in ethics, which in this context is more concerned with rightness or wrongness of actions themselves and their potential effects (rather than the actual effects of actions or omissions; Rumbold and Lesser, 1995). Hence, whether or not any harm actually follows from a nurse's actions may be ethically irrelevant, the real question being whether the nurse has behaved in a way that is professionally and morally justifiable.

REFERENCES

Beauchamp, T. L. and Childress, J. F. (1994) *Principles of Biomedical Ethics*, 4th edn, Oxford University Press, Oxford.

Benjamin, M. and Curtis, J. (1992) *Ethics in Nursing*, 3rd edn, Oxford University Press, Oxford.

Brazier, M. (1992) *Medicine, Patients and the Law*, 2nd edn, Penguin Books, Harmondsworth.

Cane, P. (1993) *Atiyah's Accidents, Compensation and the Law*, 5th edn, Butterworths, London.

Cribb, A. (1995) The ethical dimension. In: *Nursing Law and Ethics*, (eds J. Tingle and A. Cribb), Blackwell Science, Oxford.

Davies, M. (1998) *Textbook on Medical Law*, 2nd edn, Blackstone Press, London.

Davis, A. J. and Aroskar, M. A. (1991) *Ethical Dilemmas and Nursing Practice*, Appleton & Lange, Norwalk, CT.

Dimond, B. C. (1993) *Patients' Rights, Responsibilities and the Nurse*, Central Health Studies, Quay Publishing, Dinton.

Dimond, B. C. (1995) *The Legal Aspects of Nursing*, 2nd edn, Prentice-Hall, Hemel Hempstead.

Downie, R. S. and Calman, K. C. (1994) *Healthy Respect*, 2nd edn, Oxford University Press, Oxford.

Edwards, S.D. (1996) *Nursing Ethics: A Principle-based Approach*, Macmillan, Basingstoke.

Fletcher, N., Holt, J., Brazier, M. and Harris, J. (1995) *Ethics, Law and Nursing*, Manchester University Press, Manchester.

Frankena, W. (1973) *Ethics*, 2nd edn, Prentice-Hall, Englewood Cliffs, NJ.

Giddens, A. (1999) Risk and responsibility. *Modern Law Review*, **62**(1), 1–10.

Gillon, R. (1985) *Philosophical Medical Ethics*, John Wiley, Chichester.

Hart, H. L. A. (1968) *Punishment and Responsibility: Essays in the Philosophy of Law*, Oxford: Clarendon Press.

Hendrick, J. (1997) *Legal Aspects of Child Health Care*, Chapman & Hall, London.

Henry, C. (1995) An introduction to professional ethics. In *Professional Ethics and Organisational Change*, (ed. C. Henry), Edward Arnold, London.

Hunt, G. (1991) *The Concept of Moral Responsibility*. Quoted in *Ethics, Nurses and Patients*, (ed. V. Tschudin, 1996), Baillière Tindall, London.

Hunt, G. (1994) *Ethical issues in Nursing*, Routledge, London.

ICN (1973) *Code for Nurses*, International Council of Nurses, Geneva.

Jones, M. (1996) *Medical Negligence*, Sweet & Maxwell, London.

Kennedy, I. and Grubb, A. (1994) *Medical Law: Text and Materials*, 2nd edn, Butterworths, London.

Khan, M. and Robson, M. (1997) *Medical Negligence*, Cavendish Publishing, London.

Lee, R. (1995) Resources and professional accountability. In: *Nursing Law and Ethics*, (eds J. Tingle and A. Cribb), Blackwell Science, Oxford.

McHale, J. and Fox, M. with Murphy, J. (1997) *Health Care Law: Text and Materials*, Sweet & Maxwell, London.

Marks-Maran, D. (1996) Accountability. In: *Ethics: Nurses and Patients*, (ed. V. Tschudin), Baillière Tindall, London.

Mason, J. K. and McCall-Smith, R. A. (1999) *Law and Medical Ethics*, 5th edn, Butterworths, London.

Montgomery, J. (1995) Negligence: the legal perspective. In: *Nursing Law and Ethics*, (eds J. Tingle and A. Cribb), Blackwell Science, Oxford.

Nelson-Jones, R. and Burton, F. (1995) *Medical Negligence Case Law*, Butterworths, London.

Phillips, A. F. (1997) *Medical Negligence Law: Seeking A Balance*, Dartmouth, Aldershot.

Pyne, R. (1995) The professional dimension. In: *Nursing Law and Ethics*, (eds J. Tingle and A. Cribb), Blackwell Science, Oxford.

Rumbold, G. (1999) *Ethics in Nursing Practice*, 3rd edn, Baillière Tindall, London.

Rumbold, G. and Lesser, H. (1995) An ethical perspective – negligence and moral obligations. In: *Nursing Law and Ethics*, (eds J. Tingle and A. Cribb), Blackwell Science, Oxford.

Scruton, R. (1994) *Modern Philosophy*, Mandarin, London.

Sheldon, S. and Thomson, M. (1998) *Feminist Perspectives on Health Care Law*, Cavendish Publishing, London.

Singleton J. and McLaren S. (1995) *Ethical Foundations of Health Care: Responsibilities in Decision-Making*, Mosby, London.

Teff, H. (1994) *Reasonable Care: Legal Perspectives on the Doctor/Patient Relationship*, Clarendon Press, Oxford.

Tingle, J. (1998a) Legal aspects of expanded role and clinical guidelines and protocols. In: *Law and Nursing*, (eds J. McHale, J. Tingle and J. Peysner), Butterworth Heinemann, Oxford.

Tingle, J. (1998b) Patient complaints. In: *Law and Nursing*, (eds J. McHale, J. Tingle and J. Peysner), Butterworth Heinemann, Oxford.

Tingle, J. (1998c) Nursing negligence: general issues. In: *Law and Nursing*, (eds J. McHale, J. Tingle and J. Peysner), Butterworth Heinemann, Oxford.

Tschudin, V. (1994) *Deciding Ethically*, Baillière Tindall, London.

Tschudin, V. (1996) Responsibilities and rights. In: *Ethics: Nurses and Patients*, (ed. V. Tschudin), Baillière Tindall, London.

UKCC (1992a) *Code of Professional Conduct*, UKCC, London.

UKCC (1992b) *The Scope of Professional Practice*, UKCC, London.

UKCC (1992c) *Standards for Administration of Medicines*, UKCC, London.

UKCC (1993) *Standards for Records and Record Keeping*, UKCC, London.

UKCC (1996) *Guidelines for Professional Practice*, UKCC, London.

Veatch, R. M. and Fry, S. (1987) *Case Studies in Nursing Ethics*, J. B. Lippincott, London.

Young, A. (1994) *Law and Professional Conduct*, 2nd edn, Scutari Press, London.

FURTHER READING

Korgaonkar, G. and Tribe, D. (1995) *Law for Nurses*, Cavendish Publishing, London.

Montgomery, J. (1997) *Health Care Law*, Oxford University Press, Oxford.

Tschudin, V. (1992) *Ethics in Nursing: The Caring Relationship*, Butterworth Heinemann, Oxford.

4 CONFIDENTIALITY AND MEDICAL RECORDS

INTRODUCTION

Confidentiality has been described as central to preserving the human dignity of patients (Brody, 1997, p. 91) and as vitally important if we are to grow as persons and remain human (Tschudin, 1994, p. 140). Historically, health professionals have been expected to maintain confidentiality and patients have been encouraged to take this for granted.

That confidentiality has long been a part of nursing practice is also self-evident. There can be little doubt too that as the nurse's role expands – providing greater opportunities for making independent decisions about treatment – it is likely that s/he will be confronted with more and more dilemmas of confidentiality (McHale, 1993). Yet with new approaches to and more holistic frameworks of nursing, confidentiality is arguably more important than it once was (Tschudin, 1996, p. 1).

Roughly, the principle of confidentiality demands that information gained in a professional–client relationship must be kept secret, even when its disclosure might serve a greater public good (Johnstone, 1989, p. 192). Nevertheless, occasionally other important moral and legal considerations can oblige nurses to disclose information without a patient's consent. What sorts of consideration and what circumstances might be strong enough to override the duty of confidentiality are therefore the subject of this chapter. These are issues that are now more topical than ever as the spread of AIDS and the ever-growing list of demands on health professionals to disclose information to third parties (such as social workers, the police and so on) has forced all those involved in health care to reassess the ethical obligations that they owe to patients. But, as McHale points out (1993, p. 2), current concern about confidentiality has even deeper roots, reflecting the individual's increasing difficulty in keeping sensitive personal information from the scrutiny of others in an age when storage in and access to computers is so commonplace.

The chapter begins by defining what is meant by the term 'confidential' and then discusses why the requirement to protect patient confidentiality is such an important principle. It then looks at how confidentiality can be supported on moral and legal grounds before dealing with the justifications for breaching the principle. The chapter will conclude with a brief look at patients' rights in respect of their medical records.

CASE STUDY 4.1	HOW MUCH OF WINNIE'S INFORMATION SHOULD REBECCA TREAT AS CONFIDENTIAL?

Rebecca, a district nurse, has built up very good relationship with Winnie, a patient in her early seventies whom she had been treating for some time for leg ulcers. Over the months, Winnie has told her a lot about herself and her family, especially about her daughter, who lives in Australia. But some of this information is about her past medical history – the illegal abortion she had as a teenager, for example. Recently, too, she has talked a lot about her plans for the future. She is getting very frail and her eyesight is failing but she hopes to be well enough to go and spend Christmas with her oldest friend, Peggy. Her main concern, however, is her sister Annie, who lives very close by but whom she has not seen for several weeks. She tells Rebecca that she is almost certain that Annie is being abused by her son, Mark. She also suspects that he deals in drugs.

Rebecca is about to leave when Annie arrives. Rebecca decides to stop for a while as Annie appears to be very agitated and has several bruises on her arms, as well as a black eye. Rebecca suggests that she takes a look but Annie, whom she has treated in the past, refuses, telling her that she slipped on a wet floor in the kitchen. Rebecca is sure there is more to it than that but Annie insists that her injuries are accidental.

How much of the information that Winnie has provided is confidential? Who might be interested in this information? Should Rebecca report her concerns about Annie to anyone?

CASE STUDY 4.2   CAN LAURA JUSTIFY HER BREACH OF CONFIDENTIALITY?

Clive is in his early fifties and has recently been diagnosed with cancer. He has an operation, which goes well, and decides not to tell anyone in his family what was really wrong with him. Some months later Clive's health deteriorates and tests reveal that the cancer has recurred. He returns to hospital for more treatment but this time the prognosis is very poor. Nevertheless, Clive remains adamant that his family should not know how ill he is – not yet anyway. He tells one of the nurses, Laura, that he does not think his family could cope with the news and so would rather wait until the truth cannot be hidden any more. Laura thinks otherwise, or at least she thinks that Clive's wife should be told. She is sure she suspects anyway, given all the questions she has been asking recently.

Just after talking to Clive, Laura goes for a coffee break – the coffee bar is used by the people visiting patients as well as staff. In the queue is a friend of hers who works in the pharmacy. Laura starts talking about Clive, whose name she mentions as well as the details of his illness, not realizing that Clive's wife is within earshot. Clive's wife hears everything she says and rushes off in tears.

Can Laura justify breaching Clive's confidentiality? What are the likely consequences of the breach?

CASE STUDY 4.3   SHOULD BERYL BREACH JOHN'S CONFIDENCE?

Beryl is a community psychiatric nurse. For several weeks she has been visiting a patient, John, a 24-year-old chronic schizophrenic, who now lives with his parents.

The last time Beryl saw him he said he wanted to give up his medication but she managed to persuade him to continue with the injections – which she regularly gives him. He also talked a lot about his father, Paul, whom he was convinced hated him and did not want him at home. His greatest fear, however, was that his father was going to arrange for him to be sent back to hospital, where he had lived on and off for many years. Beryl managed to convince him that his fears were unfounded. But this morning when she visited him she found that his fears, far from receding, were even greater. His only solution, he told Beryl, was to get rid of his father. He was not sure how he would do it, but said: 'Don't worry, he won't be a threat for long.'

Does Beryl have a duty to warn Paul of the threats made by his son? Should she tell anyone else? What difference would it make if John's threats were made against no-one in particular, i.e. he has said that he just wanted to kill someone?

CASE STUDY 4.4 SHOULD CLAIRE SPEAK OUT?

Kathy is nearly 3 and is taken to her GP with a broken wrist. She also has several bruises, which the practice nurse, Claire, suspects may have been caused by her mother. But a more likely culprit is Kathy's stepfather, whom she knows to be violent. While examining Kathy, Claire also notices several old burns. Although she cannot be sure – they have nearly healed – she is almost certain that they have been caused by cigarettes. Kathy is also very quiet and small for her age.

Can Claire breach confidentiality and report her suspicions that Kathy has been abused? Should she?

CASE STUDY 4.5 MUST LEN'S RIGHT TO PRIVACY BE RESPECTED?

Len has been unwell for many months and finally decides to see his doctor. He has travelled abroad a lot, most frequently in Africa, and has put off having tests because he suspects that he might have AIDS. After counselling he is tested and diagnosed as HIV-positive. But he refuses to let his long-term partner, Mary, be told, even though he knows she may become infected. Len is worried that she will leave him if she finds out. The doctor, Ghita, is unable to persuade Len to change his mind and thinks his confidentiality should be respected anyway. However, she tells Gillian, the practice nurse, who thinks Mary has a right to know.

Must Len's demand for privacy be respected or can Gillian inform Mary of Len's status? Would it make any difference if Len was not HIV-positive but had another sexually transmitted disease?

CONFIDENTIALITY

An ethical approach

That patients have a legitimate expectation that the information they give health professionals will be kept secret is one of the most fundamental principles of health care, which is enshrined in virtually every code of nursing ethics (likewise in the Patient's Charter). It is therefore not surprising that the UKCC *Code of Professional Conduct* (clause 10) obliges nurses to keep their patients' confidences, as do the more recent 1996 *Guidelines for Professional Practice* (clauses 50–69; see also the 1987 UKCC advisory paper *Confidentiality: An Elaboration of Clause 9 of the Second Edition of the UKCC's Code of Conduct* and *Confidentiality: Use of Computers, Position Statement* – UKCC, 1992). According to Rumbold (1999, p. 151), the reason why the notion of confidentiality is so pervasive is because it reflects the 'special relationship' between nurse and patient, i.e. one in which the particular duties and obligations owed go beyond the scope of ordinary social intercourse.

Yet despite the widespread acceptance of the importance of confidentiality there is little, if any, clear definition of what the term 'confidential' means, i.e. precisely what information should be considered confidential. Perhaps this is due to it being in practice fairly obvious. Hence not all personal information revealed to nurses by patients is confidential. At least, not that which can be described as part of normal social intercourse or 'social chit-chat', or the things which are generally widely known about people such as their marital status, how many children they have and so forth (Rumbold, 1999). In contrast, personal details relating to the physical or mental health of a patient from which a person can be identified is certainly confidential, e.g. any symptoms they may be suffering, even though the sensitivity of these symptoms can vary enormously from, say, a cold or sore throat (which few patients would worry about disclosing) to sexual anxieties (which most patients would wish to be kept secret). Note that this information may be contained in a variety of forms, such as medical illustrations, management registers, computer or manual files, videos or in the nurse's memory.

But confidentiality is a two way process. This means that some information that is given by a nurse to the patient is also confidential. Included here would be information relating to the patient's diagnosis, treatment, nursing care and prognosis. Finally, it is worth noting Gillon's broad definition of confidentiality (1985, p. 107). He asserts that two conditions are necessary to create a moral duty of confidentiality. First, one person must undertake, either explicitly or implicitly, not to disclose another's secrets and second, that other person must disclose to the first person information that s/he considers to be secret.

A legal approach

Despite the long-recognized legal right to confidentiality – in *Wood* v. *Wyatt* (cited in *Prince Albert* v. *Strange* (1849)), publication of the diaries of George III's doctor was restrained (McHale, 1993) – there is no authoritative legal definition of 'confidential information'. Case law (see, for example, *Hunter* v. *Mann* [1974] 1 QB 767 and *A-G* v. *Guardian Newspapers (No. 2)* [1990] 1 AC 109) has nonetheless established that the courts will generally enforce a duty of confidentiality if certain conditions are satisfied. These are:

- that the information is not a matter of public knowledge, i.e. that it is of a private or intimate nature;
- that the information must have been given in a situation where there is an obligation not to disclose it – the fiduciary relationship that exists between nurses and their patients is such a situation;
- that either protecting confidentiality is in the public interest or the patient would suffer some detriment if the information is revealed;
- that the information must not be useless or 'trivial'.

Note that once an obligation of confidence has arisen it binds all those to whom the information has been given. As the Department of Health document *The Protection and Use of Personal Information* (1996) (hereinafter referred to as 'Department of Health guidance') makes clear, this potentially includes a very wide range of people, namely: all NHS bodies; everyone working for or with the NHS who records, handles, stores or otherwise comes across information; health professionals; and other individuals and agencies to whom information is passed legitimately.

It seems then that both the law and ethics recognize that some information is of a confidential nature, but why is confidentiality an important principle? It is to this we now turn.

JUSTIFICATION FOR CONFIDENTIALITY

In this section the legal and ethical foundations of the duty of confidentiality will be outlined.

Ethical sources

The most common justification given for the moral duty of confidentiality is consequentialist (Beauchamp and Childress, 1994; McHale, 1993; Stauch *et al.*, 1998). As such it focuses on the consequences (to patients and society as a whole) if confidentiality is not maintained. Briefly, the claim is that if patients cannot trust health professionals to keep their secrets they will feel betrayed and thus likely to withhold potentially significant but embarrassing details or, worse still, may not seek essential medical or psychiatric care at all. As a consequence the care they receive (if any) may be compromised, not least because, without full and frank disclosure of symptoms and so forth, accurate diagnoses may not be possible. Nor may recommended treatment and nursing care be the best available if patients have failed to be honest for fear that highly sensitive information may become widely known. A teenager, for example, who wants to go on the pill – which she knows her parents oppose – is unlikely to go to the family doctor if she thinks her parents will be told. Similarly those with a sexually transmitted disease (or with a disease such as epilepsy) are less likely to seek help or admit they are ill if confidences are not respected, thus jeopardizing not only their own well-being and health but also that of society in general.

But the duty of confidentiality can also be justified on deontological grounds (Beauchamp and Childress, 1994; Singleton and McLaren, 1995). This approach derives from several moral principles and rules but in essence asserts that the patient has a right to confidentiality. Primarily this right derives from the principle of respect for autonomy. According to Vedder (1999, p. 142), there are two sides to this autonomy. First, it has to do with considering individuals to be 'masters' of their own well-being, thereby enabling them to run their own lives by controlling what happens to personal medical information about themselves – much of which may consist of the most intimate and sensitive aspects of their personal lives. In other words, they must be entitled to decide what private information should be disclosed (if any), what should be kept secret (or revealed only to the few) and who should have access to that information. Second, respecting autonomy can be viewed as an expression of esteem for the dignity of individual persons, because in doing so they are regarded seriously, in other words as beings who are capable of making choices and acting in the morally right way (Vedder, 1999, p. 145).

A closely related deontological justification for the duty of confidentiality is sometimes grounded in another concern: to protect a person's privacy and integrity. According to Brody (1997, p. 89), privacy and confidentiality should be seen as closely linked with basic human dignity and respect for persons, as are lucidity and autonomy. But the right to privacy (which can also be defended on utilitarian grounds in that overall it benefits people by facilitating the development of meaningful personal relations) is a difficult concept to define. For Beauchamp and Childress (1994) it is a state or condition of limited access to a person. Others describe it as a collection of different spaces. The most intimate space (which only the person him/herself has access to) contains the person's most secret thoughts, feelings, hopes, fears, etc. Other wider, less private 'spaces' hold information to which a person's family, friends and so forth have access. And the widest space of all is the public domain (Brown *et al.*, 1992, pp. 96–97).

However it is defined, a right to privacy is now increasingly seen as a basic human need and an necessary condition of selfhood – hence its protection in article 8 of the European Convention of Human Rights and the Human Rights Act 1998. But despite the overlap between the right to privacy and confidentiality, they can be distinguished (see on this McHale, 1993, p. 56).

Other principles that support a duty of confidentiality include non-maleficence and beneficence. Taken together these principles require health professionals to protect patients from the harmful consequences of disclosure. But they can also be invoked to justify breaching confidentiality in certain circumstances.

Important here too is the fidelity rule. This is a rule that imposes obligations on health professionals to fulfil agreements and maintain relationships and fiduciary responsibilities (Edwards, 1996). It also requires them to keep their promises, whether these are made explicitly or, as occurs more frequently in this context, implicitly. As was noted above, one of the conditions that is necessary before the moral duty of confidentiality arises is that practitioners undertake not to divulge information about their patients' condition, care and treatment. Relying on this tacit promise, patients can feel confident that the information they give will only be revealed with their consent and then only to those with a legitimate interest in it.

Fiduciary responsibilities are also, of course, nurtured by trust. Indeed, as Murphy states (1998, p. 168), the key attraction of confidentiality is its link (albeit largely unexplored) with the concept of trust. This is because trust 'foregrounds core virtues like intimacy, commitment and risk'. But, as Murphy then explains, unfortunately in health-care attempts to unravel the virtues of trusts have been 'choked by the icy appeal of notions like contract and consent'. 'Trust' therefore remains an ill-defined concept. Yet it is one that is nevertheless now regarded as the cornerstone of the nurse–patient relationship and the reason why patients feel relaxed and safe and therefore able to disclose private information in the first place. According to Tschudin (1996, p. 7), the nurse–patient relationship is a privileged one in which 'two people trust each other to be what they appear to be, say what they appear to be saying, and believe what they appear to be believing'. Implicit in this approach is the recognition that trust is a mutual process, albeit one that is often asymmetrical. In other words both sides give, and both sides take responsibility.

However the concept of trust is defined, its central importance was acknowledged in the 1987 UKCC advisory paper on confidentiality, where it was referred to as the 'focal' word in the definition of 'confide', 'confidence' and confidentiality (Rumbold, 1999). The Guidelines too discuss trust. Hence the first clause (which explains what confidentiality means) begins by stating that 'to trust another person with private and personal information about yourself is a significant matter'. It goes on to say that patients have a right to believe that information given in confidence will only be used for the purposes for which it was given and will not be released to others without their permission (for a useful summary of the moral duty of confidentiality see the guidelines issued by the BMA in 1999: *Confidentiality and Disclosure of Health Information*).

Legal sources

Although the legal duty of confidentiality has long being recognized, there have been very few cases in which it has been directly an issue. As a consequence, the legal sources of this obligation still remain somewhat uncertain, even though there has been much academic debate on the subject (Stauch *et al.*, 1998, p. 229). Nevertheless, two sources are clear. One is equity, a system that developed hundreds of years ago to provide 'real' justice. The principles and rules of equity are much more flexible than the common law and by the 16th century equity had become a well-established source of law that recognized new rights and new remedies. In this context, equity will generally enforce an obligation to respect patients' confidences once a fiduciary relationship has arisen (such as exists between nurses and their patients).

Another source of confidentiality lies in the tort of negligence. As we saw in Chapter 3, patients are entitled to receive a reasonable standard of care. An important aspect of that care is that patients have a right to have their private affairs kept secret. Without such an assurance it is certainly foreseeable that they may suffer loss such as discrimination, social stigma and so forth – although whether such losses are legally recognized is, of course, another matter. It is also perhaps worth noting that contract law may also be a source of the duty of confidentiality for private patients who are being cared for outside the NHS. Depending on the terms of their agreement, such patients could possibly sue for breach of contract if their confidentiality was breached (Montgomery, 1997, p. 251).

In addition, contract law is the source of the duty of confidentiality nurses owe their employers (it is contained in their contract of employment). But this aspect of confidentiality – which is in issue when a nurse 'whistleblows', i.e. refuses to cover up potentially negligent or harmful practices by drawing attention to it (whether through the media or otherwise) – is not discussed in this book.

Finally, there are several statutes and other regulations that impose duties of confidentiality, in particular the Human Fertilisation and Embryology Act 1990 (in relation to infertility treatment) and the National Health Service Venereal Disease Regulations 1974 (which covers sexually transmitted diseases).

EXCEPTIONS TO THE DUTY OF CONFIDENTIALITY

This section addresses what is undoubtedly – from both a legal and ethical standpoint – the most controversial aspect of confidentiality, namely the circumstances in which it is justifiable to breach a patient's confidence. It is controversial because, although there may well be widespread agreement (at least in theory) that confidentiality is not an absolute principle, deciding when the duty of confidentiality should be overridden by other more compelling moral considerations and demands is much more difficult in practice. Nor does the fact that in some situations nurses have a choice – in the sense that they have an option to divulge confidences rather than a duty – make it any easier to make the 'right' decision.

The dilemmas that nurses typically face in relation to confidentiality were outlined in the UKCC document; Confidentiality (1987). Although written well over a decade ago, many of the situations cited are still problematic. For example, what should a nurse do when he finds a patient with a controlled drug (perhaps brought in by friends) that cannot have been obtained legally?

It is perhaps because every nursing code of ethics and the law justify breaching confidentiality (and because it is systematically and casually compromised in practice) that confidentiality has been described as a 'decrepit concept'. The phrase was coined by an American doctor (Siegler, 1982), who was astonished to learn that as many as 75 and possibly as many as 100 health professionals and administrative personnel had access to the patient's record (Gillon, 1985, pp. 109–110). It is a phrase that is often quoted but the thrust of Siegler's argument has been differently interpreted. Ridley, for example (1998, p. 97) claims that the concept emerges from his article 'alive and kicking'. This is because nothing Siegler says suggests that the goal of protecting and promoting patients' interests by the sensitive handling of personal information should be abandoned.

What then are the exceptions to the duty of confidentiality? In answering this question, two distinct approaches will be taken (although there is considerable overlap between them). One will focus on the limits to confidentiality recognized by the UKCC (i.e. those that are professionally permitted), and the other will concentrate on the law. Note that the term 'professional' is used in its broadest sense and as such is taken to reflect moral considerations.

Professional exceptions

Clause 10 of the UKCC Code makes it clear that disclosures can only be made in certain very limited circumstances. The Guidelines also, while similarly emphasizing how confidentiality should only be broken in exceptional circumstances, nevertheless acknowledge that in the following situations disclosure of information can occur:

- with the consent of the patient or client;
- without the consent of the patient or client when the disclosure is required by law or by a court order;
- without the consent of the patient or client when the disclosure is considered to be necessary in the public interest.

Taken together the Code and the Guidelines thus strongly suggest that, although the ethical obligation to keep patients' confidences is not an absolute principle, it is nevertheless a *prima facie* one. In other words, there is a very strong presumption in favour of confidentiality and any nurse who decides to divulge information must bear the burden of justifying his/her action. Each of these exceptions will now be examined in turn.

Consent

If patients consent (which can be expressed or implied) to information being disclosed nurses can act on that permission, providing it has been freely given, not obtained by undue pressure and the patient understands the consequences of the information being revealed. Although consent to disclosure is typically explicit – which is often the case, for example, when details of a patient's condition are passed on to relatives – sometimes this is impractical and it has to be implied. A common example of implied consent is when information is shared between all health professionals and other staff (such as social work practitioners) who are involved in a patient's care and treatment. The assumption is that patients realize that relevant information has to be passed back and forth between all member of the health-care team and so implicitly give consent to its disclosure.

None the less, care must be taken to ensure that only those who genuinely 'need to know' are given information and that it is used only for the purposes for which it was given. Furthermore, as the Guidelines make clear, patients must know who the information will be shared with. Note too that Department of

Health guidance on the 'need to know' exception (which it treats as a separate exception from consent) allows disclosure within the health-care team (as well as for the purposes of clinical audit, monitoring and protecting public health, coordinating health-care administration, teaching and research within the NHS, see para. 1.2). As a general rule, though, it states that patients should be told how information will be used before they are asked to provide it (for a detailed account of the 'need to know' exception see BMA, 1999).

Also sometimes included within consent exception (but often regarded as a separate exception) are disclosures that can be justified in the 'interests of a patient's own health and well-being'. Disclosures here may, it seems, even be justified if a patient refuses consent (although this is unclear). Interestingly too the UKCC 1987 advisory paper on confidentiality (but not the1996 Guidelines) recognize non-consensual deliberate breaches of confidentiality 'in the patient's interests'. In some circumstances, close relatives or some other person may legitimately need confidential information so that they can provide effective care. Obvious examples are mentally incompetent adults, those with learning difficulties or young children whose care is largely in the hands of others. While it may be more appropriate to regard this kind of disclosure as a separate category there can be little moral objection, providing, of course, the autonomy of vulnerable patients is not limited unnecessarily. This would be the case if, say inappropriate assumptions were made about their competence and understanding of confidentiality.

Disclosures under this category would also be justified if, for example, a community nurse was treating a patient at home and so would need to be given any relevant information about, for example, allergies to certain drugs and so on.

Public interest

The concept of 'the public interest' is a troublesome one, largely because no single definition of what it amounts to exists (but see BMA, 1999, which discusses the exception in detail). Given the absence of any clear boundaries and its potentially very broad scope it is therefore perhaps not surprising that this exception poses the most dilemmas in practice and has also generated the most controversy. According to the Guidelines (clause 56), public interest means: 'the interests of an individual, or groups of individuals or of society as a whole, and would, for example, cover matters such as serious crime, child abuse, drug trafficking or other activities which place others at serious risk'.

This definition is fairly broad and as a consequence provides little practical guidance to nurses. Of more help is the Department of Health guidance, which defines 'serious' as including treason, murder, manslaughter, rape, kidnapping, some sexual and firearm offences, and so forth (see Appendix D).

Inevitably, however, some situations present fewer problems than others. If a patient admitted to a nurse that he was sexually abusing a child, for example, then she would almost certainly be able to justify her action if she breached confidentiality and reported her concerns to an appropriate person, Similarly, if a nurse discovered that a rape or other serious assault had been committed he might well feel that he had a moral obligation if not to volunteer information to the police then at least to do something to help 'catch' the perpetrator. Whether or not he could justify any action he took would, however, probably depend on how far he had followed Department of Health guidance. It states that passing on information to tackle serious crime may be justified if certain conditions are satisfied: that without disclosure, the task of preventing, detecting or prosecuting the crime would be seriously prejudiced or delayed; and that information is limited to what is strictly relevant for a specific investigation. Advice in the Guidelines might also be relevant here in that they advise that, where the police are involved, say in accident and emergency admissions, it may be appropriate to involve senior staff if a nurse does not feel able to deal with the situation alone (clause 59).

There are, of course, many other situations that may require nurses to consider whether their moral obligation to keep patients' confidences are outweighed by more compelling moral considerations. Should a nurse inform the appropriate authorities if a patient (who is, say, a lorry driver) refuses to reveal his epilepsy, for example? And what if a nurse discovers that a colleague has a medical condition (or is, say, a drug addict) that could have a detrimental affect on others in the nurse's care? Although in most of these kinds of situations there is no identifiable individual who would benefit from disclosure, there are many potential victims who might suffer if confidentiality is not broken.

But in all these kinds of cases, indeed whenever nurses are faced with a 'public interest' dilemma, they will have to make choices that inevitably involve several competing moral obligations – to respect confidences or to protect 'the public' by breaching confidentiality. In reaching their decision and assessing the risk to 'others' they will have to consider not just the probability that the predicted harm will materialize but also the magnitude of the harm. So the less serious the potential harm the greater the moral obligation not to breach confidentiality. Other factors that may also have to be taken into account include the extent to which there are ways (other than breaching confidentiality) in which the potential harm can be prevented or minimized.

At this point it is worth noting a famous American case, *Tarasoff* v. *Regents of the University of California* 17 Cal 3d 425 (1976), which, as Mason and McCall Smith note (1999, p. 505), has prompted widespread debate in North America and elsewhere. It concerned a negligence claim arising out of the murder of a student, Tatiana Tarasoff. Several months before the murder, the girl's former 'boyfriend', Prosenjit Poddar, had interpreted a kiss as a symbol of betrothal. Even though he was told by Tatiana that it did not mean anything, he would not accept that the 'relationship' was over. Later he confided to a psychologist employed by the University of California that he intended to kill Tatiana when she returned home from a holiday. Although the campus police briefly detained Poddar (at the psychologist's request) he was soon released once he promised to stay away from Tatiana. The following month he murdered her. But at no time before then did anyone warn Tatiana (or her parents) of the dangers she faced.

Nor were any steps taken to commit him. The Californian Supreme Court held that, even though safeguarding the confidential nature of psychotherapeutic communication was of the utmost importance, in some circumstances this could be outweighed by an even greater concern, namely the need to protect third parties from a patient's serious intention to kill or harm them. Accordingly, the court decided that in such cases a therapist had a duty (not an option) to take reasonable care to protect the intended victim, even though s/he is not a patient – for example, by warning him/her (or others) of the danger, notifying the police, or taking whatever other steps are reasonably necessary under the circumstances. Since the psychologist failed to do anything other than alert the police, in this case he was found liable.

Not surprisingly, the Tarasoff decision was controversial, largely because it was expected to have a significant impact on the behaviour of psychiatrists in the USA who, it was assumed, would be more willing than in the past to breach confidentiality (presumably for fear of being sued in negligence; Beauchamp and Childress, 1994). It was because of this that one judge felt very strongly that imposing a legal duty on therapists would ultimately be very detrimental to potentially violent patients (yet ones who could be successfully treated) by deterring them from seeking treatment. Furthermore if they could not be sure that their confidences would be kept, even if they did seek treatment, they might not 'bare their souls' and so withhold vital information – for example, their violent fantasies. As a consequence treatment could well be ineffective. The public at large would also suffer because if patients lost confidence in their therapists violent assaults would increase.

While these arguments failed to win out in the end, they did highlight some potential problems, in particular the uncertainties associated with this kind of case. In other words, by imposing a duty on therapists to would-be victims it becomes even more important to make accurate predictions and assessments about violence and the likelihood (and seriousness) of harm. But are these always possible and who should be blamed if predictions turn out to be wrong? More importantly, perhaps, will it result in 'innocent' mentally ill people being unnecessarily detained? The answers to these questions have yet to be found but in the meantime the Tarasoff case, albeit an American one, is a powerful reminder that an absolute principle of confidentiality is a difficult one to uphold in practice. Interestingly, however, it seems that psychiatrists have not shown any increased tendency to resort to prolonged commitment in order to avoid liability (Mason and McCall Smith, 1999, p. 505).

Disclosures required by law or court order
See below.

Legal exceptions

In many instances the professional and legal exceptions to confidentiality are very similar. Nevertheless there are certain differences. Several statutes also require disclosure to be made. In outline the legal exceptions are as follows.

Consent of the patient

This exception is recognized in law and mirrors the ethical exception (see above).

Need to know

In legal texts this category (sometimes also referred to as 'the interests of the patient') is often treated as a separate one (Montgomery, 1997). The legal scope of this exception again, however, mirrors the professional one (see Consent, above).

Disclosures required by statute and police enquiries

The majority of statutory requirements deal with the collection of statistical data such as the number of births and deaths, abortions, communicable disease, substance abuse and serious accidents. There are also certain obligations to pass on information under the Mental Health Act 1983. Other statutes require disclosure of information on infertility treatment and organ transplantation. In addition, although AIDS is not a notifiable disease, health authorities have to provide certain anonymized information about patients with AIDS. Anonymized information is information from which a person's identity and other identifying details have been removed. Note that the latest recommendations from the BMA (1999) focus on the need to anonymize information.

Perhaps the most controversial of all the disclosures that are generally considered in this context are those that involve the police. Concerns here typically focus on reporting crime to the police and 'helping them with their enquiries'. This is because, in the course of their work, nurses may well acquire information or gain evidence that a patient has committed an offence or is about to commit a crime. A patient seeking treatment may, for example, admit that he received stolen goods while carrying out a burglary or some other crime. Practitioners working in the community might also come across stolen goods, perhaps, or drugs that have been obtained illegally. But do nurses have a legal duty to report these crimes? The short answer is no. Nurses are no different from any other citizen. In other words, since there is no general legal duty to report crime, nurses are not legally obliged to do anything (except where legislation specifically creates such a duty). This was confirmed in *Rice* v. *Connolly* [1966] 2 QB 414, when the judge said: '[I]t seems to me quite clear that though every citizen has a moral duty, or if you like a social duty to assist the police, there is no legal duty to this effect'.

The decision as to whether to volunteer information to the police about any 'police' matter is therefore a personal one. Note, however, that several statutes require nurses to disclose confidential information to the appropriate authorities. These include the Prevention of Terrorism Act 1989 and the Road Traffic Act 1972 (which is concerned with the identity of drivers involved in road traffic offences). Relevant here too are the provisions of the Police and Criminal Evidence Act 1984 under which personal records relating to the physical and mental health of a patient (such as medical and nursing notes, diagnostic samples and administrative records) are subject to special procedures. These procedures are designed to protect patient confidentiality and make sure that the police cannot obtain confidential health information too easily. This means that, if they want to see such records (assuming that is that the relevant NHS Trust has not already decided to disclose them), then they have to get permission from a circuit judge.

Court orders and legal proceedings

Sometimes nurses are required to produce evidence in legal proceedings – particularly in personal injury claims or those involving child protection (Dimond, 1995, Chapter 8). If they are called as witnesses then it will usually (but not always) be following a subpoena (which is a court order). Once subpoenaed to appear in court, nurses must disclose confidential information or risk being 'in contempt', which could lead to a jail sentence. The reason for this is that nurses cannot claim any special privilege that would allow them to keep information about a patient's secret.

However, in rare cases medical information may be withheld on grounds of the so-called public interest immunity. This immunity allows evidence to be excluded on public policy grounds. A good example of how it works is *D v. NSPCC* [1978] AC 171 where the NSPCC followed up a complaint about the alleged ill-treatment of a 14-month-old girl. Not surprisingly, its enquiry caused her mother a lot of distress and she sued the Society for negligence. But the House of Lords refused to order it to reveal the identity of the informant, on the basis that to do so would prevent other informants coming forward – which would ultimately be contrary to the public interest.

Public interest

This is arguably the most contentious legal exception mainly because no single and authoritative definition of the term has been provided and because in practice its scope appears to be so broad and uncertain that it can be used to justify any disclosure that is thought to be 'for the good of society' or in the interests of the community as a whole. According to Stauch *et al.* (1998, p. 221), the language of the public interest defence – which Lord Goff used in the seminal case of *A-G v. Guardian Newspapers (No. 2)* [1990] above (p. 92) – has a strong utilitarian flavour. Note that the exception does not impose any duty on nurses to disclose confidential information – it gives them the option to do so. But in what circumstances? The little case law that there is on confidentiality suggests that breaches are lawful whenever the public interest in disclosure outweighs the public interest in respecting confidences. What this means in practice is that one public interest has to be balanced against another. In other words, the interest of those claiming confidentiality has to be considered alongside the interests of others – the public generally or identifiable individuals (or an individual) who may be harmed unless confidentiality is breached.

To carry out this balancing act, however, certain very basic terms have to be clarified, in particular the meaning of 'public interest'. The most helpful cases are the following.

W v. *Edgell* [1990] 1 All ER 835 concerned a psychiatric patient, W, who was being detained indefinitely in a secure hospital as a result of a conviction for seriously injuring and shooting and killing five others 10 years previously. Following his application to a mental health tribunal a report was prepared by Dr Edgell about his mental state. This strongly opposed any transfer to a regional secure unit – which was the first step towards W's eventual release – because of his long-standing and continuing abnormal interest in firearms and home-made bombs (which he called fireworks). In short, Edgell claimed that, notwithstanding the opinion of the medical officer responsible for W that he no longer presented a danger, his view was that W was still a very dangerous man (i.e. one with an abnormal psychopathic personality) who needed further treatment.

After seeing the report, W's solicitors withdrew his application but when Edgell discovered that the report was to remain confidential – he had asked for a copy of his report to be put in W's hospital file but the solicitors refused – Edgell decided to send a copy to the director of the hospital caring for W. Finally, the report reached the Home Secretary (the person with ultimate control over W's release). W sued Edgell for breach of confidentiality but the Court of Appeal rejected his claim on the basis that the duty of confidentiality owed to W was outweighed by the overriding interest in public safety.

Undoubtedly, the court would have reached a different conclusion if Edgell had, without concealing W's identity, sold 'his story' to a newspaper or discussed the case in his memoirs. But, as one of the judges, Lord Bingham, acknowledged, Edgell acted on the basis of 'sound professional judgement' fearing a 'real risk of consequent danger to the public' unless disclosure was made. Lord Bingham also claimed that the court's decision was well in line with article 8(2) of the European Convention of Human Rights, which envisages that circumstances may arise in which a public authority may legitimately interfere with the exercise of the right of confidentiality (which is recognized in article 8(1)) in the interests of public safety or the prevention of crime.

So, what guidelines emerge from this case about the scope of 'public interest'? These can be summarized as follows.

- Before disclosure can be justified there must be a 'real' or 'genuine' serious risk of danger (which must persist) to the public, even though that danger does not have to be imminent.
- Even though disclosure can be justified it must nevertheless be both accurate and limited, i.e. only made available to the relevant person(s) or authority. In other words, disclosure to the world at large will rarely be justified since those receiving it must have a legitimate interest. Nor should more confidential information than is strictly necessary be revealed.
- Arguably, the risk to the public must be to their physical safety, i.e. danger of physical harm or disease.

Like the Tarasoff case in America the Edgell decision was controversial (but has been followed, notably in *R* v. *Crozier* [1990]). This was because many feared that if the law sanctioned disclosure in these kinds of circumstances, albeit rather rare and extreme, then patients would no longer trust health professionals to keep their secrets.

But the case generated less public interest than one that reached the courts just a few years earlier, *X* v. *Y* [1988] 2 All ER 648. This case, which was the first on breach of medical confidentiality in recent years, was (and is) arguably more significant because of its relevance to the debate about AIDS and HIV status and the acute dilemmas it can pose for all health professionals. It also raised a very important aspect of 'public interest' not dealt with in the Edgell case – freedom of the press.

Briefly the facts are these. A health service employee passed on to a tabloid newspaper details of two practising GPs who had developed AIDS. The information had been obtained from confidential medical records held by the hospital where they were being treated. The paper wanted to publish information that would almost certainly ultimately have resulted in them being identified. This was likely because, despite the existence of a court order restraining publication of the information, the paper nonetheless published an article under the headline 'Scandal of Docs with AIDS', which it intended to follow up. The health authority therefore sought another order restraining publication of the doctors' identity.

In agreeing to grant the injunction the court identified two public interests. The first was the freedom of the press and the related public interest in having an informed public debate about AIDS, and in particular on the implications of health professionals being HIV-positive. But despite accepting the importance of this public interest (which according to the court was happening in any event and would not be significantly enhanced by naming the doctors) there was another public interest that was more compelling, namely that of preserving confidentiality. Otherwise, actual or potential AIDS sufferers would be reluctant either to seek or continue treatment and counselling through fear of being identified. If that happened the public would ultimately suffer through increased spread of the disease.

While the reasons for maintaining confidentiality in this case seem clear and convincing it does raise some unanswered questions. Supposing, for example, the doctors had been surgeons rather than GPs? Would the court have reached the same decision? Should it? And even if disclosure was justified in such circumstances, how much information should be revealed and to whom? In some cases patients may need to be informed but more often it may only be necessary to inform NHS managers. Similarly, what should, for example, a nurse working in a occupational health department do on discovering that a colleague is HIV-positive? Arguably, disclosure in this kind of case would be legally justified under the public interest exception but much would depend on the particular circumstances, in particular how high the risk of transmission was and so forth and whether procedures outlined in the UKCC statement and Registrar's Letter on AIDS and HIV infection (UKCC, 1993) had been followed.

Finally, it is perhaps worth noting that, despite these two important cases, which do establish some useful guidelines about when disclosure would be lawful, the scope of public interest remains uncertain. One area in particular that is causing increasing concern is that of genetic information. Now that tests can establish much more precisely whether someone is at risk of developing or passing on an inherited disease – say, cystic fibrosis or Huntington's chorea – acute dilemmas may arise, e.g. about informing relatives that they too may be at risk. If a patient refused to give his or her consent to this kind of disclosure, could a health professional nevertheless justify breaching confidentiality? In other words, would disclosure come within the public interest exception? As yet there has been no case on this so it is only possible to speculate on what a court would decide. It is likely, however, that such a case would turn on the seriousness of the disease in question – was it life-threatening, for example? Other relevant factors would be the magnitude of the risk of the disease being inherited and so on.

In other cases it may be vital to obtain confidential information from relatives about their genetic make-up in order for a patient to be properly diagnosed or counselled. Again, the issue would be whether disclosure of that information would be in the public interest should the relative refuse to consent to the information being disclosed.

REMEDIES FOR BREACH OF CONFIDENTIALITY

Given the uncertainty surrounding much of the law of confidentiality, in particular when disclosure is justified in the public interest, it is perhaps not surprising that few patients have taken legal action to enforce their rights. In principle, however, remedies are available both to prevent a threatened breach and where a breach has already occurred. Threatened breaches can be stopped by the court granting an injunction. An injunction (like the one granted in the case of X v. Y, above) is a court order that requires someone either to do or to stop doing a particular act. An alternative remedy is for the plaintiff to claim damages, which are available for some losses, such as financial ones, but not for things such as embarrassment or upset. Usually, however, the most effective remedy is for a patient to lodge a complaint alleging professional misconduct, which could result in disciplinary proceedings. In addition, nurses who breach patients' confidentiality could find themselves disciplined by their employers and might be dismissed.

MEDICAL RECORDS

The relationship of trust and confidence between patients and nurses is a two-way process. One element is the duty of confidentiality. The other, which is equally important if patients are to have control over their health care, is the right to know what information has been compiled about them. For a long time patients' advocates have asserted the right to see medical records but it is only relatively recently that access has been granted (it is also now recognized in the Patient's Charter).

But why should access be seen as so important? First, much more information is now routinely collected and stored than ever before. As a result more confidential information – some of which is very sensitive (and thus potentially harmful if it got into the 'wrong' hands) – is widely accessible, not just to health professionals but also other health-care staff, many of whom are not bound by any professional code of practice preventing disclosure (even though their contracts of employment are likely to prohibit breaches of confidentiality). Second, information stored on record is sometimes inaccurate or misleading and patients increasingly expect to be able to set the record straight or at least check on what has been said about them, especially if they suspect that an offensive or defamatory remark has been made.

Under the common law patients do not have the right to see their health records but there are now several statutes that do grant such rights. Of these the most important in this context are the Data Protection Act 1998 (which replaces the Data Protection Act 1984) and the Access to Health Records Act 1990. Other relevant statutes are the Access to Medical Reports Act 1988, the Access to Personal Files Act 1987 and the Supreme Court Act 1981.

The Data Protection Act 1984 was the first to grant access rights. Its replacement, the 1998 Act, covers not only records kept on computer but also data that is manually stored in filing systems. The new scheme of protection is very similar to the 1984 Act and aims to protect individuals from the misuse of personal information. Like the 1984 Act it is based on several fundamental principles which, apart from giving individuals the right to find out what information has been recorded about them, also broadly aims to ensure that 'personal data' is:

- obtained and processed fairly and lawfully;
- adequate;
- accurate and kept up to date;
- held only for specified purposes;
- stored securely but only for as long as is necessary; and
- not disclosed to unauthorized people.

The term 'personal data' includes any personal information relating to the physical and mental health of an individual and so covers medical and nursing records, pathology laboratory records and any other health-related records held by (or originally recorded by) a wide variety of health professionals. The Act does not, however, guarantee access, since this can be denied in certain circumstances.

The Access to Health Records Act 1990 applies only to manual health records made since 1 November 1991. Its main purpose is to give patients the right to see their records and to have inaccurate records corrected. In the Act the term 'heath record' means any information relating to a patient's physical or mental health made by or on behalf of a health professional in respect of the patient's care. The word 'health professional' is also very broadly defined and includes doctors, dentists, nurses, midwives, health visitors, opticians and so on. As with the Data Protection Act, however, access is not guaranteed, since it can be refused if it would disclose information 'likely to cause serious harm to the physical or mental health of the patient or of any other individual' or would identify an individual who has not consented to disclosure.

Although both these Acts were welcomed, the fact that they do not guarantee access does undermine their commitment to patients' rights, especially as the grounds for refusing access are based on the principles of 'therapeutic privilege' – a concept that is well-known to encourage paternalistic practices. It is also perhaps worth noting here that the UKCC Guidelines discuss access to records for teaching, research and audit and acknowledge that these may need to be used to help students gain the skills they require. However, they make it clear that the same principles of confidentiality apply, in particular that patients should be able to refuse access to their records if they wish. Note finally the Code of Practice on Openness in the NHS, which came into force in 1995 and which aims to introduce broad principles of openness into all aspects of the operation of the NHS (Mason and McCall Smith, 1999).

CHILDREN AND CONFIDENTIALITY

Once an obligation to maintain confidentiality has arisen it is owed as much to young people under 18 as it is to any other person, providing they are sufficiently mature to form a relationship of trust. What this means is, that irrespective of a child's competence to consent (or veto) treatment, they are nonetheless owed a duty of confidence if they understand what it means to trust someone with secret information. This is, however, subject to any relevant exception (see above). Note too that even if requested treatment is refused, the confidentiality of the consultation should still be respected.

Put simply, competence and the duty of confidentiality are not necessarily connected even if in some cases, e.g. those involving very young children, they will be. In other words they will be neither competent nor mature enough to understand what keeping a promise means. In such cases, disclosure of information to parents may be an integral part of the child's care (McHale, 1998). Of course, if children are Gillick-competent then it is clear that disclosure without their consent will not normally be lawful (for further discussion about children and confidentiality, see Hendrick, 1997).

CONFIDENTIALITY AND PEOPLE WITH MENTAL HEALTH AND LEARNING DISABILITIES

The UKCC Guidelines for mental health and learning disabilities (1998) state, in the section on confidentiality, that professional practice is based upon developing a therapeutic relationship with clients; and that confidentiality within this relationship should only be broken in exceptional circumstances and only after careful consideration leading to a conclusion that this can be justified. In the absence of clear authority the extent to which an obligation of confidence is owed to people with mental health and learning disabilities is arguably much the same as in respect of children. Thus confidentiality is owed (subject to any relevant exception) if they understand what keeping a secret means. In the case of those adults who are permanently incompetent it has been suggested (McHale, 1998, p. 101) that the probable position is that information can be disclosed if it is in the patient's best interests to do so (following *Re F* [1990] 2 AC 1, see also BMA 1999).

CASE STUDY 4.1   WINNIE'S INFORMATION – A DISCUSSION

(Refer to the scenario presented on page 89.)

The initial question to resolve is what information provided by Winnie is confidential. Despite the absence of any clear professional definition, there can be little doubt that the following would be considered confidential.

First, any 'clinical' details that relate to Winnie's medical condition, care and treatment and that affect diagnosis and prognosis are confidential, i.e. her leg ulcers and the symptoms she thinks are connected to them. Details of her past medical history that are relevant to her current condition would also be included here.

Secondly, all information is confidential that, despite not being clinical, nevertheless could have an impact on Winnie's progress or recovery. Into this category would probably come her failing eyesight. Winnie's plans and anxieties about the future may be confidential but not if they fall within what can be called 'social' information. So her intention to spend Christmas with Peggy is not confidential.

Her suspicions about her nephew's drug dealing and the probable causes of Annie's injuries are also confidential, especially as Annie has made it very clear that she will not be examined by Rebecca and does not wish to discuss her bruises and black eye either with her or with anyone else.

There are several agencies or people that might have an interest in the information provided by Winnie, most obviously other members of the health-care team involved in her care and treatment, such as her GP and other nurses. Accordingly, confidential information relevant to her care and overall health, such as her failing eyesight, could be shared with them – assuming, that is, that Winnie consented to this. Winnie's past medical history should not be shared with the health-care team if it has no bearing on her current medical condition or recovery. Clearly, then, details of the abortion she had as a young woman should not be disclosed.

If Annie needs to be treated for her injuries then it would also be important for those caring for her to be informed. At the moment, however, it seems that Annie is refusing treatment and certainly has not consented to information about her injuries being shared with anyone.

Similarly, social services may need to know both about Winnie and Annie. Winnie's failing health and poor eyesight may make it difficult for her to manage much longer on her own. A social worker would need to visit her and make an assessment of her needs, and so forth. If Winnie gave her consent to this information being disclosed, then Rebecca could get in touch with them. But if Winnie refused Rebecca would have to justify breaching confidentiality on other grounds.

This she could arguably do following the UKCC Advisory Paper on Confidentiality (UKCC, 1987). In section D, it discusses deliberate breach of confidentiality 'in the interests of the patient'. According to clause 3 of that section – which confirms that information may need to be shared both with other health professionals and those in the social work field – the consent of the patient should, 'wherever possible', be first obtained. But if consent is not forthcoming it seems that sharing information may still be justifiable. Note, however, that non-consensual sharing of information in a patient's interest does not appear to have been repeated in the 1996 Guidelines from the UKCC.

As to Annie, she too may need to be supported by social services. But if she refused consent then again, if Rebecca wanted to inform the department, she would have to justify her action.

Finally, the police might well have an interest in hearing about Mark's drug activities. In addition, it seems likely that he is abusing his mother (another criminal offence). But what should Rebecca do with this information? She certainly has not got Annie's permission to divulge it. Arguably, however, she could claim that she has a moral obligation to inform the police of her suspicions – not just to protect Annie but to protect society at large as well. Before doing so, she should, however, attempt to have another word with Annie.

Let us turn now to how the law views this situation. While there is no authoritative legal definition of confidentiality it is likely that the courts would follow the professional approach. Information about Winnie's medical condition and any matter that may affect her recovery, and so forth, would therefore most probably be recognized by the common law as confidential. In other words, Winnie has entrusted 'private' information to Rebecca in circumstances where there is both an explicit and an implicit assumption that it will be kept secret. In addition, it is in the public interest to maintain confidentiality.

In legal terms too it would not be possible to justify breaching confidentiality to a fairly wide group of people. First, the law recognizes that Rebecca would be justified in sharing information with other health professionals involved in Winnie's care. But this sharing must be in the interests of the patient and so should be limited to those with a real and genuine need to know (rather than those who are merely nosy or inquisitive). Secondly, should Rebecca decide to liaise with social services given Winnie's (and possibly Annie's) probable need of support from them in the near future, she would probably be able to justify her action in law even if consent to disclosure was not forthcoming. It is worth pointing out, nevertheless, that there has been no case on the scope of either the 'need to know' exception or that concerning 'the patient's interests'. So it is not possible to know with certainty whether the law would accept Rebecca's breach (although it probably would).

As to informing the police, the legal exception that would apply here is the public interest one. Although Rebecca has no legal obligation to be a police informer – either about Mark's drug activities or his possible abuse of his mother – she may decide that, given Annie's injuries, she should consider reporting her suspicions, especially as the harm to Annie is potentially (if not already) serious. Mark's drug activities could also be a serious danger to the public. Whatever she decides, if she is questioned by the police she must not give false or misleading information nor must she conceal evidence or accept a bribe – so if she accepted money from Mark to 'keep quiet' this would be unlawful. Nevertheless, Rebecca could probably refuse to answer questions about him since her duty to maintain confidentiality would probably constitute a 'lawful excuse'. The decision as to whether to volunteer or help the police with their enquiries is thus a personal one, although if Rebecca followed Department of Health guidance on passing information to the police (see above) she would almost certainly be able to justify her disclosure in law.

CASE STUDY 4.2   LAURA'S BREACH OF CONFIDENTIALITY – A DISCUSSION

(Refer to the scenario presented on page 90.)

In this case there has clearly been a breach of confidentiality in that Clive expressly refused his consent for his family to be told the truth about his condition and yet his wife has found out in circumstances that can only be described as very distressing. The breach was not intentional – but like many breaches it was certainly careless and thoughtless to discuss Clive's case in such a public area, where patients, relatives and visitors could come and go as they liked. Indeed, it was just this type of 'indiscretion', i.e. 'wanton, often inadvertent, but avoidable exchange' that Siegler disapproved of, since it could be so upsetting to patients. Furthermore, it makes little difference even if Laura was motivated by the best of intentions – she clearly thought disclosure would be in Clive's interests, albeit relying on her own subjective assessment of his needs.

But can Laura justify her actions? The way in which she breached confidentiality would make it difficult for her to defend herself either morally or professionally – not only did she not have Clive's consent but disclosure was not made to someone involved in his care who 'needed to know' about his condition. Furthermore, even if it could be argued that Clive's wife should have been told, the way she found out was unacceptable.

Legally, Laura's actions would also be difficult to defend in law because of the way confidentiality was breached and because Laura's friend did not need to know of Clive's condition. So what consequences is she likely to face? These are difficult to predict, as much would depend on the action taken by Clive's wife. If she were to lodge a complaint then it is almost certain that Laura would be disciplined by her manager. In addition, because her breach probably meant that she had breached her contract of employment she could ultimately be dismissed or, more probably, face some other disciplinary action. Another possibility is that she could be reported to the UKCC for acting unprofessionally. It would then be up to the Professional Conduct Committee to decide whether her actions amounted to professional misconduct and if so what sanctions should be imposed.

It is unlikely that any legal claim brought by Clive would be successful unless he could satisfy a court that an award of damages was appropriate – because he has suffered physical or psychological injury, for example, or had lost his job. He could not get damages for frustration or annoyance, however, nor, given that the breach has already occurred, would an injunction achieve anything.

CASE STUDY 4.3   BERYL'S BREACH OF CONFIDENCE – A DISCUSSION

(Refer to the scenario presented on page 90.)

This case raises similar issues to the Tarasoff case, i.e. whether Beryl can justify breaching confidence and taking action to protect Paul – assuming that John refuses his consent to disclosure. The Guidelines specify that disclosure may be justified when it is considered necessary in the public interest. In other words, it recognizes that there may be circumstances when a nurse is permitted to disclose information without the consent of the patient. It further defines this to include serious crime and any activity that places others at serious risk.

The dilemma Beryl faces here, of course, is deciding whether the threats made by John should be taken seriously and whether the risk to Paul is a 'real' one. She also needs to consider how breaking John's confidence would affect her future relationship with him – would he be reluctant to trust her any more, would he hide other thoughts and fantasies, and so forth? In reaching her decision, then, she needs to assess the foreseeability of the harm Paul faces and how effective she could be in preventing it. So, the greater the risk of harm, i.e. that Paul will be seriously hurt (and the more likely it is that John will carry out his threats, i.e. that the harm will materialize), the greater Beryl's moral obligation to breach confidentiality. Before warning Paul or the police she should nevertheless, as the Guidelines suggest, discuss the matter fully with other professional colleagues and if appropriate consult the UKCC or a membership organization. It may well be that, following such a discussion, action under the Mental Health Act 1983 would be considered appropriate.

Note too that, once she has made her decision – Beryl may feel that the situation is so urgent that she must act very quickly and certainly at the very least tell Paul of the dangers facing him – then she should write down her reasons for breaching confidentiality (see clause 61 of the Guidelines). Finally, if the threats had not been made in respect of Paul but some other unidentifiable (and so unknown person) then arguably Beryl has less of a moral obligation to breach confidentiality in so far as the harm is not as foreseeable. Much would, of course, depend on the nature of John's threats, and so forth.

As far as the law is concerned, again it would be the public interest exception that would be relevant if Beryl decided to breach confidence by informing Paul and the police of John's threats. It is very likely that, following the case of W v. *Edgell*, Beryl's breach of confidentiality would be recognized in law as justifiable. But that would only be so if the threat to Paul was a genuine one that posed a real danger to his physical safety. Furthermore, to come within the law disclosure would have to be limited – which would almost certainly include telling Paul and the police, should they be able to protect him in some way or take action against John.

Whether Beryl has a legal duty to warn Paul, alert the police or take other action, such as alerting the appropriate authorities so that action can be taken under the Mental Health Act, is another matter. Most commentators doubt that the English courts would go as far as the Californian Supreme Court and impose a duty to inform in this kind of case, even when specific threats had been made against an identifiable potential victim. Ultimately, liability would turn on the law of negligence, in particular the foreseeability of serious harm to the victim – in other words whether there was a real risk that the threats would be carried out. But the biggest hurdle would be in establishing that there was a sufficiently close relationship between Beryl and Paul for the law to impose a duty of care. If Paul was also Beryl's patient then such a duty might be recognized, but even this is doubtful given the absence of any general legal obligation in English law to act as a Good Samaritan – generally, no-one is legally bound to rescue another person, even if s/he could do so with little effort or danger. As a consequence it is unlikely that any court would impose a legal duty on Beryl to inform Paul or take any other action. If John had made threats against no one in particular, it is even less likely that the law would impose a duty to take 'remedial' action.

CASE STUDY 4.4   KATHY'S POSSIBLE ABUSE – A DISCUSSION

(Refer to the scenario presented on page 91.)

Kathy is too young to enter into a confidential relationship with health professionals and thus cannot consent to information about herself being disclosed. Nonetheless, there can be little doubt that disclosure would be in her interests. Normally, non-consensual disclosure of confidential information about the health of a young child would be made to the parents and would not be difficult to justify – information would need to be shared with all those caring for the child. In this case, however, Kathy's mother and stepfather are possibly responsible for her injuries.

This raises the question of whether Claire should alert anyone else to her suspicions. In other words, is there a justification for breaching confidentiality? The most appropriate exception is again the public interest one. According to the Guidelines, public interest covers several areas, including child abuse (clause 56). In addition, the Department of Health Guidance makes it clear that in child protection cases the overriding principle is to secure the best interests of the child. Therefore if a 'health professional has knowledge of abuse or neglect it may be necessary to share this information with others – the sharing must, however, be on a strictly controlled basis so that decisions relating to the child's welfare can be taken in the light of all relevant information'. Accordingly Claire would almost certainly be able to justify her action (both morally and professionally) if she reported her suspicions to the appropriate authorities.

In law too the public interest exception would apply should Claire report her suspicions. She should take care nevertheless to follow the procedures and recommendations laid down in any relevant guidance, for example, the document *Working Together: A Guide to Inter-agency Co-operation for the Protection of Children from Child Abuse* (reissued in 1998) and its addendum: *Child Protection: Medical Responsibilities*. It is also interesting to note that, while the Children Act 1989, does not impose any legal obligation on nurses (or other health professionals) to disclose confidential information in order to protect children from abuse there is some indication that the courts may be moving towards imposing such a duty. As yet, however, there has been no case directly on this point concerning health professionals.

CASE STUDY 4.5   LEN'S RIGHT TO PRIVACY – A DISCUSSION

(Refer to the scenario presented on page 91.)

The public interest exception is at the core of this question, which raises very similar legal and ethical issues, namely whether Len's condition is such that details of it can legitimately be shared with other people. It is the kind of situation that Vedder (1999) describes as a tragic dilemma for health professionals who, on the one hand, have a duty to respect confidentiality but, on the other, a duty to prevent serious harm, a duty that can only be fulfilled by violating the confidentiality rule (p. 148).

Let us deal first with Gillian's moral obligation. There are several different approaches that she could take. One is to regard confidentiality as an absolute principle that should not be breached for any reason. Another is to treat it as a qualified principle, which would mean that confidentiality could be breached in certain circumstances – say, if another person could otherwise be seriously harmed. Another approach, which falls somewhere between the two, is for Gillian to do all she can to protect Mary but at the same time to maintain Len's confidentiality. She could, for example, try to persuade Len to take appropriate precautions and not take risks such as 'unsafe sex'.

But if, after careful reflection, Gillian decides to inform Mary of Len's HIV status, is this decision justifiable – in particular, does it comply with professional guidelines? The answer would turn on the interpretation of the term 'serious risk'. Since AIDS is a fatal disease and Mary faces a high risk of being infected unless precautions are taken, Gillian's breach of confidentiality might not be too difficult to defend, although she would, of course, have to justify her action and in particular follow recommendations in the 1994 UKCC document on AIDS and HIV infection. Note finally that guidance from the GMC (1997) advises doctors that they:

> may disclose information to a known sexual contact of a patient with HIV where you have reason to think that the patient has not informed that person, and cannot be persuaded to do so. In such circumstances you should tell the patient before you make the disclosure and you must be prepared to justify a decision to disclose information (GMC, 1997).

If Len was suffering from a disease that, although infectious, was not fatal, Gillian would probably feel less compelled to warn Mary. Nevertheless, she may decide to do so on the basis that, even though she may not have a moral duty to protect Mary, she is still morally justified in breaching confidentiality.

In legal terms the question again is whether Gillian could justify informing Mary of Len's HIV status. There has been no case directly on this issue nor any other authoritative legal guidelines that can be relied on. Nonetheless, it has been suggested (Mason and McCall Smith, 1999, p. 200) that passing on information to a patient's spouse or other sexual partner in the absence of consent is allowable so long as every effort has been made to persuade the patient to do so and there is a serious and identifiable risk to a specific individual. Disclosure to other health professionals caring for such patients would also only be justified if the risk of transmission was high. Whether a court would endorse this approach would, however, depend on the particular facts of each case and guidance from cases like X v. Y and W v. Edgell. So the questions it would ask would be, for example: How serious was the risk to Mary? Did she have a legitimate interest in receiving the information and was informing her the only practical way of protecting her? Given that AIDS is a fatal illness the answer would almost certainly be yes.

Finally, what would the position be in law if Len was not HIV-positive but suffering from another sexually transmitted disease? Again the questions that would need to be answered would be similar but it might well be that, if the disease was say easily treatable or far less harmful, then there would be less justification for breaching confidentiality.

LAW and ETHICS – a comparison

The duty to protect patient confidentiality has long been recognized in medical and nursing ethics – it was first enshrined in the Hippocratic Oath in the 5th century BC. But the relatively simple principle it describes arguably no longer exists. That this is so is evident from the increasing number of queries professional bodies receive about confidentiality (according to the BMA 1999 guidance the volume of such queries outstrips other issues of ethical concern). Nevertheless, irrespective of this debate there can be little doubt that, given the nature of contemporary health care, in particular its complexity, it would now be appropriate to reappraise traditional notions of confidentiality and focus on those aspects of the original principle that are worth retaining (Ridley, 1998, p. 95).

As was noted above, the legal sources of confidentiality are much more recent. However, the law is now well established and few would question patients' legal entitlement to have their confidences respected. Yet it is now time that the law was clarified and legislation was enacted – especially on the controversial public interest exception – that would give clear guidance to patients and all those involved in health care (as recommended by the BMA in 1999).

That said, it is worth noting how the moral, legal and professional duty of confidentiality can be justified on both consequentialist and deontological grounds. But perhaps more significant is the importance of the concept of trust, which many commentators regard as one of the most fundamental elements in the nurse–patient relationship. In law too the concept of trust has an important role to play. This is because without it the equitable obligation to keep information about patients secret (which is arguable the main source of the legal obligation of confidence) is unlikely to be recognized.

Yet even though the moral and legal basis for the duty of confidentiality is not in doubt neither in law nor ethics is it regarded as an absolute principle. In other words, in practice it is clear that not only is it sometimes inappropriate to keep patients' confidences but it is also not always in their interests. It is not surprising, then, that the law and the UKCC Code of Professional Conduct (and the Guidelines) allow exceptions to the duty of confidentiality. In broad terms this means that in some circumstances it is permissible for nurses to disclose confidential information while in others they may even have a duty to do so. The exceptions that are recognized legally and professionally include disclosure made with the patient's consent, disclosure that is required by a court (or statute) and disclosure that can be justified in the wider public interest.

While not all these 'shared' exceptions are applied and interpreted in exactly the same way, they nevertheless reflect broadly similar concerns. Indeed, they so closely resemble each other that it is very difficult to dissociate the two. Interestingly too, in the case of W v. *Edgell* the Court of Appeal in reaching its decision carefully considered the exceptions recognized by the General Medical Council's guidance on confidentiality (1995). In declaring that they – in particular the 'need to know' and public interest exception – were compatible with the law it seems that the judges made it clear that they are keen to rely on professional guidance in interpreting and developing the law of confidentiality.

REFERENCES

Beauchamp, T. L. and Childress, J. F. (1994) *Principles of Biomedical Ethics*, 4th edn, Oxford University Press, Oxford.

BMA (1999) *Confidentiality and Disclosure of Health Information*, British Medical Association, London.

Brody, H. (1997) The physician–patient relationship. In: *Medical Ethics*, (ed. R. Veatch), 2nd edn, Jones & Bartlett, London.

Brown, J. M., Kitson, A. L. and McKnight, T. J. (1992) *Challenges in Caring*, Chapman & Hall, London.

Department of Health (1996) *The Protection and Use of Personal Information*, Department of Health, London.

Department of Health (1999) *Working Together to Protect Children – Government Guidance on Inter-Agency Co-operation*, Department of Health, London.

Dimond, B. C. (1995) *Legal Aspects of Nursing*, 2nd edn, Prentice-Hall, Hemel Hempstead.

Edwards, S. D. (1996) *Nursing Ethics: A Principle-based Approach*, Macmillan, Basingstoke.

Gillon, R. (1985) *Philosophical Medical Ethics*, John Wiley, Chichester.

GMC (1995) *Confidentiality: Guidance from the GMC*, General Medical Council, London.

GMC (1997) *Serious Communicable Diseases*, General Medical Council, London.

Hendrick, J. (1997) *Legal Aspects of Child Health*, Chapman & Hall, London.

Johnstone, M-J. (1989) *Bioethics – a Nursing Perspective*, Baillière Tindall, London.

McHale, J. V. (1993) *Medical Confidentiality and Legal Privilege*, Routledge, London.

McHale, J.V. (1998) Confidentiality and access to health care records. In: *Law and Nursing*, (eds J. McHale, J. Tingle and J. Peysner), Butterworth Heinemann, Oxford.

Mason, J. K. and McCall Smith, R. A. (1999) *Law and Medical Ethics*, 5th edn, Butterworths, London.

Montgomery, J. (1997) *Health Care Law*, Oxford University Press, Oxford.

Murphy, T. (1998) Health confidentiality in the age of talk. In: Sheldon, S. and Thomson, M. (eds) *Feminist Perspectives on Health Care Law*, Cavendish Publishing, London.

Ridley, A. (1998) *Beginning Bioethics*, St Martin's Press, New York.

Rumbold, G. (1999) *Ethics in Nursing Practice*, 3rd edn, Baillière Tindall, London.

Siegler, M. (1982) Confidentiality in medicine: a decrepit concept. *New England Journal of Medicine*, **307**, 1518.

Singleton, J. and McLaren, S. (1995) *Ethical Foundations of Health Care: Responsibilities in Decision Making*, Mosby, London.

Stauch, M. and Wheat, K., with Tingle, J. (1998) *Sourcebook on Medical Law*, Cavendish Publishing, London.

Tschudin, V. (1994) *Deciding Ethically: A Practical Approach to Nursing Challenges*, Baillière Tindall, London.

Tschudin, V. (1996) Confidentiality. In: *Ethics: Nurses and Patients*, (ed. V. Tschudin), Baillière Tindall, London.

UKCC (1987) *Confidentiality: An Elaboration of Clause 9 of the Second Edition of the UKCC's Code of Conduct*, United Kingdom Central Council, London.

UKCC (1992) *Code of Professional Conduct*, United Kingdom Central Council, London.

UKCC (1994) *Acquired Immune Deficiency Syndrome and Human Immune Deficiency Virus Infection (AIDS and HIV Infection)*, United Kingdom Central Council, London.

UKCC (1996) *Guidelines for Professional Practice*, United Kingdom Central Council, London.

UKCC (1998) *Guidelines for Mental Health and Learning Disabilities Nursing*, United Kingdom Central Council, London.

Vedder, A. (1999) HIV/AIDS and the point and scope of medical confidentiality. In: *HIV and AIDS: Testing, Screening and Confidentiality*, (eds R. Bennett and C. A. Erin), Oxford University Press, Oxford.

FURTHER READING

Kennedy, I. and Grubb, A. (1994) *Medical Law: Text with Materials*, Butterworths, London.

Royal College of Nursing (1991) *Guidelines on Confidentiality in Nursing*, RCN, London.

UKCC (1994) *Anonymous Testing for the Prevalence of the Human Immune Deficiency Virus (HIV)*, United Kingdom Central Council, London.

5 JUSTICE AND ACCESS TO HEALTH RESOURCES

INTRODUCTION

One of the most pressing contemporary issues in health care is how to distribute resources fairly. Questions such as who should be treated and how priorities should be set raise fundamental legal and ethical dilemmas that have long been at the centre of health care. But now that 'rationing' is more visible, or at least more openly debated, than in the past, the ways in which decisions are made are more likely to be contested and challenged. This chapter looks at resource allocation, bearing in mind that allocation only poses an ethical and legal problem when the resources to be allocated are scarce, i.e. 'not unlimited' (Ridley, 1998). It begins by examining key concepts such as 'health', 'illness' and 'rationing' and how various competing theories of justice – the central principle in this debate – offer different guidance about how to provide comprehensive and reasonable health care on a 'just' basis. Some of the practical implications of these theories are then explored, focusing on the particular criterion of justice that each emphasizes. Legal analysis will focus on the law's role in guaranteeing access to treatment but will begin with a brief look at its contribution to health promotion and disease prevention.

CASE STUDY 5.1   HAS CAROL A LEGAL RIGHT TO TREATMENT?

Three weeks ago Carol, a 14-year-old drug addict, took an Ecstasy tablet. Without a liver transplant she will die but doctors refuse to consider her for one. Martin, a nurse working in the transplant unit, thinks this unfair – he believes Carol is being discriminated against because of her drug habit and that many 'less deserving' patients get transplants. There was Jim, for example, a famous footballer with a history of alcohol abuse who received two transplants in his forties. Martin also thinks that, given her age, Carol should at least be given a chance to live. Carol's father is threatening legal action if she is denied a transplant.

Has Carol a legal right to treatment? Is it morally justifiable to treat Jim rather than Carol?

CASE STUDY 5.2   HOW CAN ARUNDHATI DIVIDE HER TIME AND CARE FAIRLY?

Arundhati works on a children's cancer ward. Over the last year or so she has got to know 16-year-old David very well. David has leukaemia. As his condition has deteriorated he has become increasingly dependent on Arundhati. She has tried to spend as much time as possible with him but has other patients to look after, in particular William, a 10-year-old who has just been diagnosed with bone cancer. He is very frightened and cries a lot of the time. His parents are finding it difficult to come to terms with his cancer and with the likelihood that his leg will have to be amputated.

How then should Arundhati divide her time and nursing care? Whose interests should she prioritize – William's or David's? Does the law have any role to play in this type of situation?

ISSUES OF DEFINITION

These case studies represent only some of the difficult choices that have to be made about the allocation of scarce resources. They have been chosen not because they are necessarily typical of the daily situations that nurses face but because they involve patients with life-threatening diseases. As such, they are the most morally agonizing and require complex and profound analysis. This means that they can not normally be dealt with instinctively (as is the case in routine small-scale resource decision-making). Note too that the case studies focus on decision-making at the 'micro' or individual level, i.e. deciding which patients will obtain particular treatments or services where only a limited amount is available (Hendrick, 1998). Deciding who should have priority in a accident or emergency department and who should get the last bed in an intensive care unit are examples of such decision-making as are decisions about allocating nursing skills and time (Dickenson, 1994).

Furthermore, while the case studies focus on the clinical role of nurses, it should be noted that nurses in administrative positions also commonly have to make difficult decisions about resource allocation (Dimond, 1995). Nor can nurses ignore how decisions are made at the macro level. Macroallocation involves deciding how much of a society's resources should be allocated to health care (which has to compete with education, housing, defence and other social goods) and how these resources should be divided between community and institutional settings (Singleton and McLaren, 1995). But they concern nurses, not just because the distinction between microallocation and macroallocation is rather a crude one – both obviously interact, notably at the meso or intermediate level (which deals with distribution of resources at regional or hospital level) – but also because they can influence macroallocation as health professionals and as citizens (Edwards, 1996, p. 119).

But before looking at the ethical and legal implications of resource allocation, certain preliminary concepts need to be clarified. These are as follows.

Health-care resources

According to Buchanan (1997), who defines the term expansively, health-care resources are any goods or services that can reasonably be expected to have a positive effect on health. As such they include, but are not restricted to, medical resources. Nor are they limited to those produced by health professionals or even just medical drugs, procedures and treatments, but include the many resources used for pollution control, shelter and food required for normal growth and functioning (Buchanan, 1997, p. 322). This broad definition is echoed by Edwards, for whom 'health care' covers its provision in hospitals and in the community as well as health education and promotion, disease prevention and all related resources, e.g. personnel (medical, nursing, administrative and so on), equipment, research projects and buildings (Edwards, 1996, p. 106).

Rationing

This term derives from the Latin word *ratio* (meaning 'reason'). Originally, it referred to one's ration (or portion). In this primary sense it implies a method of distributing limited goods and services according to a 'rational' plan so that everyone will receive a fair portion (Veatch and Fry, 1987). 'Ration' is thus both a 'rational and a moral concept and a practical correlate of justice' (Baker, 1995, p. 58). More recently, however, it has become a pejorative term associated with denying health resources to those who are legitimately entitled to them. It is not surprising therefore that it has been replaced in much of the literature by the less threatening phrase 'priority setting' or 'the allocation of scarce resources' (Newdick, 1995, p. 18).

For a number of reasons, a general consensus has developed – indeed the conventional wisdom now is – that health-care rationing is inevitable (but see, for example, White and Waithe, 1995, who suggest otherwise). The main reasons advanced are, first, the ageing population. As more people live longer so does the cost of supporting them increase, from the treatment of acute and chronic conditions to providing long-term care. A second reason advanced for the inevitability of health-care rationing is the impact of sophisticated medical and pharmaceutical developments. Medical 'miracles' and new life-saving and life-enhancing technologies that were once only dreamt about can now be used to diagnose, cure and keep alive patients with conditions that were once untreatable or from which they would almost certainly have died. In short, the very success of modern health-care systems raises expectations that result in ever-increasing demand (Ridley, 1998).

Illness and disease

While these are now very familiar and commonly used terms (typically used as synonyms) that play a vitally important role in our daily lives, there is surprisingly little agreement on their precise meaning. Why is this?

For Greaves and Upton (1996) it is simply because none of them can be objectively defined. They are, in other words, influenced by prevailing values and norms of a given society. As value-laden concepts their meaning will therefore change according to medical advances and changes in social and cultural attitudes. That the term 'illness' is by definition subjective and thus specific to time, place and culture is, for Caplan (1997, p. 65), beyond dispute. To illustrate the way values influence the definition of health and disease, he cites the 'disorder' of drapetomania, which, according to 19th-century US medical texts, afflicted an astounding number of black men and women. It was 'a horrible plague that denoted an obsessive desire on the part of a slave to run away from his or her owner' (1997, p. 69).

The role played by values is perhaps most obvious in the mental health contexts. As Engelhardt notes (1996, p. 192), for example, the 'disease' of masturbation, from which individuals were thought to die in the 18th and 19th centuries, led to 'treatment' for female masturbators that included the excision of the clitoris with scissors. This 'treatment' was necessary to 'terminate the long continued peripheral excitement, causing frequent and increasing losses of nerve force'.

If we accept, then, that values influence the way we think about illness and disease (note that many think otherwise, i.e. that determinations of illness and disease are matters of empirical fact and nothing more – Caplan, 1997, p. 64), it is perhaps not surprising that people with diseases or illnesses that were once accepted as incurable (or which were instead simply regarded as unpleasant or disabling) now expect to have their lives prolonged or at least their symptoms alleviated.

Health

The ever-expanding demand for health care is further complicated by the fact that there is little consensus on what it means to be 'healthy'. The World Health Organization, for example, describes 'health' as 'a state of complete physical, mental and social well-being and not merely the absence of disease and infirmity'. But, as Gillon implies (1985, p. 150), the idea of health it propounds is so broad and flexible that it is almost worthless. There is uncertainty too as to whether health should be described in medical (or biological) terms or in social (or functional) terms. Should infertility and arthritis, for example, be defined in biological terms, meaning the absence of illness, or in functional terms, as departures from normal physiological states? If the latter, who is to define what is 'normal' (Newdick, 1995, p. 6)?

JUSTICE – AN INTRODUCTION

For most philosophers who have searched for a single principle to justify the fair allocation of scarce health resources, the starting point has usually been the principle of justice (Baker, 1995). But, despite its pervasive use in the rationing debate, justice is a concept that is far from easy to define. This is partly because it is a quality or moral value that almost everyone considers desirable – in the sense that everyone claims to want justice and to know what is morally the 'right' thing to do – but that few understand or interpret in the same way (Riddall, 1999). Also, even though the notion of universal justice is described in the Bible and has exercised the minds of great thinkers from Plato onwards, conceptions of justice vary from age to age and from culture to culture. It is not therefore surprising that it has been said that 'to invoke justice is like banging on the table' (Ross, 1958).

Commonly, justice is thought of in two ways: justice as fairness and justice as appropriate punishment for wrongdoing (Seedhouse, 1988). These correspond to the two categories of justice identified by Aristotle: distributive justice, which was concerned with the distribution of goods such as honour and money in society, and corrective justice, which was concerned with ensuring that people did not profit from their crimes (Solomon and Murphy, 1990). Note that, because this chapter deals with the allocation of health resources, it focuses only on distributive justice. What then do we mean by this phrase?

Justice and equality

Central to Aristotle's notion of distributive justice is the principle that equals should be treated equally and unequals unequally. This did not mean that each should receive equal shares but rather that individuals should receive 'goods' in proportion to their merits. The notion that justice requires (or is linked to) equality of treatment is widely accepted as a formal or basic principle of justice – in the sense that like shall be treated as like, so that everyone who is classified as belonging to the same category, for a particular purpose, is to be treated in the same way.

But once attempts are made to interpret and apply this principle there is less consensus. One of the most fundamental problems is that this formal principle is rather an empty concept. Thus, although it is of some help in ensuring equity in health care, since it identifies the unfairness of the maldistribution of resources by, for example, geographical region, it tells us nothing about which differences are relevant in deciding health-care priorities (Campbell *et al.*, 1997, p. 184), nor does it provide much help on how people should be categorized. With no guidance on this how are we to establish what makes one individual equal to another? Or to put it another way, how do we decide which characteristics are relevant in judging individuals as equals?

Of course one way of doing this is to determine which characteristics do not count. Hence most would agree that a person's race, gender, height and employment status should be ignored in deciding who should get medical treatment (Fletcher *et al.*, 1995, p. 85). On the other hand, some characteristics or considerations are likely to be much more morally significant – factors such as medical need, the likely outcome and cost of treatment, and in some cases age too.

However, as we shall see, many of these concepts are problematic. Take need, for example – how should two people who are both suffering from cancer or heart disease be compared so as to arrive at a conclusion that they are equal (and hence entitled to equal treatment)? And what if patients are competing for beds in the ITU or for organ transplants? Again, treating patients equally and giving them equal treatment requires very subjective judgements to be made of the ways in which such individuals are equal.

Justice and merit

Given the difficulties of linking justice with equality, in particular the fact that on the basis of equality alone we do not know whether or on what basis we have to ignore or regard certain differences, is there any other way in which the concept of justice can be understood? In other words, what other principles can be used for determining what differences should be regarded as relevant in delivering health care?

One approach is to claim that justice consists of giving to each person his or her due. According to Aristotle, distributive justice was primarily concerned with what people deserve (Solomon and Murphy, 1990). At a simple level, a desert-based approach is appealing since it assumes that people are responsible for their actions and as a consequence it seems only fair to praise or blame them according to how they behave. So, if a student nurse studies hard few would argue with a system that rewards her with relevant benefits – a student prize, perhaps. On the other hand, the student nurse who spends much of his time partying instead of studying is likely to be seen as getting what he deserves if he fails his exams.

But what do we mean by 'due' and how should merit or worth be assessed? In health care a desert-based criterion involves deciding what kinds of things people have to do to merit medical treatment and perhaps even more importantly what kinds of activity should disqualify them. Praiseworthy behaviour could include anything that benefits society, such as fighting for one's country, working hard and so on. Yet, assessing the value of contributions is inherently problematic, not least because of the difficulty of reaching agreement on what each particular society values. Furthermore, although there is no reason why this desert criterion should not in principle be broad enough to include financial contributions – say, taxes – as well as other socially useful actions, i.e. those involving the expenditure of time, effort or personal resources, it may automatically (and unfairly) disadvantage certain groups, the young in particular (because they have had little time to make their contributions; Edwards, 1996, p. 112).

As to the actions that might result in individuals forfeiting medical treatment (or at least certain types of treatment), this could extend to anything potentially detrimental to health or well-being such as smoking or drinking too heavily. Especially hazardous activities (e.g. certain dangerous sports) could also be included here, as well as other pastimes. But, as Mason and McCall Smith point out (1999, p. 301), it needs no profound philosophical analysis to make one appreciate instinctively that it is right to use a helicopter to rescue a man on a drifting pleasure raft, despite the fact that his danger is of his own making, despite the expense and despite the fact that the helicopter is designed to carry 10 persons. Note too that to exclude (or in some way limit) health care in respect of those whose ill-health is caused by their own actions would not only be very difficult to monitor – everyone's activities or lifestyles would need to be centrally recorded – but is also ethically questionable because it would necessitate unacceptable interference with individuals' liberty in respect of actions that arguably harm no-one but themselves. To be workable there would also need to be some consensus (which would be very difficult to achieve) on what should count as a forfeit.

One other important question that is typically raised in connection with the desert-based approach is whether it is it fair to reward individuals for 'unearned' factors and initial advantages – such as intelligence, great athletic ability, privileged upbringing and so forth – that are outside their control but are likely to have enhanced their chances of 'succeeding' in life.

THEORIES OF JUSTICE

Let us turn now to how some theories of justice approach the question of resource allocation. Do they offer any useful guidance on the best way to allocate health care?

We begin with a consequentialist approach, in particular **utilitarianism**. According to its most famous formulation, namely 'the greatest good for the greatest number', the allocation of health care should be carried out in a way that ensures the best outcome, i.e. that maximizes benefit or utility. As Beauchamp and Childress observe (1994, p. 335), this approach to justice involves trade-offs and balances – as public and private benefits are compared, cost savings are predicted and risks and probability of failure are assessed. It also means that more emphasis is placed on basic health care and public health measures (such as health promotion and disease prevention) because these are the most socially useful and cost-effective. They are socially useful in the sense that they are more likely to prevent future costly illness and are also more likely to generate the most beneficial 'returns' for society (to the extent that they would favour, for example, the economically productive). Given too the utilitarian's concern to use funds in a way which helps the most people, resources would have to be channelled into treating the most common and least costly diseases. This would inevitably result in expensive or rare conditions being given low priority.

Not surprisingly, the consequentialist approach has been cricitized (see, for example Beauchamp and Childress, 1994, Ch. 6), First, it would almost certainly mean that the young would get preferential treatment, given that their health and well-being is most likely in the long term to be in society's interests – in employment as well as in other terms (Edwards, 1996, p. 107). It would also mean that certain groups, such as those with a stigmatizing or rare illness or those who are not socially valued, could be excluded (Kopelman, 1995, p. 209). Second, a problem for all utilitarians is not only the impracticality (if not impossibility) of accurately predicting the consequences of health-related actions but also of calculating what is best for the greatest number, given that the concept of health itself is such an elastic concept (Brock, 1982).

Another theory of justice adopts a deontological approach (although it is more often referred to as egalitarian). This holds that the 'goods' in society should be provided to everyone on the same basis. According to Kopelman (1995), what this means in terms of the principle of justice is that we should try to make people's objective net well-being as equal as possible (p. 210). In emphasizing equality, however, egalitarians do not want exactly the same treatment for everyone as a condition of justice. Rather, they want everyone to have access to the same health benefits on the same footing. So, what is provided to one person should be provided to all others similarly situated.

But in holding that health benefits should be distributed equally, egalitarians face several difficulties, in particular what kind of equality is important. As we have seen above, equality is a problematic concept in this context. Thus, if equality is to be interpreted in terms of equal treatment on the basis of common need, some consensus on the meaning of 'need' is necessary (but is difficult to achieve, see below). Nor is understanding equality in terms of outcome much less problematic (see below). Moreover, as Buchanan points out (1997, p. 350), it would be irrational for anyone, including the worst-off, to insist on equality if allowing certain inequalities would improve everyone's situation. Thus if higher salaries would encourage more people to become health professionals – with the result that a higher quality of care would become available to all – it seems unlikely that such a system would be considered to be objectionable (assuming, that is, that health professionals' increased incomes did not have negative effects outweighing the gain in the quality of care for the least well-off).

Another conceptual difficulty is the egalitarian claim that the right to health care requires that no one is to have access to any health care that is not available to everyone else in similar need. If we accept this then there are two options. One is to set the level of health care so high (so as to satisfy everybody's need) that almost all available resources will be consumed, thereby placing an unacceptable strain on overall social resources. The other is to set the level of care below that which is the technically possible optimum. But this is also problematic – assuming, that is, that those with additional resources are prohibited from purchasing better quality care. This is because such a system would not only involve an unacceptable interference with an individual's right to buy the health care he or she desires but it would also be inefficient (Buchanan, 1997, p. 351).

One very influential egalitarian theory of justice is that of the modern philosopher John Rawls. His approach – which identifies justice with fairness – is rooted in the idea of the social contract (which explains why it is sometimes called a **contractarian** theory). In the limited space available it is not, of course, possible to do justice to Rawls's intricate theory (a useful introduction is *Reading Rawls* (ed. N. Daniels, 1975)). Yet its implications for the distribution of scarce resources are important, not least because, even though Rawls does not specifically mention health, his analysis has been applied to the allocation of resources by others, notably Norman Daniels (1985).

Rawls approaches the idea of justice through an imaginary situation. Using the device of a hypothetical social contract he asks us to choose the principles (or rather terms of a contract) by which the good society should be organized. In other words a society whose 'social primary goods' are distributed equally. Social primary goods are the things that all rational individuals are presumed to want because they are useful whatever a person's rational plan of life. They include rights, powers, opportunities, wealth, income and self-respect (Rawls, 1971, p. 62). But in choosing the relevant principles, how do we make sure that we get the best possible deal for ourselves, i.e. the highest possible amount of the primary goods? The answer lies in the so called 'veil of ignorance' behind which all decisions must be made and as a consequence of which no-one knows anything about themselves – their status or class, fortune, level of natural ability, intelligence and the like. The reason for making choices 'in the dark' is that, without knowing in advance one's position in society we would – being rational and self-interested – select impartial principles that benefit everybody. To do otherwise, i.e. to suggest a 'selfish' set of principles that would disadvantage particular groups would be irrational given the risk that we might very well find ourselves in that very group we have chosen to discriminate against.

Rawls proposes two principles. First, we should choose a society in which there is the maximum individual freedom compatible with the freedom of others (1971, p. 60). Note that Rawls is concerned here with a set of basic liberties such as the right to vote, freedom of speech, assembly, thought and conscience, and so on. The second principle is based on equality and is two-pronged, covering equality of opportunity – positions within society should be open to all equally – and equality of distribution (Rawls, 1971, p. 60). Recognizing that in every society there are people of different abilities and that some inequalities (such as wealth) will benefit everyone, Rawls requires the benefits and burdens in society to be distributed in such a way that the position of the most disadvantaged is as good as it can be. In other words, whatever inequalities (whether social or economic) are countenanced they should result in those at the bottom of society, i.e. the worst off, getting the best deal they can (Elliott and Quinn, 1998).

To illustrate how this aspect of Rawls's theory works, consider the following example (taken from Fletcher et al., 1995, p. 92). Two patients, one a surgeon, the other a waiter, require treatment for renal disease. The options are dialysis, which is effective but limits lifestyle, and a transplant, which almost guarantees that the patient can return to a normal life. But there is only one kidney available. Applying Rawls's theory, the surgeon should have the transplant, the reason being that with the better treatment she will be able to return to work and so will be able to benefit any person in society needing surgery. The resulting inequality – the waiter being treated with dialysis – is tolerated because it would be easier to find a replacement for him than it would be to replace the surgeon. And this will not affect the worst off as much as if the surgeon cannot continue to work.

Rawls's theory of justice is, of course, much more sophisticated and comprehensive than this very brief outline suggests. It has, however, been extensively criticized. An obvious problem is the artificiality of the veil of ignorance. How can meaningful and rational choices be made about social arrangements if the 'choosers' are stripped of everything – experiences, backgrounds, values, race and so forth – that make such choices possible in the first place? Secondly, what proof is there that liberty would be regarded by all societies as such an important principle? Might some not chose an authoritarian society or one in which Rawls's social primary goods are replaced by other desired goods? And, as Dworkin notes in Taking Rights Seriously (1977), principles chosen behind the veil of ignorance might no longer be followed once some individuals discovered that they were advantaged and so were able to enhance their own position at the expense of others. Is it thus the case that Rawls appears to view human beings as rather more perfect than they have in fact shown themselves to be?

Such objections do not, however, concern Robert Nozick (a former student of Rawls) who rejects one of Rawls's basic assumptions – that everyone's well-being in society depends upon social co-operation so that talents are pooled for everyone's benefit. Nozick is the best known defender of the **libertarian** theory of justice (see his influential text *Anarchy, State, and Utopia*, 1974). He, like other libertarians, generally believes that justice means respecting peoples' rights, in particular rights to property. Provided individuals have obtained their property in a just manner (i.e. through, for example, inheritance or just transfer) its distribution throughout society is just. As a consequence, individuals should not be forced to do anything unless it prevents harm to third parties, and certainly should not be made to redistribute wealth, even for health care. The state's role should therefore be limited to (1) protecting citizens from assault, theft and so forth; (2) providing those services that the free market has not produced; and (3) enforcing individual rights – such as to property – providing these have been justly obtained (Beauchamp and Childress, 1994).

In applying their theories to health care, libertarians would put the primary responsibility on individuals themselves, who should be able to freely choose what kind of arrangements suit them best, e.g. private health insurance or other health investments. Given that libertarians reject paternalistic interference and the idea that society is morally obliged to provide funds for health care (although they concede that special protection may be necessary for incompetent people such as children), it seems that they would not object to market forces facilitating the sale of kidneys. Note too that libertarians do not necessarily object to redistributing health care (although their preference is for a privately purchased scheme) providing the redistribution is contractually agreed to – in other words it has been freely chosen. (Nozick's theories have also of course been criticized – see, for example, Harris, 1997, chapter 20.)

PRACTICAL APPROACHES

In this section we will look briefly at some of the practical implications of the theories of justice outlined above.

Need

Providing health care to those who need it seems, at least initially, to be the simplest and most preferred way of allocating scarce resources. Not only does it reflect the commitments made in the Patient's Charter – that every citizen has the right to receive health care on the basis of clinical need – but it also corresponds with what many regard as the basic function of the National Health Service, namely to provide equal access to health care for those in equal need (Mason and McCall Smith, 1999, p. 290).

Yet despite frequent use of the term 'need' and widespread acceptance that it is a necessary criterion for the fair allocation of resources, its meaning is far from clear (Gillon, 1985). Thus if a very broad definition is adopted – for example, that a person can be said to need something if without it s/he will be harmed or detrimentally affected (Beauchamp and Childress, 1994, p. 329), then the term is so expansive that it becomes difficult to distinguish need from desire, demand or mere wants. Furthermore, as was noted earlier, just as perceptions of illness, health and disease (which are subjective concepts) vary from person to person and from time to time, so too are our perceptions of need culturally and socially determined. It is not surprising, then, that there has been little agreement to date on a set of consistent and objective principles that can be used to assess the basis of need (Newdick, 1995, p. 16).

Another difficulty is, as Baker points out, that there are two different models for the determination of need: the market conception of patient or consumer demand and the professional conception of expert-determined health-care need (Baker, 1995, p. 62). If the patient-led model is adopted, then whatever patients demand and believe they have a legitimate right to claim – be it cosmetic surgery, counselling or infertility treatment – can be construed as an unmet need if it is not satisfied. But nor is the professional conception of need any more precise, not least because as new treatments, services, knowledge and technology become available so do 'expert' perceptions of need change (and invariably expand).

It is also worth pointing out that the task of defining need is made no easier if, as some suggest, the State's role should be limited to satisfying peoples' basic health needs, since this raises the question as to what counts as basic (Beauchamp and Childress, 1994). Few would accept that only life-threatening conditions should be included, but where would the line be drawn? In particular, would it inevitably include treatment for conditions – say, hip replacements – that, while not life-threatening, are nevertheless life-enhancing? And finally, perhaps one of the biggest problems of all with a needs-based approach is noted by Gillon (1985, p. 96): what happens when there are too many 'needy' patients chasing the same scarce resource? How should choices be made between these competing patients (who are agreed to be in need). Who, in other words, should get priority? This is a question which brings us back almost to where we began.

Outcome

An alternative but nevertheless related approach is to look at the outcome of treatment, in particular to allocate resources according to the probability of medical success (Gillon, 1985, p. 96). Note that medical benefit is sometimes treated as a separate criterion but is often combined with need – in the sense that patients can plausibly be said only to need treatment if it will benefit them. But what do we mean by outcome?

'Outcomes' were initially defined in limited terms to include mortality, complication and readmission. Now, however, the concept is more broadly defined to include such quality of life measures as emotional health, social interaction, degree of stability and so on (Ranade, 1994). Increased emphasis is also now being placed on obtaining the views of patients themselves. 'Outcome', therefore, is clearly a value-laden and relative term that cannot be objectively defined.

Similar conceptual problems plague the phrase 'medical success'. How do we determine it? What criteria are appropriate and how is success to be measured? As Newdick notes (1995), there is really no objective way of determining the effectiveness of treatment given the different perceptions people have of illness and health. But even supposing there was agreement on the appropriate criteria for measuring success, there are other problems. If treatment is only palliative should it nevertheless be considered to be successful?

Relevant also is the issue of cost and efficiency. This is particularly important when treatment is very expensive and can help just a minority of patients. In such cases, diverting funds from ITUs and organ transplants, for example, to cheaper treatments (or even preventive measures) that could potentially benefit far more people may seem to be a much fairer way of allocating scarce resources.

Maximization of welfare

One utilitarian solution that claims to overcome at least some of the difficulties outlined above has been developed by health economists. It is utilitarian because it seeks to produce the greatest amount of a particular benefit that it values. Often described as 'scientific', the concept of quality-adjusted life years (QALYs) adopts a cost–benefit analysis to the allocation of resources. This form of analysis brings together as many of the costs and benefits as possible and may include intangible things such as the value of improvement in health (Downie and Calman, 1994).

Developed by Alan Williams in 1985, QALYs aim to calculate the most efficient use of resources – that which will most improve the quality of people's lives over the longest period of time. Very crudely (for a more detailed analysis see Newdick 1995), the QALY principle is that a year of healthy life expectancy scores 1 and a year of unhealthy life is taken as less than 1, its value diminishing as quality of life decreases in the unhealthy. The QALY principle compares the cost (in financial and other terms) of different treatments, procedures and health 'problems'. For example, the cost of achieving one QALY for renal dialysis might be equal to 19 hip replacements or 190 preventive advice sessions on smoking by GPs (Ranade, 1994, p. 41).

Questions typically asked in assessing health benefits include: How much does a particular treatment cost? For how long and to what extent will it improve the quality of a patients life? Note that benefits are defined as improvements in life expectancy adjusted for changes in four key indicators of quality of life: physical mobility, capacity for self-care, freedom from pain and distress, and social adjustment (Ranade, 1994).

Patients who score well on the so-called healthy–death scale are those who are the cheapest to treat and who will achieve the best quality of life over the longest period of time (i.e. the cost per QALY is low). In contrast, patients who are expensive to treat and whose life expectancy is short or whose quality of life is not likely to increase significantly score low marks on the scale (i.e. the cost per QALY will be high).

Questions of cost and efficiency are therefore central to the QALY approach, which many welcome, not least because they encourage open discussion on what are undoubtedly very relevant factors in any rationing debate. But the approach has been extensively criticized (almost every text on nursing and medical ethics discusses QALYs in detail but see in particular Seedhouse, 1988 and Singleton and McLaren, 1995). The most common criticisms and moral arguments against QALYs are as follows.

- As QALYs are based on utilitarian calculations of benefit, some individuals/ groups – such as the elderly (whose life expectancy is short), wheelchair-bound patients (whose mobility would not improve after treatment) and those whose treatment is very expensive – will automatically be discriminated against (Mason and McCall Smith, 1999).
- The criteria chosen to measure quality of life are not only far from scientific (because they contain a large subjective component) but are also excessively narrow in that they assume that the only purpose of health care is to maximize health (which is largely defined in quantitative terms), thus ignoring, for example, non-health factors that may nevertheless significantly affect a person's life. Note too that, because health is a complex concept, it can mean different things to different individuals. Hence a disabled person may not necessarily view himself or herself as less healthy (Singleton and McLaren, 1995).
- By focusing on the end-point of treatment QALYs neglect the proportional loss or gain in a person's quality of life. QALYs also assume that it is possible to be certain about the outcomes of treatment – that we know how long people live (Seedhouse, 1988).
- The use of QALYs imposes the subjective values of others on an individual's life plan. In other words they fail to take into account who is experiencing them. As Mason and McCall Smith note: 'It is hard for a middle class doctor not to see a middle class life as being of higher quality than one sustained on social security' (1999, p. 303).
- QALYs implicitly assume that some people's lives are less worthy than others – in the sense that those with a poor quality of life are regarded as less entitled to health care.

It seems clear then all the criteria that have been outlined are problematic in one way or another. This is perhaps why Edwards suggests (1996, p. 114) that the most pragmatic approach to limited resources is the following: as a general rule resources should go to those who need them, but where this is not possible, other sorts of consideration should be taken into account. So, needing a health-care resource 'marks one as a possible candidate for the receipt of resources, and then other criteria may be brought in to play in the assessment of one's claim'.

A similar 'mixed' approach that focuses on need has also been proposed by others. Campbell *et al.*, for example, suggest that a basic framework for a just system of health-care provision should consist of several core principles. These include:

- accepting that the only basis for discrimination is the degree of need for health care;
- in trying to put different needs into some order of priority, paying particular attention to the disadvantaged, since their liberty to improve their own health is likely to be most limited;
- when society has decided that a health-care need should be met, all those with that need should be treated equally;
- a minimum entitlement to health care should be defined and applied without discrimination (1997, p. 193).

Whether such frameworks would lead to a fairer distribution of resources in practice is, of course, another matter. Nevertheless they are arguably likely to be more just than a system that relies on the random selection of patients (sometimes referred to as a lottery, or the first-come, first-served method (Mason and McCall Smith, 1999, pp. 305–307)). These latter options may have the advantage of being apparently more objective but in failing to take account of the patient's condition or medical benefit they are unlikely to be widely accepted.

RESOURCES AND THE LAW

This section will look mainly at the law's role in guaranteeing access to health care but it will begin with a brief account of its impact on health promotion and the control and prevention of disease.

Health promotion and disease prevention

The European Social Charter of 1961, to which the UK is a signatory, imposes several health related obligations, notably:

- to remove as far as possible the causes of ill-health;
- to provide advisory and educational facilities for the promotion of health and the encouragement of individual responsibility in matters of health;
- to prevent as far as possible epidemic, endemic and other diseases.

Well before 1961, however, public health measures to control the spread of infectious diseases had been in place. In fact the current law – which is largely to be found in the Public Health (Control of Disease) Act 1984 – has its roots in the 19th century. Under the 1984 Act public health officials have extensive powers of compulsory medical examination, removal to hospital and detention in hospital. These measures are designed to control the spread of infectious diseases (in the Act these are referred to as notifiable diseases and include cholera, plague, smallpox, typhus and relapsing fever, among others). Although these provisions also apply to AIDS, duties of notification in this case are governed by the AIDS (Control) Act 1987.

In addition to these 'control' powers there are a range of other provisions in the Act that can be used to exclude people with notifiable diseases from certain public places and prevent them from working. Criminal offences can also be committed by those who knowingly expose others to risk of infection (these provisions do not apply to AIDS). Taken together these powers are very draconian (for a more detailed account see Montgomery, 1997, Ch. 2). They are also controversial, not least because although they are designed to promote the welfare of society and protect the public they can nevertheless significantly limit the autonomy and civil rights of infected people. Furthermore their deterrent effect and their ability to control behaviour and protect potential 'victims' is difficult to assess. Other 'control' measures include the duty imposed on doctors to provide appropriate authorities with details of those with notifiable diseases or food poisoning.

Also relevant in this context are several statutes that are concerned with limiting environmental damage. These include measures to ensure that water is 'wholesome', air is 'clean' and pollution is 'controlled'. Another preventive measure that has been widely adopted despite libertarian objections that it denies people the 'right to be ill' (or rather the right to have tooth decay) is fluoridation. But even though fluoridation is undoubtedly paternalistic it is usually defended on the grounds that it promotes the general public good. Less easy to defend perhaps, at least in civil liberty terms, are the compulsory care provisions of the National Assistance Acts under which certain people – those who might well be competent but because they are 'suffering from grave chronic disease' or, being 'aged, infirm, or physically incapacitated', are living in insanitary conditions and are unable 'to devote to themselves proper care and attention' (and are not receiving it from others) – can be removed to hospital against their will. Since these provisions do little to protect elderly, disabled or vulnerable people from abuse or neglect their legitimacy can at the very least be questioned and reforms proposed by the Law Commission in 1995 have generally been welcomed.

Finally it is worth noting briefly the law's contribution (whether indirectly through taxation or otherwise) to the promotion of 'healthy' lifestyles. For example, not only are tobacco and alcohol heavily taxed but the sale, advertising and consumption of certain harmful products and substances (such as cigarettes) are restricted and controlled (in part to protect children). Other harmful products, may be temporarily banned (such as certain cuts of beef during the BSE crisis), and legislation such as the Misuse of Drugs Act 1971 seeks to control the use of illicit drugs. Doctors are also required to counsel patients about the significance of diet, exercise, tobacco, alcohol and the misuse of drugs and solvents.

Access to health services – is there a right to health care?

Central to the debate about access to health care is the notion of a right to health. But, as Ridley points out (1998, p. 243), a right entails an obligation. In other words, to say that someone has a right to health means that someone else has an obligation to provide it. This section therefore begins by looking at what rights people can claim to have in the health sphere.

Several sources strongly suggest that such rights do exist. One is the World Health Organization, which was established in the aftermath of the Second World War. As was noted earlier, it defines health so broadly that few if any governments could ever have the resources to achieve it. The WHO's commitment to human rights in health care was reinforced in 1995 with the publication of the document *Promotion of the Rights of Patients in Europe*, in which it affirmed that 'everyone has the right to such protection of health as is afforded by appropriate measures for disease prevention and health care, and to the opportunity to pursue his or her own highest attainable level of health'. Another source is article 2 of the European Convention of Human Rights (now incorporated in the Human Rights Act 1998), which states that 'everyone's right to life shall be protected in law. No one shall be deprived of his life intentionally...'. In addition, article 25 of the Universal Declaration of Human Rights asserts that: 'everyone has the right to a standard of living adequate for health and well-being of himself and his family, including food, clothing, housing and medical care and necessary social services....'

Treating rights to health care as basic human rights is very persuasive but raises important questions as to how attainable these rights actually are in practice, especially as the courts are very unlikely to recognize a legal right to health care if that means telling health authorities how to assess priorities and allocate scarce resources.

Before looking at the case law, however, we need to look at the legal framework of the NHS, which was established in 1946. The law is now contained in the National Health Service Act 1977, which imposes on the Secretary of State a broad general duty to continue the promotion in England and Wales of a comprehensive health service to secure improvement (1) in the physical and mental health of the people of those countries and (2) in the prevention, diagnosis and treatment of illness' (s. 1). Furthermore, services must be provided 'free of charge' unless the law expressly allows charges to be made (for example, for treatment following road accidents). Other sections impose more detailed duties, in particular to provide hospital accommodation, medical, dental, nursing and ambulance services, and facilities for the care of expectant and nursing mothers and young children; the prevention of illness and care (and aftercare) of those who are or have been ill (s. 3); the medical and dental examination and treatment of state school children; and family planning services (s. 5).

While the duties contained in the Act seem fairly comprehensive, almost all of them are qualified in that they only have to be provided 'to the extent that the Secretary of State considers necessary to meet all reasonable requirements'. As such, those exercising them have considerable discretion in how they are implemented. Other statutes governing the provision of health-related services include the National Health Service and Community Care Act 1990 and the Chronically Sick and Disabled Persons Act 1970. But given the limited space available the extent to which a comprehensive health service is, in practice, provided under these various statutes will not be considered. Nor, for similar reasons, will the way in which the duties imposed by the National Health Service Act 1977 are carried out – such as by contracting out primary care services or establishing NHS Trusts (Fletcher and Buka, 1999).

We turn instead to consider the role of law in enforcing the duties imposed by the National Health Service Act 1977. Essentially that means looking at how aggrieved patients can use the law to gain access to health care. There are two types of legal action. One is judicial review. Patients are most likely to use this option to force a health service body to provide a particular service that has been denied. Alternatively it can be used to challenge how clinical priorities have been set. Either way, the claim is that the NHS has failed to perform its statutory duties and has acted irrationally or illegally, or that there were serious procedural irregularities. The second legal option is one based either on breach of statutory duty or common law negligence. In both the claim is for compensation – based on the allegation that a patient has suffered damage as a result of a failure to provide services. Rarely, however, do such claims succeed.

The classic case in R v. *Secretary of State for Social Services* ex p. *Hinks* (1980) 1 BLMR 93. It concerned four orthopaedic patients who alleged that they had waited far too long for hip-replacement surgery and certainly longer than was medically advisable. But their claim – that they had not been provided with a comprehensive health service, in particular with orthopaedic services as required under section 3 of the National Health Service Act 1977 – was rejected by the Court of Appeal. It held that the Act did not impose an absolute duty to provide health services irrespective of the government's economic policy. Instead, the Minister had a discretion in the allocation with which the court would only interfere if he had acted 'unreasonably' (which in that case he had not). As Lord Denning said:

> *It cannot be supposed that the Secretary of State has to provide all the latest equipment ... all the kidney machines which are asked for ... or heart transplants in every case where people would benefit from them ... it cannot be said that [he] has to provide everything that is asked for in the changed circumstances, which have come about. That includes the numerous pills that people take nowadays: it cannot be said that he has to provide all these free for everybody.*

A similar decision was reached in R v. *Central Birmingham HA* ex p. *Walker* (1987) 3 BLMR 32. Here a premature baby needing heart surgery had his operation postponed five times because of the nursing shortages in a neonatal intensive care unit. Even though beds did become available, these were repeatedly allocated to more urgent cases. But the Court of Appeal refused the mother's claim that the surgery should be carried out for much the same reason as in the Hinks case, namely that it would not substitute its own judgement for the judgement of those responsible for the allocation of resources (unless they had acted unreasonably, which again they had not).

In both the above cases the patients' lives were not in danger. This raises the question of whether a court would reach a different decision if a patient's health was in jeopardy. It seems not, at least not according to R v. *Central Birmingham HA* ex p. *Collier* (1988) 6 January (unreported). This case concerned a 4-year-old boy suffering from a hole in the heart who was said by the consultant to be 'in desperate need' of life-saving surgery and who would probably die without it. His operation had been postponed three times because of lack of intensive care beds. But yet again the court refused to order the health authority to carry out the operation as it decided that the relevant legal principles were no different from previous cases that sought to challenge the allocation of resources. In other words, patients facing death could not expect a court to interfere with a health authority's decision unless that authority had made a decision that no reasonable person or body would have made. As the judge, Stephen Brown LJ, said: '[T]he courts of this country cannot arrange the lists in the hospital ... and should not be asked to intervene'.

In recent years several other cases have also come to court that have indirectly been concerned with resource allocation as well as other issues, notably the appropriateness of treatment. In *Re J* [1992] 4 All ER 614, for example, the central issue was what life-saving treatment a 16-month-old baby should have. Following an accidental fall when he was 1 month old, J was profoundly handicapped, both mentally and physically. He was microcephalic and had a severe form of cerebral palsy, cortical blindness and severe epilepsy. His life expectation was uncertain but unquestionably short. J's mother wanted his life to be saved as long as possible, using all life-saving measures, but the consultant paediatrician considered such life-prolonging treatment to be futile and so, if J were to suffer a life-threatening event, he recommended that it would be appropriate to offer ordinary resuscitation with suction, physiotherapy and antibiotics, but not prolonged life support. The Court of Appeal rejected the mother's claim. In so doing it implicitly accepted that resource allocation formed a proper part of medical decision-making. As Balcombe LJ said:

> [M]aking an order which may have the effect of compelling a doctor or health authority to make available scarce resources ... to a particular child ... might require the health authority to put J on a ventilator in an intensive care unit, and thereby possibly to deny the benefit of those limited resources to a child who was much more likely than J to benefit from them.

Later he also noted:

> ... the sad fact of life is that health authorities may on occasion find that they have too few resources, either human or material or both, to treat all patients whom they would like to treat in the way in which they would like to treat them. It is then their duty to make choices.

Regrettably the court failed to make clear whether it would have ordered further treatment if resources had not been so limited. This raises the question as to whether the concept of futility is being used to disguise arbitrary rationing of resources (Mason and McCall Smith, 1999, p. 379).

The issue arose again in a case that attracted a great deal of publicity, not least because it was widely reported as one of the most explicit examples of rationing in the 'new' NHS. *R* v. *Cambridge HA* ex p. *B* [1995] 2 All ER 129 concerned a 10-year-old girl suffering from leukaemia with a life expectancy of about 2 months who had been refused a second bone marrow transplant and further chemotherapy (she had already had one transplant and two courses of chemotherapy) on the basis that 'no further treatment could usefully be administered'. But B's father sought other medical opinions, one of which suggested a more hopeful prognosis but this depended on further expensive treatment costing in all about £75 000.

The health authority refused to fund this treatment, claiming it was not in B's interests and was not an appropriate use of the authority's limited resources. B's father challenged this refusal and somewhat surprisingly (in the light of cases like Hinks, Walker and Collier) the authority was ordered by the High Court to reconsider its decision. But within 24 hours the Court of Appeal predictably overruled the High Court, repeating once again that the courts had no right to interfere with a health authority's funding decisions providing they were rational and fair. Of particular interest was the court's account of the pressures facing health authorities:

[I]t is common knowledge that health authorities of all kinds are constantly pressed to make ends meet. They cannot pay their nurses as much as they would like; they cannot provide all the treatments they would like; they cannot purchase all the extremely expensive medical equipment they would like; they cannot carry out all the research they would like; they cannot build all the hospitals and specialists units they would like.

Even more significant was the court's explicit reliance on utilitarian arguments as the moral basis for its decision. According to Sir Thomas Bingham: 'difficult and agonizing judgements have to be made as to how a limited resource is best allocated to the maximum advantage of the maximum number of patients. That is not a judgement which a court can make.'

In contrast to the court's utilitarianism, the physician who had been treating B since her illness was first diagnosed was more concerned with B's therapeutic needs, and in particular the very poor prospects of success and the suffering that B would undergo if she had further treatment (which the physician described as experimental). For her, then, it seemed that the cost of treatment (and the overall benefit to society of using the money on other patients) were of little relevance in considering B's moral claims to treatment.

Finally it is worth noting the decision in *A, D and G* v. *North West Lancashire HA* (1999) *Medical Law Monitor*, 8 September. The case concerned three patients who wanted gender reassignment treatment. They had been refused treatment because the health authority had made a policy decision to place such treatment low on its list of priorities, because it did not regard it as a procedure considered to be capable of providing any clinical gain to patients – it was in fact ranked as of a similar standing as cosmetic surgery, reversal of sterilization and homeopathy. The court held that the health authority had failed to take relevant considerations into account, in particular what treatment was appropriate for the condition or illness involved in transsexualism. Accordingly, the authority's policy was unlawful.

The health authority appealed but lost. The Court of Appeal, although accepting that rationing was inevitable and necessary, nevertheless agreed that the authority's policy was flawed. Furthermore, by refusing to deal with trans-sexualism as an illness – regarding it instead as a state of mind, which did not deserve medical treatment – the authority had unlawfully imposed almost a blanket policy of refusing treatment.

But despite the success of this case – which turns on its own special facts, notably the decision to refuse all treatment for an illness – it is only rarely, if ever, that patients will be able to enforce the legal duties contained in the National Health Service Act 1977 when treatment is denied. This is partly because the courts are reluctant to make orders they cannot supervise but also because of their unwillingness to be drawn into policy questions about the distribution of finite resources, which they have consistently regarded as questions for Parliament not the courts.

Failure to provide a statutory service may, nevertheless, lead to a private law action for compensation. If the claim is based on breach of statutory duty such a claim will rarely succeed. But a negligence action is more likely to be successful – even if resource constraints are mainly to blame – provided it can be shown that the plaintiff's injuries were caused by the failure of a health authority or NHS trust to carry out its functions properly. A good example of this type of case is *Bull* v. *Devon HA* [1993] 4 Med LR 117 (for details see Chapter 3), where the health authority's argument that they had provided the best maternity service they could given available funds was rejected by the court and it was found liable for the injuries suffered by Mrs Bull's son at birth.

CASE STUDY 5.1   CAROL'S LEGAL RIGHT TO TREATMENT – A DISCUSSION

(Refer to the scenario presented on page 118.)

In this case it is necessary to consider what principles justify refusing Carol a liver transplant and in particular whether she and Jim have been treated equally. From the standpoint of need there can be little doubt that Carol should receive a liver transplant, since without one she will almost certainly die in the very near future. But is need alone a sufficient criterion, given that the demand for liver transplants far exceeds supply and that there are almost certainly going to be other patients who are equally needy?

Arguably it could be deemed unfair not to consider other factors, in particular the potential medical benefit to Carol of a transplant. Will treatment improve Carol's quality of life and how long is she likely to live after a transplant? How much pain and suffering will she have to endure? And as a teenager does she have a stronger claim to health care than an older person? Hence a utilitarian might, for example, justify preferential treatment for Carol because of her potential future contributions to society.

A further complicating factor is whether Carol would continue to take drugs following treatment and if so how that would affect her long-term prognosis. In other words, would scarce resources be wasted on her? Some might consider her an 'undeserving' patient who has forfeited her right to treatment (likewise the attempted suicide, the drug addict who develops AIDS or the smoker with lung cancer, for example). And why should Jim have two transplants if his liver failure has been caused by excessive drinking?

Giving both Carol and Jim lower priority than other patients who have developed liver failure through no fault of their own (or even denying them transplants altogether) could be justified on several grounds. First, it might be considered that it is fair to hold people responsible for their own actions and decisions and to require them to acknowledge that they have a chronic disease by seeking effective treatment before it is too late. Secondly, effective transplant programmes require public support. This will be significantly reduced if patients with, for example, alcohol-related liver disease, are given equal treatment to children born with liver defects.

The issue of individual responsibility to avoid the need for health care is a controversial one. While many would defend the right to be unhealthy – a liberty that can be justified on both Kantian and utilitarian grounds – fewer would claim that the actions of those whose lifestyles or behaviour result in or contribute to their ill-health should be totally ignored, even though the Patient's Charter states that patients have a right to treatment irrespective of lifestyle. However, while it might seem unfair (and financially unwise in terms of the overall cost and efficiency) to ignore the effect of, say, smoking, drinking and drug use, especially if treatment is likely to be ineffective in the long term because of the patient's continued unhealthy 'habits', there are nevertheless several difficulties with such an approach.

One is the implicit assumption that individuals are wholly to blame for the self-inflicted conditions they suffer or unhealthy lifestyles they lead. But are they? According to Beauchamp and Childress(1994, pp 358–361), this is a crucial question because withholding health care from those who appear to take risks voluntarily can only be justified if they are fully autonomous, i.e. are aware of the risks and accept them. However, as they point out, individual risk-taking sometimes has genetic or sociocultural roots. Of relevance here too is the increasing evidence of the close link between poverty and ill-health, in particular that problems with smoking, drinking and diet occur more frequently in lower social groups (Newdick, 1995). The addictive nature of some conditions ought also to be a consideration, perhaps.

Given these contributing factors – which strongly suggest that at least some apparently voluntary actions are caused by factors outside the 'risk-takers' control – the notion that they should bear full responsibility for their self-harming behaviour becomes more difficult to defend. What too of the fact that some occupations are inherently more hazardous or stressful than others or that some activities are more dangerous? Again, to deny such individuals certain forms of treatment (or to expect them to pay for it) would require some very subtle and controversial judgements to be made (Fletcher *et al.*, 1995).

The second ethical objection to depriving the 'undeserving' of various forms of health care is based on the difficulty of accurately identifying the causes of ill-health. Unlike injuries caused by, say, rock climbing, the causes of many diseases or illnesses are much more difficult to establish. Moreover, they are likely not to have one single cause but several, including in particular genetic predisposition. Nor can environmental and social considerations be ignored. With so many potentially competing causes it is difficult to isolate any one as the primary cause – even with smoking-relating diseases, where a causal link has long been known. This is because, while some smokers will develop lung cancer, all do not. Similarly, some individuals develop lung cancer who have never smoked. Accordingly in some cases explanations may have to be sought from elsewhere – heredity, for example, or occupational factors.

Let us turn now to Carol's legal rights. It is again very unlikely that Carol's father would succeed in persuading a court to override a doctor's refusal to consider her for a liver transplant providing the decision was based on reasonable clinical grounds. This is because this case study is largely based on a recent Scottish fatal accident inquiry (the Scottish equivalent of an inquest) in which the mother complained that her 17-year-old daughter (who was admitted to hospital after experimenting with Ecstasy but died 3 weeks later) was denied a liver transplant because the doctor had made a moral judgement and was concerned about 'wasting a liver' on someone who had taken drugs. The inquiry exonerated the consultant surgeon – who was said to have acted with 'immense professionalism'. Other health-care staff were nevertheless criticized for not carrying out blood tests at a crucial time and for being influenced by the fact that the teenager had taken Ecstasy.

CASE STUDY 5.2	ARUNDHATI'S DIVISION OF TIME AND CARE – A DISCUSSION

(Refer to the scenario presented on page 118.)

This case study raises the question of nursing care and in particular the special knowledge and expertise of nurses in the rationing debate. Few health professionals know as much about or are as skilled in meeting patients' daily needs – be they physical, emotional or spiritual – as nurses. But nurses cannot achieve the impossible and be in two places at once. How then should Arundhati divide her time?

If Arundhati decided to divide her time and energy equally between David and William, i.e. to spend the same amount of time with each of them, she could claim that she had satisfied a widely recognized criterion of justice, namely that she had given them equal treatment. However, to do so might result in an unfair outcome. This is because there is a distinction between the claim to equal treatment and the claim that individuals should be treated as equals. The difference can be explained by another, more dramatic example. Suppose a nurse comes across a car accident. One victim has been very badly hurt and the other much less seriously. But she only has emergency medical supplies with her – which she decides to use exclusively on the most needy victim. As result she saves her life. The other victim is left in pain, however. By giving priority to the victim in most need it is certainly true both have not received equal treatment. Nevertheless, they have both been treated as equals because equal respect and concern has been shown to them. That is because both their lives have been regarded as of equal value and worth saving. If on the other hand they had received equal treatment, one of them might have died (see further Fletcher et al., 1995, pp. 86–88).

Applying this example to William and David, Arundhati would be justified in treating them differently. But how should she choose between them?

Who is the most needy – David, who is dying, or William, who has just been told of his cancer? Ranking their needs is far from easy. Arguably, David has the greatest need because he is facing death, but William has to be helped to come to terms not only with cancer but also with the amputation of his leg. His needs too are likely to last much longer than David's. Another complicating factor is the effect of the diagnosis and proposed treatment on William's parents, who may be unable to give their son the necessary support. But should the 'shortfall' be made up by Arundhati? Relevant too in assessing need is the pain and other physical and emotional effects of their illnesses.

If the criterion of need fails to provide many easy answers, perhaps Arundhati should consider who would most benefit from her time. As William is younger and has a chance of recovering it could be argued that he will derive the most medical benefit (society too could benefit from his potential future contribution to society). But against this must be considered the incalculable benefit to David of Arundhati's care during his last few months. Will her support help him to face death more easily? If the answer is yes it would be morally difficult to deny him her time.

It seems then that there are no simple answers to the dilemma Arundhati faces – the only consolation, perhaps, being that however she divides her time and whatever criteria she applies she will almost certainly be able to justify her action according to one or other principle of justice.

As far as the law is concerned the most appropriate action, if any, would be one based on negligence. Its chance of success is nonetheless remote because, as with all negligence claims, several elements would have to be proved. While there is no doubt that Arundhati owes William and David a duty of care, showing that it has been breached would be very difficult unless the standard of nursing care she provided fell below the standard that could reasonably be expected in such circumstances. Note, however, that a court is unlikely to accept a defence of pressure of work (even if it is caused by inadequate resources), since patients are entitled to receive a reasonable standard of care. Finally, of course, it would have to be proved that Arundhati's actions (i.e. her lack of nursing care) have caused William and David harm. This is yet another hurdle which would be very difficult, if not impossible to prove in practice.

LAW and *ETHICS* – a comparison

Comparing law and ethics in relation to the allocation of scarce resources is not an easy task. This is because at one level the idea of law has always been associated with justice – in the sense that achieving justice can be said to be the ultimate goal of the law. Indeed the whole of the law is said to be concerned with justice, not least because judges are appointed to do justice according to the law. In other words, whether they are administering civil or criminal law, their function is to serve the interests of justice (Raphael, 1994, p. 68). But justice is a much wider conception than law since it can apply whenever there is a set of rules, legal or non-legal. Nevertheless, when the idea of justice is used in the law it is a powerful reminder that the law has an ethical purpose and is at the very least expected to use ethical methods. How then do the principles of justice inform the legal framework that governs the provision of health care? Or to put it another way, what common concepts underpin both law and ethics in this context?

The first is the formal principle of justice: equality, i.e. that equals must be treated equally and unequals unequally. As we have seen, while this principle lacks any substantive content it is widely accepted and features in many theories of justice. It is also one of the founding principles of the NHS in so far as it was intended to provide a comprehensive health service irrespective of age, sex and occupation. The NHS is now governed by the National Health Service Act 1977, which, in imposing a wide range of duties on the Secretary of State, can be said to enshrine the principle of equality and give it legal force.

The concept of need is another common fundamental principle in that all the legislation governing the provision of health care – e.g. the National Health Service Act 1977, National Health Service and Community Care Act 1990 and the Health Act 1999 – seeks to ensure that access to health care is determined not by wealth, privilege or advantage but by need alone. That does not mean, of course, that the law will guarantee that everyone who 'needs' treatment will be able to enforce a claim through the courts. As we have seen the courts are in practice unlikely to do so because they will almost always accept clinical judgement and refuse to order any treatment that health professionals consider inappropriate. It seems then that the law – notably in cases like *Re J* [1992] and *R* v. *Cambridge HA* [1995] – appears to recognize the morality of medical utility: in other words, of denying treatment to those who will not benefit.

Sometimes, however, patients who could benefit from treatment are denied it. But it seems – from cases such as *Hinks, Walker* (1987), *Collier* (1988) and *A, D and G* v. *North West Lancashire HA* (1999) – that only exceptionally will the courts intervene and take a more active part in the rationing debate. Unless this changes, the law will increasingly be seen as a blunt tool – in other words, of little use to those who wish to enforce their rights to health care through the courts.

Of course, the fact that the courts tend to rubber-stamp how health authorities allocate resources and similarly rarely challenge the decisions made by health professionals about who (and how) to treat patients could signify that current practice is fair and just. This will not always automatically be the case, however. Take the QALY principle, for example. It is certainly arguable that to give it prominence in practice would not be lawful under the National Health Service Act 1977. This is because the NHS was set up to ensure that everybody in the country, irrespective of age, means, sex or occupation, should have equal opportunity to benefit from the best and most up-to-date medical and allied services available. But under the QALY principle entire areas of care might have to be excluded. Similarly the needs of certain individuals – the old, for example, or the disabled – would inevitably be given very low priority. Such a scenario would be wholly incompatible with the 1977 Act, which describes a broad range of services, some of which it is the duty of the Secretary of State to provide, others of which 'may' be provided. Nowhere, in other words, does the Act talk in terms of priorities.

With the dearth of case law on issues of rationing it is not, of course, possible to predict how the courts would react if the QALY principle was applied in practice and then questioned by an aggrieved patient who had been denied health care. Nor is it possible to anticipate the impact of the Human Rights Act 1998, which is not yet in force. In so far as it recognizes a right to life it may well be, however, that patients denied life-saving treatment might invoke it. Certainly such applications will be possible. Whether they will be successful is another matter, given that the courts seem currently willing to accept rationing under the guise of medical futility and so are likely to do so in the future.

REFERENCES

Baker, R. (1995) Rationing, rhetoric, and rationality. In: *Allocating Health Care Resources*, (eds J. M. Humber and R. Almeder), Humana Press, Totowa, NJ.

Beauchamp, T. L. and Childress, J. F. (1994) *Principles of Biomedical Ethics*, 4th edn, Oxford University Press, Oxford.

Brock, D. W. (1982) Utilitarianism. In: *Justice For All*, (eds T. Regan and D. Van De Veer), Rowman & Allanheld, Totowa, NJ.

Buchanan, A. (1997) Health care delivery and resource allocation. In: *Medical Ethics*, 2nd edn, (ed. R. Veatch), Jones & Bartlett, London.

Campbell, A., Charlesworth, M., Gillett, G. and Jones, G. (1997) *Medical Ethics*, 2nd edn, Oxford University Press, Oxford.

Caplan, A. L. (1997) The concepts of health, illness, and disease. In: *Medical Ethics*, 2nd edn, (ed. R. Veatch), Jones & Bartlett, London.

Daniels, N. (1985) *Just Health Care*, Cambridge University Press, Cambridge.

Dickenson, D. (1994) Nurse time as a scarce health care resource. In: *Ethical Issues in Nursing*, (ed. G. Hunt), Edward Arnold, London, pp. 207–217.

Dimond, B. C. (1995) *The Legal Aspects of Nursing*, 2nd edn, Prentice-Hall, Hemel Hempstead.

Downie, R. S. and Calman, K. C. (1994) *Healthy Respect*, 2nd edn, Oxford University Press, Oxford.

Dworkin, R. (1977) *Taking Rights Seriously*, Duckworth, London.

Edwards, S. D. (1996) *Nursing Ethics: A Principle-based Approach*, Macmillan, Basingstoke.

Elliott, C. and Quinn, F. (1998) *English Legal System*, 2nd edn, Addison Wesley Longman, Harlow.

Engelhardt, H. T. (1996) *The Foundations of Bioethics*, 2nd edn, Oxford University Press, Oxford.

Fletcher, L. and Buka, P. (1999) *A Legal Framework for Caring: An Introduction to Law and Ethics in Health Care*, Macmillan, Basingstoke.

Fletcher, N., Holt, J., Brazier, M. and Harris, J. (1995) *Ethics, Law and Nursing*, Manchester University Press, Manchester.

Gillon, R. (1985) *Philosophical Medical Ethics*, John Wiley, Chichester.

Greaves, D. and Upton, H. (eds) (1996) *Philosophical Problems in Health Care*, Avebury, Aldershot.

Harris, J. W. (1997) *Legal Philosophies*, 2nd edn, Butterworths, London.

Hendrick, J. (1998) Legal and ethical issues. In: *Textbook of Children's Nursing*, (eds T. Moules and J. Ramsay), Stanley Thornes, Cheltenham.

Kopelman, L. (1995) The injustice of age bias against children in allocating health care. In: *Allocating Health Care Resources*, (eds J. M. Humber and R. Almeder), Humana Press, Totowa, NJ.

Mason, J. K and McCall Smith, R. A. (1999) *Law and Medical Ethics*, 5th edn, Butterworths, London.

Montgomery, J. (1997) *Health Care Law*, Oxford University Press, Oxford.

Newdick, C. (1995) *Who Should We Treat?*, Clarendon Press, Oxford.

Nozick, R. (1974) *Anarchy, State, and Utopia*, Basic Books, New York.

Ranade, W (1994) *A Future for the NHS: Health Care in the 90s*, Longman, Harlow.

Raphael, D. D. (1994) *Moral Philosophy*, 2nd edn, Oxford University Press, Oxford.

Rawls, J. (1971) *Theory of Justice*, Oxford University Press, Oxford.

Riddall. J. G. (1999) *Jurisprudence*, 2nd edn, Butterworths, London.

Ridley, A. (1998) *Beginning Bioethics*, St Martin's Press, New York.

Ross, A. (1958) *On Law and Justice*, Stevens & Sons, London.

Seedhouse, D. (1988) *Ethics – the Heart of Health Care*, John Wiley, Chichester.

Singleton, J. and McLaren, S. (1995) *Ethical Foundations of Health Care: Responsibilities and Decision Making*, Mosby, London.

Solomon, R. and Murphy, M. C. (1990) *What is Justice? Classic and Contemporary Readings*, Oxford University Press, Oxford.

Veatch, R. and Fry, S. (1987) *Case Studies in Nursing Ethics*, J. B. Lippincott, London.

White, L. and Waithe, M. (1995) The ethics of health care rationing as a strategy of cost containment. In: *Allocating Health Care Resources*, (eds J. M. Humber and R. Almeder), Humana Press, Totowa, NJ.

FURTHER READING

Butler J. *Ethics of Health Care Rationing: Principles and Practices*, Cassell, London

Fairbairn, G. and Fairbairn, S. (1988) *Ethical Issues in Caring*, Avebury, Aldershot.

6 BIRTH AND ITS REGULATION

INTRODUCTION

The reproductive choices that are now available have made decisions – such as when to have children and in what circumstances – much more complex than they were only a few decades ago. Assisted reproduction, for example, offers the chance of parenthood to the infertile – believed to include approximately 10% of married couples (McLean, 1999, p. 26; Mason, 1998, p. 207) – as well as single people and those living in gay relationships. But the technology that has made this possible has not been universally welcomed, especially by those who want to preserve traditional family structures or who find the idea that everyone has the right to rear or have children however or whenever they choose morally objectionable.

There are, of course, opposing views that, while broadly supportive of the 'reproductive revolution', nevertheless acknowledge that it raises fundamental questions about the nature of the family and the concept of parenthood (see Liu, 1991 Ch. 4 for a useful summary of the moral arguments against artificial reproduction). The 'rights' of women to control their fertility (through sterilization and contraception, for example) are also relevant in this context.

This chapter will focus on abortion, surrogacy and the management of pregnancy and childbirth. These aspects of birth and its regulation have been chosen for the following reasons:

- **abortion** because it continues to arouse passionate debate even though the Abortion Act 1967, which liberalized abortion, was passed over 30 years ago;
- **surrogacy** because it touches on what many claim to be a basic human right, namely to found a family;
- **the management of pregnancy and childbirth** because they highlight the potential for conflict between the interests of the mother and those of her unborn child.

CASE STUDY 6.1   **DOES KATIE HAVE THE RIGHT TO REPRODUCE?**

Katie was sexually abused by her stepfather and ran away from home when she was 14. She spent several years on the streets and has a criminal record (for soliciting and theft). She was also a drug addict but since meeting Jack, whom she married 5 years ago, she has been 'clean'. Katie and Jack have always been very keen to have children but so far have been unsuccessful. They decide to seek infertility treatment. But Katie, who is 32, is refused IVF services. With no other option available Katie decides to ask her sister Mary to be a surrogate. Mary agrees and soon becomes pregnant (following 'DIY' insemination with Jack's sperm). As the pregnancy proceeds the relationship between the two sisters deteriorates. This is partly because Katie does not think that Mary is being careful enough about her diet – she loves soft cheeses (which carry a listeriosis risk). But even more worrying, she has started to smoke again despite promising Katie she would not while she was pregnant. She also has begun drinking heavily. Last week Mary, who is very near to term, confided in the midwife, Sharon, that she does not think she will be able to give up the baby.

Should Katie have been accepted for treatment? In other words, does she have a right to reproduce? What moral and legal aspects of surrogate motherhood are most relevant here; in particular, should Mary be obliged to give up her child and who would be its 'parents'? Can (and should) Mary be prevented from smoking and eating what she likes during the pregnancy?

CASE STUDY 6.2   CAN LUISA BE FORCED TO HAVE A CAESAREAN SECTION?

Luisa is 8½ months pregnant with her first child. The pregnancy has been going well but she has just been told that, because her baby is in breech position, a caesarean section is likely to be necessary. Luisa rejects this advice, as she has always wanted a 'natural' birth. Furthermore, her closest friend gave birth some years ago by vaginal breech despite being advised against it. Despite being fully informed of all the possible consequences both to her and her baby, Luisa remains adamant. She will not have a caesarean section. Her partner, Manjit, is, however, having second thoughts. He is not only worried about the baby but fears for Luisa's well-being. Fran, the midwife, is also very concerned since, although she wants to respect Luisa's wishes, she wonders whether in the interests of the baby she should be compelled to have a caesarean. A few hours ago Luisa's labour started but she is still refusing to change her mind.

Can she be forced to have a caesarean against her wishes? Does Manjit have any say?

ABORTION

More than 30 years after the Abortion Act 1967 became law, arguments about the rights and wrongs of abortion continue to rage (Mason, 1998, p. 107). This is perhaps not surprising, given the fundamentally different approaches towards abortion that contemporary ethical literature distinguishes (Szawarski, 1996, p. 37). Nor are attitudes to abortion likely to be less polarized in the future, despite Dworkin's attempt (1993) to identify common ground between the 'pro-life' and 'pro-choice' lobbies.

There are several reasons for the continuing debate. First, there are the questions that abortion raises about the moral and legal status of the fetus, the nature of personhood and when human life begins. Second, at the heart of the debate is the issue of the right to life – a claim that has generated an enormous amount of literature but little consensus. And third, advances in medical technology, better diagnostic procedures and more sophisticated antenatal genetic care enable much more to be known about the fetus than was possible in the past (McLean, 1999).

Because it is common to hear abortion discussed in terms of rights – of the fetus, the mother and other 'interested parties' (Clarke, 1990, p. 163) – a similar approach will be adopted here.

Fetal rights

Moral aspects

The right to life

The claim that the fetus has the same moral status as a human being and therefore the same right to life as any other human being has a long history in Judaeo-Christian thought. Expressed another way, the right to life claim means a right not be deliberately killed. It is based on the belief that life is divine and sacrosanct and thus that God alone has the authority both to give life and to take it away. This sanctity of life doctrine – which is essentially a religious notion – is usually summed up in the following way: It is wrong to kill innocent human beings; A human fetus is an innocent human being; Therefore it is wrong to kill a human fetus (Johnstone, 1989, p. 238).

It is the second premise of this argument that proponents of a more liberal view of abortion challenge. They claim that, even though the fetus is undeniably genetically human it does not have a right to life because it does not have the same status as a human being. This is because, unlike an adult, it lacks the characteristics that qualify it as a person. What is emphasized here, therefore, is the concept of a person – a term that is often used interchangeably with 'human being', suggesting that they both mean the same thing. But many philosophers are very careful to distinguish between them. Singer, for example, who claims that a person is not by definition a human being, has little doubt that a gorilla (which he describes as 'thinking intelligent being that has reason and reflection') is a 'nonhuman person' (Singer, 1995, p. 182). But the more pressing concern here is to identify the capacities that are normally associated with personhood, i.e. what it is to be a person. Or, as Harris puts it, identifying what it is that is so different about a person that justifies valuing such a creature above others (Harris, 1985, p. 14).

What is a person?

One of the most well-known definitions of personhood is that of John Locke, the 17th-century philosopher. For him its distinguishing features were a combination of rationality – which did not have to be of a very high order – and self-consciousness, which basically meant the awareness of one's own existence. Since then, of course, there have been many attempts to refine the concept, although most analyses suggests that persons are beings who possess higher mental capacities such as rationality and self-awareness. Thus for Harris a person will be 'any being capable of valuing its own existence' – a capacity that he describes as fairly low-level since it merely requires the ability to want to experience the future, or to not want to experience it, and the awareness of those wants (Harris, 1985, p. 18). Similarly, Warren (1997, p. 84) suggests that the following characteristics are central to the concept of personhood: sentience, emotionality, the capacity to communicate, self-awareness and moral agency (see also Tooley, 1972, p. 44).

But despite the many attempts to formulate precise criteria of personhood no agreement has been reached. This is perhaps not surprising in that, while we may all roughly agree that people are conscious beings who are capable of some degree of thought and some kind of emotional response and of having some sense of their own identity, we are much less likely to agree on that one special feature that is the essential ingredient of personhood (Glover, 1977, p. 122). Another difficulty is that it remains unclear why cognitive capacities should be considered more morally significant than biological characteristics unless, as seems plausible, these are the capacities that enable one to be a moral agent, i.e. someone who is responsible for his or her own actions, who can be held accountable, praised and blamed.

Given the difficulties associated with establishing what the term 'person' means, some have suggested an alternative criterion of moral status by which to distinguish those entities that have full moral rights, in particular the right to life, and those that have lesser rights or even none at all. Thus for some philosophers (such as Singer, 1995) it is not the higher mental capacities that are important but something more basic, namely sentience – in other words the capacity to feel pain or pleasure – that marks the point at which something acquires an independent moral status and so begins to matter. But how can we know for sure which living organisms are sentient and which are not? Furthermore, as Singer notes (1995, p. 208), if sentience is seen as a sufficient reason to grant a being a right to life then we will have to grant the same right to every vertebrate animal, since there is more evidence of a capacity to feel pain in a frog than there is in a fetus of 10 weeks gestation.

In conclusion, then, it seems that whatever criterion of moral status is chosen there are difficulties. But even if consensus could be reached another question would still need to be resolved, namely, when does life begin?

When does life begin?
Those who regard abortion as an absolute moral wrong, i.e. they adopt the most conservative position, generally consider conception (when sperm and ovum join together and form a zygote) to be the moment when life begins. It is at this time that the new human being receives its genetic code and also when, or so many Catholic theologians believe, ensoulment occurs, i.e. it is the moment at which the body is endowed with a soul (Mason, 1998, p. 109). But, as Singer notes (1995, p. 95), there is no moment of conception at all. Rather, conception is a process lasting in all about 24 hours.

This explains why some choose instead implantation of the fertilized egg as the moment when the embryo acquires moral status. Others attach significance to the time when fetal movement can first be felt by the mother. But since 'quickening' has little to do with fetal maturity (it depends largely on how active the fetus is), it too has been challenged as a measure of life (Brown *et al.*, 1992, p. 130). Nor is viability any more acceptable as a moral landmark because it is no more a 'natural' stage in the development of the fetus than quickening, in that it is determined by the state of medical science rather than gestational age. Thus, as Glover observes, it is absurd to say 'last year this fetus would not have been a person at this stage, but since they re-equipped the ICU, it is one' (Glover, 1977, p. 125).

Finally, what about birth itself as the beginning of human life? In the search for the 'moment' when life begins, birth has much to commend it, not least because it marks the time when the baby can first be seen and when it first becomes possible to interact with it, to ascribe it feelings and emotions and get a sense of its unique characteristics and personality. But while this is undeniably so, we still need to explain the moral significance of these developments. Isn't a fetus just before birth the same entity, i.e. one with all the same characteristics, features and so forth, as the baby once it is born? As Glover says (1977, p. 126), 'if we could see the fetus from outside the womb would we be so sure about the immense difference between the fetus/baby just before and just after birth?'

It seems, then, that every stage in the development of the fetus that is chosen as morally significant is problematic. This is perhaps why many now adopt what has been described as a gradualist position, i.e. one that recognizes that the fetus has intrinsic value but rejects the notion that it acquires human status at any specific point in time. Instead the fetus's humanity evolves over time. In other words, it has a kind of intermediate moral status. Consequently, as it matures so its moral worth increases until it reaches birth – at which time it acquires the same moral status as a person. As McHale *et al.* point out, this is a view that many British commentators share (1997, p. 705).

Alternatively we can avoid the problem of pinpointing the moment when life begins by adopting the potentiality argument.

A potential life?

Briefly, the basic idea behind the potentiality argument is that because the fetus has the potential for personhood or humanhood it has the right to life. In other words, even although the fetus is not a person now and is certainly unrecognizable as a human being – at least during the early stages of its development – it does have the potential, following conception, to develop characteristics such as rationality, self-consciousness and so on. As a consequence, it should have the same basic rights and protections as actual human beings, in particular the right not to be deliberately killed (see further on this approach Warren, 1993, p. 312; Ridley, 1998, p. 116).

What the potentiality argument requires us to do, therefore, is to value not the fetus itself but rather what it will develop into. Accordingly, we are expected to treat something that only has the potential to achieve a certain status – and therefore acquire certain rights – as if it had already acquired that status. But in no other context do we do that. We do not, for example, treat children of 6 as though they were 18 just because they may reach that age eventually, and so on. So why should we treat the fetus as if it was already a baby? Or, to take Harris's example even, though we will inevitably die that is no good reason for treating us now as if we were already dead (Harris, 1985, p. 11).

Another difficulty with the potentiality argument is that it is not only the fetus or fertilized egg that is potentially a human being. The unfertilized egg and the sperm are equally potentially new human beings (Harris, 1985, p. 11). Does this therefore mean that they should have the same moral status as persons – and thus the right to the same protection or at least the same right to fulfil their potential? There are, of course, other reasons for rejecting the potentiality argument (see, for instance, Steinbock, 1992, p. 59). Yet its emphasis on what the fetus may become is one that Marquis accepts. For him, abortion is seriously immoral because of its effect on the victim. This is because by being 'killed' one is deprived of all the experiences, activities and so forth that would otherwise have constituted one's future. In short, it deprives the fetus of 'a valuable future just like ours'. Hence it is *prima facie* wrong (Marquis, 1997).

Legal aspects

It has been established beyond doubt that English law does not recognize the fetus as a legal person. It is not, in short, a person in its own right. What this means is that it is only after birth, i.e. once a baby is born alive and has a separate existence from its mother, that any rights it might have acquired as a fetus crsytallize. This was made clear in *Re F* [1988] 2 All ER 193. The case concerned a 36-year-old women who had a history of mental health problems and drug abuse. The local authority became very anxious about the safety of her unborn child – the mother had left her flat and her whereabouts were unknown – and attempted to take wardship proceedings in respect of the fetus, which would, if successful, have required her to live in a specified place and attend hospital. The Court of Appeal rejected the application, mindful not just of the practical difficulties of enforcing such orders but also of their implications for the liberty and privacy of the mother. It therefore decided that until it was born and had an independent existence the fetus had no legal personality.

But despite the fetus's lack of legal status, some legal protection is given to it before birth. Thus if it is harmed *in utero* as a result of a criminal act committed against its mother the perpetrator can face criminal charges (providing the fetus is born alive). This was established in *A-G's Reference (No. 3 of 1994)* [1997] 3 All ER 936. And, as we shall also see below under the Congenital Disabilities (Civil Liability) Act 1976, a fetus injured *in utero* might also be able to sue in tort (see Mason, 1998, Ch. 6 for an analysis of the legal protection of the fetus). Finally, it is worth noting that deliberate non-treatment of a living abortus might result in manslaughter or murder charges (McHale, 1998, p. 192).

Maternal rights

Moral aspects

A right to choose
The slogan 'a women's right to choose' first came to prominence during the rise of the women's liberation movement in the 1970s. It was a popular slogan because it conveyed in simple terms the essence of what can broadly be called the feminist approach to abortion, namely that pregnancy is a 'uniquely female experience which must be controlled by the individual woman concerned ... free from the intrusion by third parties, including the state' (McHale, 1998, p. 704). Those who claim that a woman's right to control her own body is one of the most basic of human rights (and one to which the rights of the fetus must normally be subordinate) typically appeal to a variety of 'rights' to support their approach.
These are:

- a right to self-defence;
- autonomy;
- ownership; and
- consequentialist arguments.

A right to self-defence
This maintains that a woman is entitled to defend herself against an intruder who threatens her in some way (Davies, 1998, p. 268). The self-defence argument is most often invoked when the pregnancy threatens the mother's life, i.e. she would die unless the pregnancy was terminated. In this kind of situation, no-one, except perhaps an ultraconservative, would deny that the mother's right to life comes first and overrides any right the fetus may have not to be deliberately killed. Similarly the right of self-defence is invoked when the pregnancy was non-consensual (if the mother was raped, for example) or if during the pregnancy she is diagnosed as suffering from a progressive debilitating disease, which the pregnancy will aggravate (Rumbold, 1999, p. 113).

But in cases where the risk to the mother's physical or mental health is less serious, the self-defence argument becomes harder to justify, especially if the reason for the abortion is the inconvenience of an unwanted pregnancy or some other minor or vague threat to the mother's health or well-being (Mason, 1998, p. 123).

Autonomy
In their most extreme form, autonomy arguments assert that a woman's right to self-determination, liberty and bodily integrity means that she should be able to decide not to continue with a pregnancy at whatever stage in the pregnancy and for whatever reason. Thus the termination might be sought to maintain current lifestyle or economic stability, not to interrupt career plans, and so on. But, as Warren points out, it is one thing to have a right and another to be morally

justified in exercising that right (1993, p. 306). This raises the question as to whether autonomy-based arguments can ever support abortion on demand, especially if the reasons seem trivial.

Ownership

A variant on autonomy is based on the notion that women have rights to ownership of their bodies. It is a view that is often associated with the American philosopher Judith Jarvis Thomson. In her seminal article 'A Defense of Abortion' (1971) she claimed that since a woman 'owns' her body she has the right to reject any 'occupant' she is unwilling to shelter. It is only, therefore, if a woman has accepted special responsibility for a fetus – by, for example, not trying to prevent its existence – that she is morally obliged to continue with the pregnancy. If on the other hand the woman has used all reasonable contraceptive precautions, then she cannot be assumed to have accepted responsibility for the unwelcome fetus who accordingly has no right of occupation!

Thomson's arguments are, of course, much more subtle and complex than this and have generated much debate and criticism. Glover, for example (1977, p. 134), objects to her central assumption that we only owe duties towards those for whom we have voluntarily assumed a special responsibility. He contends that it is not plausible to maintain such a sharp distinction between people to whom we owe moral duties and those to whom we may or may not be chari-table (see also Stauch et al., 1998, p. 410; Ridley, 1998, p. 140). But irrespective of the merits of Thomson's argument there is arguably a more compelling justifi-cation for liberal abortion laws, namely the consequences of too restrictive a regime.

Consequentialist arguments

As Warren notes (1993, p. 303), there is ample evidence throughout history that without access to safe, effective and accessible abortions women will resort to backstreet abortionists (almost always unqualified) or folk remedies. Either way they put their health at risk and some will die. Nor are the consequences of forcing women to continue with unwanted pregnancies any more acceptable. Not only will they have too many children too often – thus facing the risks of pregnancy and the perils of childbirth – but their choices following birth may be very limited.

Legal aspects

Women's rights under the Abortion Act 1967

It is a mistake to assume that women have any legal right under the Abortion Act since it does not entitle them to demand an abortion, even during the earliest stages of pregnancy. Instead it gives doctors the right to decide whether a woman's particular circumstances meet the terms for an abortion specified in the Act (Clarke, 1990, p. 163). But before outlining the Act's provisions it is worth noting that sections 58 and 59 of the Offences Against the Person Act

1861, despite being well over 100 years old, are still the basis of the law of abortion, as the Abortion Act 1967 did not repeal the 1861 Act but rather provided that in certain circumstances abortion would be lawful.

The 1967 Act states that abortions are lawful provided they are carried out by a registered medical practitioner – a term that includes nursing staff acting under the directions of such a doctor (i.e. one who has overall responsibility) after two registered medical practitioners have decided in good faith that one or more of the grounds specified in the Abortion Act apply. These can be summarized as follows (for further detail see Davies, 1998, pp 276–279).

- **The social ground** – to avoid adverse effects, albeit relatively minor ones, to the woman's physical or mental health or that of her family. Note that abortions in this category (which accounts for roughly 95% of all abortions) can only be performed if the pregnancy has not exceeded its 24th week.
- **The preventive ground** – to prevent grave permanent injury to the physical or mental health of the pregnant woman. There is no definition in the Act of the word 'permanent'.
- **The life-saving ground** – this ground is very limited as there has to be a risk of death before it can be invoked.
- **The eugenic ground** (or **fetal disability ground**) – to prevent the birth of 'seriously handicapped' infants. It seems that this ground can be used irrespective of when the 'handicap' will occur, i.e. at birth, during childhood or later in adult life.

The Act also specifies that, except in emergencies, i.e. 'when a termination is immediately necessary to save the woman's life or prevent grave permanent injury to her physical or mental health', abortions must be carried out in NHS hospitals or other licensed places (e.g. private clinics). In emergencies too the requirement to get the opinion of a second doctor is relaxed.

Paternal rights

Moral aspects
Little has been written about the moral claims of fathers (or 'putative fathers' as they are usually called) in the abortion debate. Yet if it is accepted that both women and men have a legitimate interest in procreation it is at least arguable that a father should have some right to intervene in respect of a fetus that has half his genetic make-up and may well have been willingly conceived.

But even supposing a set of father's rights could be agreed, how could they be enforced? In other words if men and women were to have a say, how could their conflicting claims be reconciled? Supposing, for example, a father opposed an abortion that his partner wanted? Should (or could) she be forced to continue with the pregnancy? Nor would the reverse scenario be any easier to resolve, i.e. when the woman wanted to give birth but the father wanted her to have an abortion. Nevertheless, to deny fathers any rights whatsoever does seem, at the very least, questionable. As Mason has noted (1998, p. 127):

[T]here is a world of difference between on the one hand, grave danger to a woman's health and, on the other, some of the relatively trivial conditions which will satisfy the conditions of the Abortion Act 1967. It is suggested that more consideration might well be given to the hurt done to a man whose fatherhood is denied in the latter circumstances.

Legal aspects

There have been a steady trickle of cases in the English courts where fathers – it makes no difference whether they are married or not – have attempted to prevent an abortion. None of these has been successful.

The first of these, for example, was *Paton* v. *British Pregnancy Advisory Service* [1978] QB 276. A father who failed to get an injunction went to the European Commission of Human Rights to argue his case. But he lost there too as the Commission held that, even though the fetus enjoyed a qualified right to life, that right was subordinate to the mother's health and welfare (*Paton* v. *UK* (1981) 3 EHRR 408). More recently, in *Kelly* v. *Kelly* [1997] 2 FLR 828, a father claimed that the fetus was a legal person whom he was entitled to represent in order to prevent a legal wrong (the abortion) being committed. Not surprisingly the father's claim failed, with the court reiterating again that the fetus was not a legal person until birth. As a consequence, the father had no claim on behalf of the fetus (see also *C* v. *S* [1988] QB 135).

From these cases it is now clear that English law (like most other jurisdictions) gives fathers no rights to challenge or veto an abortion. Nor do they have the right to be consulted or informed that an abortion is to be performed.

Third party rights – nurses

Moral aspects

As is well known, abortion is one procedure to which many nurses hold a conscientious objection. A nurse who refuses to participate in carrying out an abortion will usually justify her decision by claiming that she is following her conscience. But what does having a conscience mean?

In simple terms it involves being conscious of the moral quality of what one has done or intends to do. In the Christian tradition, conscience can be viewed as 'the voice of God within' each of us (Routledge, 2000, p. 167). Similarly, Beauchamp and Childress describe conscience (1989, p. 387) as 'a form of self reflection on one's acts and their rightness or wrongness, goodness and badness'.

As a guide to moral actions, however, conscience has its limitations, not least because, without knowing the convictions and principles upon which it is based, it is ultimately just an empty concept. Or, to put it another way, conscience alone cannot tell us what is right or wrong. Furthermore, a nurse who uses conscience to guide her decision-making in relation to abortion may find not only that she compromises her career but that she may also be accused of acting unprofessionally – by increasing the workload of other health professionals, for example, or failing to respect the autonomy of patients (Rumbold, 1999, p. 250).

That said, the right to make a conscientious objection is recognized in clause 8 of the UKCC Code of Professional Conduct (UKCC, 1992). Subsequent guidelines (UKCC, 1996) also make it clear that except in emergencies – when nurses would be expected to provide care – those who do not wish to carry out treatment or care because of personal morality or religious beliefs should declare their objection soon after taking up employment in time for managers to make alternative arrangements. Interestingly the guidelines conclude the section on conscientious objection with a reminder that refusing to be involved in the care of patients because of their condition or behaviour is unacceptable (clause 49).

Note too guidance from the Royal College of Midwives Ethics Committee, which states how and when conscientious objection should be raised (RCM, 1996). It also discusses what amounts to 'participation in treatment' and states that the conscience clause 'solely covers being involved in the immediate preoperative and operative care of women, as well as caring for women during induction of labour, and that [it] is morally unacceptable to refuse to care for women at any other time' (RCM, 1996, p. 4). How this guidance is interpreted in practice, however, will vary from one NHS trust to another.

Legal aspects

According to Lord Denning, nurses are expected to be mobile throughout the hospital system (*Royal College of Nursing of the United Kingdom* v. *Department of Health and Social Security* [1981] AC 800). In the light of this expectation and bearing in mind the increasing use of modern non-surgical methods of inducing abortion such as prostaglandins (in which nurses are much more likely to be involved), the extent to which the law recognizes rights of conscience is an important concern. According to section 4 of the Abortion Act 1967, no person is legally obliged to participate in any treatment authorized by the Act to which they have a conscientious objection. In emergencies, however, i.e. when the life of the pregnant woman is at stake or she faces grave permanent injury, the exemption does not apply.

At one time there was some uncertainty as to the meaning of the word 'participate' but this was clarified in *Janaway* v. *Salford AHA* [1989] AC 537. The case concerned a doctor's receptionist (a devout Roman Catholic) who refused to type a letter of referral for an abortion, claiming that she was covered by section 4. As a consequence, she was dismissed from her job at a health centre. Her claim was rejected on the basis that the word 'participate' was not intended to be interpreted too broadly but was limited to its ordinary and natural meaning. In other words, to be able to rely on section 4 a person had to be actually taking part in treatment – which did not extend to writing letters.

SURROGACY

Although surrogacy has an ancient history going back to biblical times it is only relatively recently that the practice has caused so much controversy (Freeman, 1999, p. 1). Much of the hostility provoked by surrogacy, the incidence of which it is almost impossible to gauge (Morgan, 1990, p. 66), can be explained by the commercialization of the practice whereby the surrogate (and possibly a third party) receives some financial benefit from the arrangement. Given that surrogacy is now often combined with artificial reproductive techniques it is also perhaps not surprising that it is attacked for being an 'unnatural' practice that threatens 'normal' marital relationships and undermines the family (Singer and Wells, 1984; Liu, 1991, Chs 4 and 6). Yet it is arguably because surrogacy challenges traditional assumptions about the institution of motherhood and the role of women that it arouses such moral indignation.

Before looking at some of the moral and legal aspects of surrogacy, however, we need to define what surrogacy is.

Essentially surrogacy covers any situation in which a woman (the surrogate) agrees to bear a child for another. The intention behind all surrogacy arrangements is that the child should be handed over at birth to the 'commissioning parties', but they can take several different forms. In 'partial surrogacy' the surrogate mother is the child's genetic mother. But if the surrogacy is a 'full' or 'total' one (also known as womb-leasing), the commissioning couple provide the gametes, which are then fertilized *in vitro* and implanted in the surrogate. This method produces a child genetically related to the commissioning couple (for other less common variants of total surrogacy see Hendrick, 1997).

Moral aspects

One of the most compelling arguments in support of surrogacy is that it may be the only way some forms of infertility can be alleviated. If it is accepted that the inability to have a child can be a traumatic and destructive experience, it is difficult to justify denying infertile men and women what may be the only chance they have to reproduce or found a family. This is so irrespective of whether or not the desire to be a parent is biologically driven or is caused by social pressures (or is a combination of both; Chadwick, 1987, p. 13). That infertility may be socially determined is a perspective that McLean takes up when she looks at infertility as a social construct, i.e. one that is intimately bound up with our perceptions of women and what it is to be female, or a 'real' woman (McLean, 1999, p. 27).

Another persuasive moral argument in favour of surrogacy is based on the concept of autonomy. According to this view a woman's right of self-determination includes the right to use her body to have a baby for another. Surrogacy, in other words, is a legitimate reproductive choice that a woman is entitled to make as part of her life plan. As an expression of autonomy, surrogacy, whatever form it takes, should therefore not be prohibited.

The autonomy argument is of course rather more complex than is suggested here (Dodds and Jones, 1989). For one thing, we have to be sure that a women who decides to be a surrogate is really making an autonomous decision. And what of her right to keep the child she has borne? While this is clearly contrary to the whole idea of surrogacy, it is certainly arguable that it is one of the rights that a surrogate mother with a genetic link to a child can claim to possess.

Finally, it is worth pointing out that it is not uncommon for surrogacy to be defended on the basis that it is very similar to adoption (Liu, 1991, p. 98). While in some respects this may well be true, in that both may involve a child being brought up by a couple who are not genetically related to it, there are fundamental differences. One is that in adoption a child has already been born and adoption is deemed the best option for its welfare. In contrast, surrogacy involves the deliberate creation of a child. More importantly, modern adoption procedures ensure that the child's best interests are the paramount concern. As a consequence, prospective parents are rigorously vetted. In contrast, except in those cases where surrogacy is combined with artificial reproductive techniques – in which the child's welfare is only nominally taken into account – there is much less scrutiny of the commissioning couple.

Turning now to the main objections to surrogacy. For Freeman the most substantial argument against surrogacy is its detrimental effect on children. He contends (Freeman, 1989, p. 175) that, whether a child is born as a result of altruism (whereby a fertile sister 'gives' her infertile one a child) or the child's birth follows a commercial arrangement, a potential consequence is that children may come to be seen as commodities. In others words, they will treated like other consumer durables such as a TV or fridge, i.e. those that are essential for a family to be 'complete'.

The idea that surrogacy may turn babies into a market commodity purchasable if the price is right may seem a little far-fetched. Nor will everyone agree with Freeman's contention that surrogacy poses a threat to our notion of childhood and the ideal of children for which the children's rights movement strives (Freeman, 1989, p. 176). Nonetheless, it is clear that the spectre of baby-selling (or baby-buying) in which low-income baby breeders sell their gestational services (with or without the help of commercial agencies) has been one of the major obstacles to the acceptability of surrogacy as a solution to infertility. Indeed, evidence about comparative levels of income and education suggesting a significant disparity of bargaining power between surrogate and couple was one of the three particular factors highlighted in the surrogacy review (Department of Health, 1998; see also Brazier, 1999, p. 181). However, once a distinction is made between paying the surrogate reasonable compensation for her expenses during pregnancy (such as loss of earnings and so on) and paying her or an agency a fee (i.e. the profit element), fears about baby selling seem less compelling (Liu, 1991, p. 101). Nevertheless they can not be dismissed altogether, since any surrogacy arrangement that involves the payment of money may result in the surrogate feeling more pressurized to hand over a child she wants to keep than would have been the case had no money changed hands.

Other potential harms to surrogate children include the risk of the commissioning couple rejecting an 'imperfect' baby or the child being the subject of a traumatic dispute if the surrogate mother wants to keep the baby. Much has also been made of the psychological and emotional problems surrogate children may experience when finding out about their true identity, i.e. that parents who have brought them up are not their 'real' mother or father. They may also be confused about the circumstances of their conception and birth. Yet these problems may also be experienced by adopted children. This is not to say that they can therefore be ignored but rather that the needs of surrogate children can be anticipated and sensitively dealt by policies that are now well established in relation to adopted children, such as counselling before access to birth records and so on (Freeman, 1989, p. 176).

Another argument against surrogacy contends that it is inconsistent with human dignity because it degrades and dehumanizes women and treats them as breeding machines. Some would even go far as to say that it is like slavery in that a surrogacy arrangement will normally try and exert considerable control over the life of the surrogate (Freeman, 1989, p. 169). While this comparison can be easily dismissed – for example the surrogate can break the arrangement at any time and so is hardly subject to the kinds of restrictions that typically characterized slavery – it is certainly true that poor women are much more likely to be paid surrogates.

Does that mean then that surrogacy is inherently exploitative, i.e. that the surrogate is coerced (through poverty, unemployment and so on) into doing something (which many would claim is akin to prostitution, in so far as it involves women unwillingly selling their bodies for profit) that she would not otherwise do? Or is this a paternalistic approach that denies women the right to use their bodies as they wish? Whatever the answers to these questions and regardless of financial dimension it is certainly arguable that to the extent that surrogacy objectifies the surrogate it offends the Kantian principle that people should never be treated simply as means to an end but always at the same time as ends in themselves.

This at least was the philosophical position adopted by the Warnock Report in 1984 (Warnock, 1985), the findings of which formed the basis of the Surrogacy Arrangements Act 1985, to which we now turn (for further discussion of the risks and issues surrounding surrogacy see Department of Health, 1998, Ch. 4; Mason, 1998, Ch. 10; Mason and McCall Smith, 1999, Ch. 3).

Legal aspects

The Surrogacy Arrangements Act 1985

Almost all surrogacy arrangements come within the Surrogacy Arrangements Act 1985. Usually described as a panic measure, the Act was passed within a few months of the 'baby Cotton' case, which concerned an American couple who arranged a surrogacy in England through an American commercial agency. The agency was paid approximately £10 000, half of which went to the surrogate – which was hyped up by the media into a sordid tale of baby-selling and profit-making.

The Act does not make surrogacy in the UK illegal or unlawful but instead tries to discourage it. First, it makes surrogacy arrangements legally unenforceable. The effect of this is that the surrogate cannot be forced to give up the baby if she changes her mind and a court thinks it is in the baby's best interests for it to stay with her. Secondly, it criminalizes the commercial exploitation of surrogacy. This basically means outlawing commercial surrogacy agencies but not non-profit-making voluntary agencies. Payments made to the surrogate for e.g. loss of earnings or reasonable expenses are also lawful.

Put simply, paid surrogacy is not criminalized providing it is of the homespun type, i.e. no broker or agency gets a fee for arranging it. Accordingly, negotiating surrogacy arrangements on a commercial basis and several other related activities (e.g. advertising by or for a surrogate) are criminal offences.

Since the Act was passed, surrogacy has increasingly become an acceptable means of overcoming infertility (see, for example, BMA, 1996). It is perhaps not surprising, therefore, that the legal framework it set up is now in need of reform. Those suggested by the surrogacy review (Department of Health, 1998) focused on payments to surrogates, the regulation of surrogacy and new legislation to replace the 1985 Act (on which see Brazier, 1999 and Freeman, 1999).

PREGNANCY AND CHILDBIRTH

Several well published cases in the late 1990s involving pregnant women refusing to have caesareans have been interpreted by some commentators as convincing evidence that an ever-increasing number of women would rather sacrifice their unborn children than undergo treatment they do not want. In *Norfolk and Norwich Healthcare (NHS) Trust* v. *W* [1996] 2 FLR 613 and *Tameside and Glossop Acute Services Trust* v. *CH* [1996] 1 FLR 762, for example, the courts imposed caesarean sections on women against their will. But conflicts like these are rare, since the vast majority of women are willing to accept very significant risks, pain and inconvenience to give their babies the best chance possible. Indeed, as Steinbock says (reporting the words of an obstetrician), 'most women would cut off their heads to save their babies' (Steinbock, 1992, p. 147).

Yet because conflicts do sometimes arise it is worth examining the moral and legal issues they raise. As McLean notes, however, use of the word 'conflict' in this context is arguably inappropriate, in so far as it suggests a battle of sorts, yet there can be no conflict because there is only one person (McLean, 1999, p. 51). Also examined here is the question of whether women should be free to adopt whatever lifestyle they want during pregnancy – in other words, whether there is any justification for regulating behaviour that puts the fetus at risk. Finally, we examine the respective rights of fetuses and women during pregnancy and childbirth.

Moral aspects

Although there is now clear evidence of what is 'good' for a fetus, i.e. what will most promote its health and development, it is quite another thing to say that as a consequence a pregnant women has a moral duty to provide such an environment and so must avoid taking any risk that could compromise her child's future health. Yet if a pregnant woman neglects her own health by abusing drugs, smoking or drinking excessively, or ignores advice about diet – the potential hazards of which are now well-documented – then in so far as these risks are unnecessary and unreasonable it is at least arguable that taking them is morally wrong (Steinbock, 1992, p. 128). In so far too as pregnant women are now the legitimate targets of health promotion campaigns it seems clear that society accepts that the decision to have a baby brings with it certain moral obligations to the child who will be born.

But although the idea may be relatively uncontroversial that pregnant women have moral obligations to their fetuses – or at the very least the duty to consider the impact of their behaviour on the developing fetus – there is likely to be much less agreement about the precise scope of these moral obligations, in particular what sacrifices women must undergo 'for the sake of the baby'. Should they stop drinking and smoking and eat only 'healthy' foods as soon as they know they are pregnant or even before then when trying to conceive? Should they immediately give up any activity, even their current employment, just because it may, however remotely, endanger the fetus? To require mothers-to be to conform to such a high standard may be considered morally responsible yet given the contradictory advice pregnant women often receive, the uncertainty about what is 'safe' during pregnancy and variations in the quality of antenatal care and access to it, it is unlikely that an appropriate standard of care could ever be agreed, let alone enforced (Brazier, 1997, p. 273).

Ensuring that the fetus is safely delivered is arguably an altogether different issue, however, which raises several questions, in particular whether it is ever morally justifiable to force a women to have a caesarean or other invasive medical treatment against her wishes in the interests of the fetus. The main argument used to support such interventions is that a duty to care (and thus a duty to do all that is possible to promote the baby's safe delivery) arises because of the 'special relationship' between mother and child. In other words, just as pregnancy imposes moral obligations on mothers-to-be so does the voluntary act of continuing a pregnancy to term create special obligations over and above those that are normally expected. In particular, it means that a pregnant woman is morally and physically responsible for the life within her and so must do more than the minimum to promote its welfare, even if this entails submitting to medical procedures she would otherwise reject.

Yet despite the claim that pregnancy imposes a moral responsibility on the mother for the health and well-being of her fetus, there are nevertheless strong arguments that it is not morally wrong for a pregnant woman to refuse medical treatment at the time of birth. The strongest, or at least the most commonly used, is the value society places on autonomy – which in this context means the right to decide what medical treatment to accept or reject. It is assumed here, of course, that respecting a woman's refusal of treatment actually does uphold her autonomy. It is also assumed that autonomy is an absolute value and so does not have to be balanced against other important values, such as the life and health of the 'nearly born' fetus.

Second, doctors may be too alarmist and are also fallible. In short, doctors can get things wrong. Another argument is that although the risks associated with caesareans are very low they do nevertheless carry some risk to the mother and may result in lasting physical harm and sometimes, albeit rarely, death. Thus to impose such a risk on an 'unwilling' woman means that a different and much higher moral standard is expected of pregnant women. Moreover, forcing women to undergo major surgery, even relatively safe surgery, would in effect mean imposing on them a duty to rescue – which, as McLean points out (1999, p. 56), would not be imposed under any other circumstances on any other person.

Finally, however tempting it may be in individual cases to ignore a mother's refusal and use coercive measures, the more they are used the more it is likely – as the Royal College of Midwives points out (1996) – that pregnant women will be alienated. As a consequence they may well avoid developing any relationship with health professionals during pregnancy at all.

Legal aspects

The case of *Re F* [1988] outlined earlier, in which the court decided that a fetus could not have any rights of its own until it was born and had a separate existence from its mother, makes it clear that for the moment at least it is very unlikely that the civil law will be used to control the behaviour of pregnant women, however harmful it may be to the fetus.

As Brazier argues (1997, p. 275), there are sound reasons for not using tort law to enforce a moral responsibility on women for fetal welfare. One is that even if it was possible to identify a reasonable standard of prenatal conduct, enforcing such a standard would impose an unreasonable limitation on women's liberty and privacy and ability to lead a normal life, given the range of conduct that is potentially prejudicial to the health of the fetus. Another is that the ability of women to take care of themselves during pregnancy is very much determined by their social and personal circumstances. To impose the same standard on all women irrespective of the diversity of their lives would therefore not only be unreasonable but also unjust. Nor would jailing pregnant drug addicts – as has happened in America – be much more effective, in that it would neither benefit the health of their future children nor society itself (Steinbock, 1992, p. 141). It is more likely as Brazier points out (1997, p. 290) that, fearing criminal sanctions while addicted, they would not seek medical help.

Congenital Disabilities (Civil Liability) Act 1976

But despite the law's reluctance to regulate behaviour during pregnancy, a fetus can sue for certain prenatal injuries if it is born disabled. There are several categories of prenatal injury: the parents' reproductive capacity could have been damaged; the fetus could have been harmed *in utero* (by, say, drugs taken by the mother during pregnancy or negligent infertility treatment); or injuries could have occurred during childbirth itself. Claims for prenatal injuries brought on behalf of children will usually be made under the Congenital Disabilities (Civil Liability) Act 1976 (another option is the Consumer Protection Act 1987, but this only applies to injuries caused by defective drugs).

The 1976 Act is complex and has only rarely been successfully used. It does have implications for nurses and other health professionals, however, because if their negligence harms the fetus they may face a substantial compensation claim. Briefly, the Act's main provisions are as follows.

- It applies only to children born 'alive' (i.e. those that survive for at least 48 hours).
- Children's legal rights under the Act are derivative. In other words, children can only sue if a duty of care owed to either parent was breached.
- Liability generally does not arise if the parents knew of the risk of their child being born disabled.
- Mothers, but not fathers, are given extensive immunity, the legal effect of which is that they cannot be sued by their children even though they may have caused their disabilities (except when a child is born disabled as a result of its mother's negligent driving).

Another point worth noting is that, where a parent is partly to blame for a child's disabilities, compensation can be reduced. The Act retains the fault principle. As with all negligence claims, both these elements can in practice be almost insurmountable obstacles (see Chapter 3).

Claims for prenatal injuries under the 1976 Act are essentially claims that the defendant was responsible for the child's disabilities, i.e. the defendant's negligence caused the damage. A different kind of claim, albeit one that is also caused by a negligent act or omission, is one that asserts that, although the defendant's behaviour did not directly damage the fetus, it nevertheless resulted in a birth of a disabled child who would never otherwise have been conceived or, having been conceived, would not have been born alive. This kind of claim – in which the child is basically claiming that it would have been better off not to have been born at all – is called a '**wrongful life**' action. It is likely to arise out of negligent genetic counselling (either pre- or postconception) or prenatal screening and, less frequently, negligent infertility treatment. For example, *McKay* v. *Essex AHA* [1982] 2 All ER 771 concerned a child's claim that she was born partially blind and deaf as a result of the negligent testing of her mother's blood during pregnancy – the mother suspected that she had caught rubella but was told that neither she nor her baby had been infected. To date the courts have not allowed these claims, for the following reasons.

- To recognize a wrongful life action would, in effect, impose on doctors a duty to abort.
- Such a legal duty would compromise the value of human life by implicitly suggesting that a disabled child has the right to be born 'whole' or not at all. It would mean in effect that a court would be saying to the child: 'Yes, it would have been better had you not been born.'
- It would be impossible to assess the amount of damages because this would involve assessing the difference between the value of a life with disabilities and non-existence (see Mason and McCall Smith, 1999, pp. 160–166; Mason, 1998, p. 161–164).

An alternative claim that is recognized in English law is the 'wrongful birth' action. It arises out of exactly the same circumstances as the wrongful life claim, notably negligent prenatal screening and so forth, but is brought by parents. Thus in *Salih* v. *Enfield AHA* [1991] 3 All ER 400, the facts of which were very similar to the McKay case, compensation was awarded that included an amount for the additional cost of raising a disabled child over and above the cost of raising a healthy child. However, such claims can only succeed if the ordinary principles of breach of duty and causation are established. This perhaps explains why so few have been successful (for further discussion of wrongful life and wrongful birth claims, see Beaumont, 1996).

Birth plans and place and manner of birth

Birth plans are now commonplace but what is their legal effect? Briefly, a birth plan is a statement of a woman's wishes about labour, delivery and postnatal care and is usually agreed well before labour. It is thus not only an expression of her autonomy but is also a significant legal document, which in essence is an 'advance directive' in that it may contain refusals of treatment – such as for example, drugs for pain relief or episiotomy – as well as positive preferences about treatment during labour and delivery.

Whether a birth plan is legally binding depends on several factors. Thus the plan can only be valid in law if it is based on the woman's consent (see Chapter 2). But as with any other form of treatment it is most unlikely that the courts would force health professionals to provide treatment requested by the woman that is either unavailable or in their view contraindicated. Note too that any refusal of treatment would have to be respected whatever its consequence. In other words, if a competent woman refuses treatment then that refusal must be respected (an advance refusal of treatment by a woman under 18 can, however, be overruled).

As Harpwood has noted (1996, p. 113), birth plans are important in so far as they present a perfect opportunity to formalize informed consent. Yet there are disadvantages in introducing rigid birth plans, not least their resourcing implications. A further problem arises when a baby is damaged as a result of such a plan. Could a health professional who had followed the plan be liable in negligence? (For a discussion of this see Harpwood, 1996, Ch. 3.)

As to the place and manner of birth, although a woman cannot be compelled to go to hospital to give birth (except in cases where the Mental Health Act 1983 applies), it is a criminal offence under the Nurses, Midwives and Health Visitors Act 1997 for a person other than a registered midwife or registered medical practitioner to attend a woman in childbirth. The only exception to this rule is in cases of 'sudden or urgent necessity'.

But the birth process itself is regulated by common law, notably the law of consent. As was noted above, several high-profile cases in the 1990s have brought childbirth sharply into focus. Basically, the central issue is whether a competent woman who refuses a caesarean or other medical intervention without which she and/or the fetus would die or be seriously harmed can be treated without her consent. It now seems clear (following *Re MB* [1997] 2 FLR 426, see Chapter 2) that, although a court declaration can be granted to save the life or prevent a deterioration in the physical or mental health of an incompetent patient, if the patient is competent then she is entitled to refuse treatment, including a caesarean, even when this places her life and her baby's at risk.

The woman only has this 'right' if she is competent, however, and given that the pain-relieving treatment used in labour – for example, gas and air – may in itself cause the patient to become temporarily incapable or at least cast doubt on her competency, it is not surprising that in all but one of the cases that reached the court declarations were granted authorizing caesareans on the basis that the women were in fact incompetent – a finding that may well have been justified in some of the cases but by no means in all of them.

It was initially assumed that *Re MB* had settled once and for all the law in this context but *St George's Healthcare NHS Trust* v. *S (No. 2)*; *R* v. *Collins* ex p. *S (No. 2)* [1998] 3 WLR 936 revealed a new twist. This case arose out of the treatment of a 36-weeks pregnant woman who had been diagnosed with pre-eclampsia and advised that she needed urgent attention, bed-rest and admission to hospital for an induced delivery. She fully understood the potential risks but rejected the advice as she wanted her baby to be born naturally. She was then seen by a social worker and two doctors, who repeated the advice, which she again rejected. As a consequence she was sectioned under the Mental Health Act 1983 and admitted to hospital for assessment. Her baby was then delivered by caesarean section without her consent, even though her detention under the Act was terminated a few days later.

The Court of Appeal held that S's admission under the Mental Health Act had been unlawful – since she had been detained because of her pre-eclampsia, not because of mental disorder as required by the Act – and awarded her damages. According to the court it was wrong to detain S against her will 'merely because her thinking process was unusual, even apparently bizarre and irrational, and contrary to the views of the overwhelming majority of the community at large'. Thus the fact that S had said that she did not want the baby, that she did not care if she died and that if the baby died too it would serve the father right did not make her incompetent in legal terms. As the court stressed:

[W]hile pregnancy increased the personal responsibilities of a woman it did not diminish her entitlement to decide whether or not to undergo medical treatment. She was entitled not to be forced to submit to an invasion of her body against her will, whether her own life or that of her unborn child depended upon it. Her right was not reduced or diminished merely because her decision to exercise it might appear morally repugnant.

Paternal rights
Issues of law and morality in relation to pregnancy and childbirth almost always focus on the mother's rights and responsibility. Yet, just as in the abortion debate, the father's position should perhaps not be ignored. It could be argued,

for example, that as more emphasis is placed on the caring role of fathers in the upbringing of their children so their moral standing should also increase. Whether this should bring with it some legal control over pregnancy – which current law denies – is another matter. Nevertheless, more consideration of the interests of the father may not be inappropriate (Mason and McCall Smith, 1999).

CASE STUDY 6.1	KATIE AND MARY'S SURROGATE RELATIONSHIP – A DISCUSSION

(Refer to the scenario presented on page 144.)

Dealing first with Katie's claim that she has a right to reproduce – a phrase that can be understood in several different ways: the right to have one's own biological children (whether by natural or artificial means); the right to be a social parent, in other words to rear a child and found a family; or the right to choose to reproduce.

Many regard the desire for children as a basic human need and a fundamental human right. Others have suggested that it is an absolute right to be exercised by anyone who is capable of reproduction. Whether infertility constitutes an 'illness' (rather than a symptom) under the National Health Service Act 1977 and so is something that the Secretary of State for Health has a duty to treat, is however, unclear. Nevertheless the importance of the family unit is recognized in various international declarations on human rights and the Human Rights Act 1998. Taken together they arguably constitute a recognition of the freedom to procreate, even though the extent of this right has yet to be determined (Douglas, 1991, p. 22). Nor is it yet clear whether the 'rights' recognized imply a positive right to have a child (Stone, 1990, p. 67). Indeed, as Grubb and Pearl point out (1987), international documents on human rights only protect a right to choose whether or not to reproduce rather than an absolute right to do so.

As far as the law is concerned, the courts have yet to recognize a right to reproduce. The closest they have come to even considering such a concept was in Re D [1976] I All ER 326, which concerned an II-year-old girl with Soto's syndrome. This is a rare condition characterized by epilepsy, clumsiness, unusual facial appearance, behavioural problems, aggression and impairment of mental function. D was described as having an IQ of 80, some reading and writing skills, good conversational skills and the understanding of a 9- or 9½-year-old. Her mother, who was anxious that, given her 'precocious' physical development, she might get pregnant, gave her consent to sterilization. But the girl's educational psychologist opposed the procedure and made her a ward of court. The court refused to authorize the sterilization for several reasons, one of which was that the operation would involve 'the deprivation of a basic human right, namely the right to reproduce'.

A different but related question is whether Katie can challenge the fact that she has been refused treatment (bearing in mind that if she were fertile she could get pregnant if and when she chose without anyone questioning whether she would make a 'good' mother). The Human Fertilisation and Embryology Act 1990 makes it clear, however, that the screening of those requesting infertility treatment is not just appropriate but essential. This is because access to treatment is mainly governed by the welfare test contained in section 13(5). It states 'that a woman shall not be provided with treatment services unless account has been taken of the welfare of any child who may be born as a result of the treatment (including the need of that child for a father), and of any other child who may be affected'. Effectively this means that clinics operate a 'fit parent' test and thus can refuse treatment to women they consider 'unsuitable', although in making their assessment they are bound by a code of practice (issued by the Human Fertilisation and Embryology Authority, 1995) as well as any particular treatment criteria that individual clinics may operate.

It is, of course, possible to challenge how these criteria have been interpreted, but anyone doing so is unlikely to succeed unless a clinic acted unreasonably or irrationally – in other words, based its decision on irrelevant or unlawful criteria or discriminated unfairly, i.e. refused treatment on the basis of an applicant's race or religion (see R v. Ethical Committee of St Mary's Hospital ex p. Harriott [1988] 1 FLR 152).

A more pressing problem for Katie, however, is the surrogacy arrangement. Such arrangements are more common than in the past and are now recognized generally as an acceptable option, albeit, as guidance from the BMA (1996) notes, 'one of last resort'. Guidance from the Ethics Committee of the Royal College of Midwives (RCM, 1996) also acknowledges that such arrangements are increasing and states that irrespective of any reservations midwives might have in relation to the ethics of surrogacy it is 'not their role to condemn or condone, but to ensure that the surrogate mother is treated with the same respect as any other women in their care'. Mindful of the special needs of surrogate mothers the guidance further notes that they may require more information and support, particularly in making plans for the organization of antenatal care and preparation for birth.

This raises the question as to whether Mary fully understands the effect of her current lifestyle, especially her drinking and smoking. If not, Sharon, the midwife, may be the best person to advise her. But whatever the moral implications of Mary's behaviour, any attempt by Katie or Jack, her husband, to use the law to force Mary to change her lifestyle would be futile. This is because it is extremely unlikely that a court would ever compel Mary to keep to her side of the bargain, even if she clearly was in breach of all the 'prenatal' terms she had agreed to. Nor is a court ever likely to recognize that Jack has any rights he could enforce.

As to handing over the child at birth, it seems likely that Mary will renege on that too. But even such a fundamental breach as this cannot be enforced, according to the Surrogacy Arrangements Act 1985. In other words, the so called 'transfer term', namely the one that states that Mary will hand over the baby to Katie and Jack, is legally unenforceable. But this does not mean that Mary will automatically be able to keep the child because, once the courts become involved, they will decide its future care by applying the 'best interests' test. What's best for a child will always turn on the facts of each case (see, for example, *Re P (minors)* [1987] 2 FLR 421; *Re W* [1991] 1 FLR 385), but it seems that maternal bonding is by far the most influential factor and will in practice usually outweigh all other considerations.

Finally, who in law are regarded as the baby's parents? According to section 27 of the Human Fertilisation and Embryology Act 1990, the woman who carries and gives birth to the child is its legal mother. This means that Mary is the legal mother. As to the legal father, this is covered by several complex provisions but it is likely that Jack, the sperm donor, would be considered the legal father. But whatever the effect of these provisions, Katie and Jack would be able to jointly acquire legal parentage by applying for a parental order under section 30 of the Act.

CASE STUDY 6.2   LUISA'S CAESAREAN SECTION – A DISCUSSION

(Refer to the scenario presented on page 145.)

The central issue here is whether Luisa has the right to refuse treatment, a decision that will compromise both her life and that of her baby. It is an issue that has prompted several sets of ethical guidelines, including guidance from the NHS Executive (Department of Health, 1999). But the main focus of guidance from the Royal College of Midwives is the concept of autonomy.

The College notes how many definitions of autonomy infer that if an individual's actions harms others then the right to act autonomously should not be seen as absolute. But despite acknowledging that 'this harm to others is a powerful argument when caring for pregnant women because most decisions on the management of labour will affect the well-being of the fetus and the mother', and also that the moral pressure to save and protect life is very great, the College nonetheless emphasizes that 'it is not within the remit of medical or midwifery staff to act against the wishes of women'. In other words patient autonomy must be respected. It also goes on to say that 'to do otherwise, i.e. to accept that women lose the right to make autonomous decisions once they are pregnant, is to accept the slippery slope towards total medical/midwifery control over management of care'.

In adopting this position it is also worth noting how the College perceives the midwife's advocacy role, in that it states that, even if the midwife and obstetrician do not agree with the woman's decision, 'it is the woman's choice that the midwife must represent. Only if a woman is not competent can her treatment choices be challenged.' It seems, therefore, that, unless Luisa is incompetent, her decision to have a vaginal birth must be respected whatever the consequences to her and the fetus. In short, Luisa's right of self-determination prevails over any moral claims her fetus may have.

As to Luisa's legal rights, it is now clear following the case of *Re MB* [1997] and *St George's Healthcare NHS Trust* v. *S (No. 2); R* v. *Collins* ex p. *S (No. 2)* [1998] 3 WLR 936 (referred to hereafter as *Re S*) that, providing she is competent, she has the right to refuse medical treatment, including a caesarean, even if that decision puts her life and that of the fetus at risk. In addition, in Re S the court issued guidelines about how future similar cases should be dealt with, i.e. treatment of patients of doubtful capacity (see Department of Health, 1999, appendix B). If there is any doubt about Luisa's competence, therefore, a declaration can always be sought from the court.

Much will therefore turn on Fran's assessment of Luisa's capacity, in particular the effect of shock, fatigue, confusion, pain or drugs. But, as Brazier has commentated (1997, p. 341), 'all [of which] are in so many cases an inevitable part of childbirth'. It is worth noting, however, that as the guidelines in Re S effectively allow health professionals to decide on the issue of competence and only approach the court if there is doubt, they are, in practice given very wide discretion to treat women in labour in the way they feel is in their best interests.

Finally what legal rights does Manjit have? Current law denies him any. Thus he has no legal right to make decisions on Luisa' s behalf nor can he take any action to protect the fetus. This means that health professionals could not rely on his consent to perform a caesarean section.

LAW and *ETHICS* – a comparison

It is not surprising that abortion and surrogacy provide such a good context in which to explore the interdependence between law and morality. Not only have both prompted specific so-called 'moral-issue' legislation, notably the Abortion Act 1967, the Surrogacy Arrangements Act 1985 and the Human Fertilisation and Embryology Act 1990, but the legal and ethical problems they raise have much in common.

Perhaps the most fundamental problem both face is how to reconcile and accommodate diametrically opposed positions. In relation to abortion, for example, we have seen how the debate between the 'pro-life' and 'pro-choice' group has become increasingly polarized. As a consequence the likelihood that agreement will ever be reached as to the moral status of the fetus seems remote. It is thus not surprising that, whatever the law's response it will inevitably conflict with the strongly held moral position of some parts of society.

Hence the Abortion Act 1967 may be seen by some as a necessary and pragmatic response to the problem of abortion (in so far as legislation prohibiting abortion would be almost impossible to enforce and would inevitably drive the practice underground). Yet for those who claim that the fetus has the same moral worth and status as a human being, the Abortion Act 1967, which seeks to set out the circumstances in which an abortion is permissible rather than appropriate, is tantamount to 'legal murder'. For others, however the Act does not go far enough – not only because it limits the circumstances in which abortion is permitted but more importantly because, rather than give women the legal right to demand an abortion whenever they choose (or even if they consider that their circumstances fit those specified in the Act), it instead gives doctors the upper hand and the discretion to decide who should have an abortion.

So it seems that, even though law and morality ask many of the same questions in relation to abortion – What is the status of the fetus? Who, if anyone, ought to be permitted to have an abortion? Under what circumstances? – they invariably come up with different answers or at least answers that are unlikely to please everyone. Hence in denying that the fetus has any legal status (and thus no legal right to life) its moral claims are of little practical significance, in that they cannot be legally enforced.

As for surrogacy, it can be argued that here too law and morality attempt to answer common questions. These include under what circumstances or conditions surrogacy might be allowed, whether anyone should be permitted to profit from surrogacy and who should be allowed to be a surrogate mother. Yet despite common concerns the legal and ethical responses to surrogacy do not coincide. This is perhaps not surprising, since the Surrogacy Arrangements Act 1985 was passed largely to appease surrogacy's most vociferous critics and long before its moral and legal implications had been worked out. As a consequence, the stance taken by the Act may well have eliminated what many regard as the most morally objectionable aspects of surrogacy – its commercial exploitation – but left unresolved several other fundamental concerns, in particular the role that could or should have been played by a central supervisory body such as the Human Fertilisation and Embryology Authority, which regulates and monitors the provision of infertility services.

The absence of such a body means that surrogacy arrangements are left largely to the individuals concerned. In many cases this may not be problematic and although it is far from certain that such a body would be able to eliminate all the legal and moral dilemmas associated with surrogacy – such as, for example, when a surrogate refuses to surrender the child or when surrogacy is sought for convenience rather than medical reasons – it would at least come some of the way towards preventing the risks associated with uncontrolled and amateurish arrangements.

Finally we turn to the legal and moral framework of pregnancy and childbirth. It seems self-evident that current ethical and legal debates between health professionals, who contend for the life of the unborn child, and feminists, who contend for the rights of a pregnant woman to determine treatment, are passionate and seemingly irreconcilable. Yet, as was noted above, although the fetus is not a legal person in its own right it has increasingly been awarded legal protection, in particular rights under the Congenital Disabilities (Civil Liability) Act 1976. But so far the law has stopped short of giving the fetus rights separate from its mother that could be used to protect its welfare *in utero* when the mother's behaviour threatens it in some way.

When there is conflict between the safety and wishes of the mother and the safe delivery of the baby it seems too that, in theory at least, the law upholds the absolute right of a competent woman in labour to consent to or refuse consent to treatment, irrespective of the consequence to her and the fetus. In other words, she has the same common law rights as any other competent patient. The fact that the law has chosen to protect women's rights to self-determination and bodily integrity over the right to a 'safe' delivery for the fetus should not, however, be interpreted as implying that pregnant women have no moral responsibilities and obligations towards their unborn children. Rather it acknowledges the limitations of the law in enforcing such obligations and the fact that there is a world of difference between moral claims on the one hand and legal claims that can be enforced by the courts, i.e. between how a pregnant woman ought to behave and how she must behave (and so can be compelled to behave by the State).

REFERENCES

Beauchamp, T. L. and Childress, J. F. (1989) *Principles of Biomedical Ethics*, 3rd edn, Oxford University Press, Oxford.

Beaumont, P. (1996) Wrongful life and wrongful birth. In: *Contemporary Issues in Law, Medicine and Ethics*, (ed. S. McLean), Dartmouth, Aldershot.

BMA (1996) *Changing Conceptions of Motherhood: The Practice of Surrogacy in Britain*, British Medical Association, London.

Brazier, M. (1997) Parental responsibilities, foetal welfare and children's welfare. In: *Family Law Towards the Millennium*, (ed. C. Bridge), Butterworths, London.

Brazier, M. (1999) Regulating the reproduction business. *Medical Law Review*, 7(2), 166–193.

Brown, J. M., Kitson, A. L. and McKnight, T. J. (1992) *Challenges in Caring*, Chapman & Hall, London.

Chadwick, R. F. (1987) Having children: an introduction. In: *Ethics: Reproduction and Genetic Control*, (ed. R. F. Chadwick), Routledge, London.

Clarke, L. (1990) Abortion: a rights issue. In: *Birthrights: Law and Ethics at the Beginnings of Life*, (eds R. Lee and D. Morgan), Routledge, London.

Davies, M. (1998) *Textbook on Medical Law*, Blackstone, London.

Department of Health (1998) *Surrogacy: Review for Health Ministers of Current Arrangements for Payments and Regulation, CM 4068*, Stationery Office, London.

Department of Health (1999) *Consent to Treatment, HSC 1990/031*, Stationery Office, London.

Dodds, S. and Jones, K. (1989) Surrogacy and autonomy. *Bioethics*, 3, 1–17.

Douglas, G. (1991) *Law, Fertility and Reproduction*, Sweet & Maxwell, London.

Dworkin, R. (1993) *Life's Dominion: An Argument about Abortion and Euthanasia*, Harper Collins, London.

Freeman, M. (1989) Is surrogacy exploitative? In: *Legal Issues in Human Reproduction*, (ed. S. McLean), Dartmouth, Aldershot.

Freeman, M. (1999) Does surrogacy have a future after Brazier? *Medical Law Review*, 7(1), 1–20.

Glover, J. (1977) *Causing Death and Saving Lives*, Penguin, Harmondsworth.

Grubb, A. and Pearl, D. (1987) Sterilisation and the courts. *Cambridge Law Journal*, 439.

Harpwood, V. (1996) *Legal Issues in Obstetrics*, Dartmouth, Aldershot.

Harris, J. (1985) *The Value of Life: An Introduction to Medical Ethics*, Routledge, London.

Hendrick, J. (1997) *Legal Aspects of Child Health Care*, Chapman & Hall, London.

Johnstone, M. J. (1989) *Bioethics: A Nursing Perspective*, Baillière Tindall, London.

Liu, A. (1991) *Artificial Reproduction and Reproductive Rights*, Dartmouth, Aldershot.

Marquis, D. (1997) An argument that abortion is wrong. In: *Ethics in Practice*, (ed. H. LaFollette), Blackwell, Oxford.

McHale, J. (1998) Reproductive choices. In: *Law and Nursing*, (eds J. McHale, J. Tingle and J. Peysner), Butterworth Heinemann, Oxford.

McHale, J. and Fox, M., with Murphy, J. (1997) *Health Care Law: Text and Materials*, Sweet & Maxwell, London.

McLean, S. (1999) *Old Law, New Medicine: Medical Ethics and Human Rights*, Pandora, London.

Mason, J. K. (1998) *Medico-legal Aspects of Reproduction and Parenthood*, 2nd edn, Dartmouth, Aldershot.

Mason, J. K. and McCall Smith, R. A. (1999) *Law and Medical Ethics*, 5th edn, Butterworths, London.

Morgan, D. (1990) Surrogacy: an introductory essay. In: *Birthrights: Law and Ethics at the Beginnings of Life*, (eds R. Lee and D. Morgan), Routledge, London.

RCM (1996) *Proceedings of the Ethics Committee*, Royal College of Midwives, London.

Ridley, A. (1998) *Beginning Bioethics*, St Martin's Press, New York.

Routledge (2000) *Routledge Encyclopedia of Philosophy*, Routledge, London.

Rumbold, G. (1999) *Ethics in Nursing Practice*, 3rd edn, Baillière Tindall, London.

Singer, P. (1995) *Rethinking Life and Death*, Oxford University Press, Oxford.

Singer, P. and Wells D. (1984) *The Reproduction Revolution*, Oxford University Press, Oxford.

Stauch, M. and Wheat, K., with Tingle, J. (1998) *Sourcebook on Medical Law*, Cavendish Publishing, London.

Steinbock, B. (1992) *Life Before Birth*, Oxford University Press, Oxford.

Stone, J. (1990) Infertility treatment. In: *Ethics and Law in Health Care*, (ed. P. Bryne), John Wiley, Chichester.

Szawarski, W. (1996) The debate on abortion. In: *Philosophical Problems in Health Care*, (eds D. Greaves and H. Upton), Avebury, Aldershot.

Thomson, J. J. (1971) A defense of abortion. *Philosophy and Public Affairs*, 1, 147–166.

Tooley, M. (1972) Abortion and infanticide. *Philosophy and Public Affairs*, 2, 37–65.

UKCC (1992) *Code of Professional Conduct*, United Kingdom Central Council, London.

UKCC (1996) *Guidelines for Professional Conduct*, United Kingdom Central Council, London.

Warnock, M. (1985) A Question of Life (the Warnock Report), *Cmnd 9314*, Blackwell, Oxford.

Warren, M. A. (1993) Abortion. In: *A Companion to Ethics*, (ed. P. Singer), Blackwell, Oxford.

Warren, M. A. (1997) On the moral and legal status of abortion. In: *Ethics in Practice*, (ed. H. LaFollette), Blackwell, Oxford.

FURTHER READING

Beauchamp, T. L. and Childress, J. F. (1994) *Principles of Biomedical Ethics*, 4th edn, Oxford University Press, Oxford.

Harris, J. and Holm, S. (eds) (1998) *The Future of Reproduction*, Clarendon Press, Oxford.

Locke J. (1964) *An Essay Concerning Human Understanding* (1690), Oxford University Press, Oxford.

7 MENTAL HEALTH

INTRODUCTION

It is estimated that one in six adults in Britain will suffer from mental illness every year – about 250 000 people are admitted to psychiatric facilities per year (Bartlett and Sandland, 2000, p. 85). And although psychotic illnesses are rare, depression will affect roughly half of all women and a quarter of all men before the age of 70 (Department of Health, 1998). There can therefore be little doubt that mental illness is a huge social problem, which can have a profound effect on an individual's life. Under the Mental Health Act 1983, for example, people can be compulsorily admitted, detained and treated against their will. Detention can last for several months if not years and treatment, which can be both invasive and hazardous and have adverse effects, may significantly curtail a person's quality of life.

To say that such Draconian powers need to be justified is thus to state the obvious. Legally, the concern must be to ensure that people should only be deprived of their liberty providing the most stringent legal procedures have been followed. As to the moral issues, these focus primarily on the conflict between autonomy and paternalism, i.e. in what circumstances it is justifiable to limit a person's autonomy and right to run their own lives by making decisions on their behalf.

But in concentrating on the Mental Health Act 1983 and its ethical framework, other aspects of the care and treatment of those who are just as vulnerable, e.g. people with mental handicap or learning disability, can all too easily be neglected. As they are often given medical treatment without their consent – treatment that raises broadly similar legal and ethical issues as non-consensual treatment under the Mental Health Act – it is appropriate also to cover these aspects in this chapter. Because of limited space, however, it is not possible to look at the role of the criminal law, nor the effect of the Mental Health (Patients in the Community) Act 1995, which governs the supervision in the community of patients who have been released from detention (on which see Dimond, 1997).

As in previous chapters, we begin with some case studies.

CASE STUDY 7.1   CAN JANE BE FORCE FED?

Life has not been kind to Jane, who is 22 and suffering from anorexia nervosa. Her mother died when she was 4 and her father, who was successfully caring for her and her twin brother, Alistair, was killed in an accident at work just a few years later. Since then she has lived in several foster homes but all the placements broke down for one reason or another. At her last home she was sexually abused by her foster brother, as a result of which she ran away and lived rough for several months until she moved in with Alistair. For a while that arrangement worked well and Jane seemed to thrive. But last year Alistair died of a drug overdose. This affected Jane very badly. She took an overdose and was unconscious when admitted to hospital.

In recent weeks her weight has become dangerously low and anorexia nervosa has been diagnosed. There is little doubt that if she continues to refuse to eat or take any fluids her health and possibly her life will be in danger. A decision is therefore taken that she should be 'sectioned' under the Mental Health Act and force-fed.

Is such non-consensual treatment lawful under the Mental Health Act 1983?

Can force-feeding be morally justified?

CASE STUDY 7.2   SHOULD ALVA BE STERILIZED?

Alva is 19 years old and has lived for several years as a voluntary patient in a mental hospital. She has been assessed as having the intellectual development of a 6-year-old. Several staff at the hospital are concerned about Alva's welfare because, even though she has all the physical sexual drive and inclinations of a physically mature young woman, she would not be able to give informed consent to any act of sexual intercourse. Although Alva can manage the necessary hygienic mechanics of menstruation it is thought that she could not cope with contraception. There is therefore a significant danger of pregnancy, which would be potentially disastrous for Alva because she would be unlikely to agree to an abortion but would be very distressed if the baby was taken away from her.

A decision is taken, therefore, that Alva should be sterilized. But Basil, a nurse, who has cared for Alva for several years believes that such drastic action is unnecessary.

Is sterilization of a mentally incompetent adult lawful? In what circumstances can such an operation be morally justified?

DEFINING MENTAL ILLNESS AND MENTAL DISORDER

To understand the role of the law in relation to mental health and the moral presuppositions on which it is based, it is important to define terms such as mental illness and mental disorder. But to do so in a clear and universal way is not easy despite attempts by several international bodies. For example, the United Nations' *Principles, Guidelines and Guarantees for the Protection of Persons Detained on Grounds of Mental Ill-Health or Suffering from Mental Disorder* (1986) defines mental illness as 'any psychiatric or other illness which substantially impairs mental health'. And a mentally ill person is taken to mean 'a person who, because of mental illness, requires care, treatment or control for his own protection, the protection of others or the protection of the community, and who for the time being is incapable of managing himself or his affairs'.

The Mental Health Act 1983 (hereafter referred to as 'the Act') and the Code of Practice which accompanies it (the Code) avoid defining the concept of mental illness, thus leaving the courts to come up with their own interpretation, which they did in W v. L [1974] QB 711. This case concerned a 23-year-old man who had put one cat in a gas oven and made another inhale ammonia after which he cut its throat with a cup. He also hanged a puppy and strangled a terrier with a wire. Finally he began to focus on his wife, threatening her with a knife and that he would push her downstairs as a way of getting rid of the baby she was expecting. In finding that he was mentally ill the court defined mental illness as follows:

> [T]he words [mental illness] are ordinary words of the English language. They have no particular medical significance. They have no particular legal significance ... [they] should be construed in the way that ordinary sensible people would construe them ... what would the ordinary sensible person have said about the patient's condition in this case if he had been informed of his behaviour to the dogs, the cat and the wife? In my judgement such a person would have said: 'Well, the fellow is obviously mentally ill'.

This definition, which Hoggett describes as the 'the man must be mad test' (1996, p. 32), has been much criticized. The main criticism is that it relies too heavily on the ordinary person's, i.e. society's, perception of what is 'normal' rather than a psychiatric assessment. As such, it assumes (wrongly) that there is a known and consistent view among lay people as to what constitutes mental illness (Cavadino, 1991, p. 299). More worryingly perhaps, it is also all too easy to use it to impose conformity to societal norms upon anyone whose behaviour is in some way unusual, eccentric or simply inconvenient. Furthermore, it is certainly questionable whether mental illness is an 'ordinary' concept. If it was, it would by now have been possible for Parliament, the courts, philosophers and psychiatrists to have been able to agree on a working definition at least, which to date they have failed to do.

As to the term 'mental disorder', this is defined broadly in the Mental Health Act 1983 as 'mental illness, arrested or incomplete development of mind, psychopathic disorder or any other disorder or disability of mind' (section 1(2)). Specifically excluded from this definition are promiscuity, immoral conduct, sexual deviancy or drug abuse (section 1(3)). This means that under the Act a diagnosis of mental disorder can never be founded solely on these grounds.

The Act's limited definitions of mental illness and disorder are perhaps not surprising, given, first, the reluctance of practitioners to attempt any formal definition and, second, the controversy that surrounds the diagnosis and treatment of these 'conditions'. Thus some psychiatrists believe that because some mental disorders are caused by bodily defects it will eventually be possible to trace all mental disorders to physical or organic causes. But others reject this 'organic' approach and focus more on how patients interact with their families or cope with social pressures. Yet another approach ignores the causes of mental disorder altogether and focuses instead on how it manifests itself, i.e. it concentrates on developing systems of behaviour modification (Hoggett, 1996, p. 27).

Finally there is the antipsychiatry movement, which questions whether mental illness and insanity exist at all and asserts that these notions are at best confused and arbitrary and are in essence no more than devices that can be used to detain people whose values or ways of life differ from those prevailing in society. Thomas Szasz (1970), for example claims that 'mental illness is a myth' and is no more real than witchcraft. He maintains, in short, that there is no such thing as mental illness and that to hold otherwise is to imply (falsely) that mental illness is like physical illness, i.e. something that has a physical cause with objective symptoms. But for Szasz, whereas there are certain diseases of the brain, e.g. tumours, that do cause people to behave strangely, 'functional diseases' like 'schizophrenia', 'depression' and 'mania' are simply inventions. So in describing such 'states' as illnesses psychiatrists are misdescribing as medical problems what are actually 'moral problems in living'. Put another way, these 'states of being' are basically forms of deviant behaviour that people who are powerful (and so can influence public debate and policy) find morally objectionable.

Szasz's views are less popular than in the past but even though few would now accept that mental illness is a myth it is nevertheless difficult to deny that ascriptions of mental illness do rest, at least in part, on value judgements – about what are desirable and undesirable attitudes and conduct. That this is so is perhaps most obvious in relation to the diagnosis of schizophrenia. Despite being one of the most frequent diagnoses under the Act its reliability has certainly been problematic in the past. Although the diagnosis is more reliable now, given the many different causal theories that seek to explain it (which include biochemical and social factors), Bartlett and Sandland (2000, p. 40) question whether the definition actually refers to anything or whether, like Santa Claus, it is a definition devoid of reality.

Also worth noting here is the approach taken by labelling theorists such as Thomas Scheff (1966), who claims that terms such as 'delinquent', 'mentally ill', 'schizophrenic and so on are catch-all labels for 'residual deviance' – a term that is applied whenever there is no specific name for describing the way in which a social rule has been broken. According to Scheff these labels should not be used because they are unscientific and inhumane and ignore the processual aspects of labelling. What he means by this is that many people who show what could be regarded as the 'symptoms' of mental illness never get labelled as mentally ill because whether this happens or not depends on the responses of others. In other words, attaching the label mentally ill to someone is not so much a state of affairs as a social process that depends on others making judgements (Gomm, 1996, p. 81).

Ethical Justifications for Compulsory Intervention

One of the main reasons why compulsory hospitalization needs to be justified is the practical consequences that can follow from a diagnosis of mental illness. Because of the general ignorance about mental illness, the crude assumptions that are made about it, the personal, legal and social stigma the label carries and society's prejudiced attitude towards the mentally ill, it is probably not surprising that there is extensive evidence that the mentally ill are discriminated against. This discrimination, which is widespread, routine and pervasive, affects not only the labour market, housing, leisure and social services but the health services too (Campbell and Heginbotham, 1991). Moreover, it is also likely to be long-term because once someone has been labelled 'mentally ill' there is almost nothing s/he can do to overcome the 'tag'. It is, in short, so tenacious and enduring that it is likely to profoundly influence perceptions of the patient and may even act as a self-fulfilling prophecy (Rosenhan, 1996, p. 77)

That compulsory admission, detention and treatment needs justification is thus self-evident. Yet even John Stuart Mill, the great libertarian thinker (see Chapter 1), acknowledged that it was legitimate to limit the autonomy of certain people. He thus qualified his 'harm principle' (i.e. that people should have the freedom to run their own lives free from interference as long as they do not harm others) by stating that:

> it is perhaps, necessary to say that this doctrine is meant to apply only to human beings in the maturity of their faculties ... those who are still in a state to require being taken care of by others, must be protected against their own actions as well as against external injury.

So what moral justification is there for restricting the liberty of people with mental illness? One is to protect the public and the other is to protect the mentally ill person from himself. Each of these will now be dealt with in turn.

The protection of others

Traditionally, this justification asserts that compulsory intervention is legitimate to protect the community at large from the threat posed by the mentally ill. In some cases, albeit rarely, this is because they have committed a serious crime but in the vast majority of cases it is because of the fear that the patient will do so unless s/he is detained in hospital and/or compulsorily treated.

Whether or not the protection of others is a sufficient criterion for limiting the autonomy of the mentally ill depends, of course, on establishing the kind of danger or harm they have to present before compulsory intervention in their lives can be triggered. How 'dangerous' do they have to be, for example and how 'serious' must the harm be that they pose? Dangerousness is after all a social construct rather than a psychiatric phenomenon and thus not just difficult to define objectively but also almost impossible to predict with any accuracy. But even if we can assume that most people would agree that society had the right to be protected from conduct that the law defines as criminal there would be much less agreement on what other kind of harm it had the right to protect itself from. Thus some would want to define harm very broadly and so include protecting families from the physical and mental strain of caring for the patient. And what about the emotional and sometimes financial suffering that may be caused by living with someone who is mentally ill? It may also be that children in the family will need protection, for example, from the developmental damage suffered when a patient cannot adequately cater for their needs. It would, in short be very difficult to decide on where the boundaries should be drawn (Hoggett, 1996, p. 45).

In attempting to answer this type of question a compromise has clearly to be found, one that balances the conflicting interests of the mentally ill and the public who are entitled to be protected from unacceptable risk. In reaching any compromise, however, several myths need to be dispelled. Perhaps the most significant one is the assumption that mentally ill people who commit crimes, especially violent ones, are very likely to reoffend. In fact, evidence suggests otherwise. In other words, mentally ill offenders are no more likely to reoffend than are 'mentally normal' offenders. To detain the former on the basis of their potential dangerousness but not the latter is thus at the very least morally questionable. Equally questionable is the assumption, in respect of which again there is little evidence, that the mentally ill (who have committed no crime) threaten the safety of the community. The actual threat posed by psychiatric patients is actually very small. In fact, evidence indicates that the vast majority of those with psychiatric difficulties are simply not dangerous (Bowden, 1996, pp. 17–22; Cavadino, 1989, pp. 99–102).

The protection of self

The other justification for the compulsory admission and detention of the mentally ill is that it is in their own best interests. In other words, without paternalistic intervention they will harm themselves in some way. But again, what does the word harm mean in this context? Or, to put it another way, what different kinds of paternalism are typically invoked here? As we saw in Chapter 2, paternalism is the belief that it is right to make decisions for other people 'for their own good' irrespective of their own wishes or judgements.

Three versions of paternalism are usually distinguished in this context, notably physical paternalism, which is aimed at safeguarding an individual's own physical health and safety; psychological paternalism, which is concerned with preventing psychological harm coming to the individual (i.e. his or her mental health); and moral paternalism, which is aimed at the individual's moral welfare, the concern being to make the individual a morally better person and ensure s/he does not come to moral harm (Cavadino, 1989, p. 133). The extent to which these three different kinds of paternalism can ever justify the compulsory detention and treatment of the mentally ill is, of course, debatable. Thus those who support a more liberal approach to mental health law – and who therefore place value on the liberty of the individual – would only consider compulsory action to be justified in order to protect the patient's physical health and safety.

In contrast, those who think professionals should be allowed wide discretion in dealing with the mentally ill with minimal legal scrutiny would use their flexible powers to 'save' patients from all types of harm – physical, psychological and probably moral too.

But even supposing it was possible to agree on which version of paternalism was appropriate it would still be necessary to come up with a convincing argument as to why the mentally ill should be subject to compulsory action for their own protection. This is arguably necessary because other people, such as smokers, heavy drinkers, sky divers and mountaineers, are free to act as they please irrespective of the potential harm to their health. It is usually argued that the crucial moral distinction lies in the inability of some mentally ill people to make rational choices. Thus, even though there may be little agreement among philosophers as to what it means to make a rational decision, it is plausible to suggest that people with 'severely irrational beliefs' are more likely to harm themselves and act in ways that are not in their own interests. As Lindley notes (1978, p. 42), a man who thinks he is Superman and thus indestructible, for example, can justifiably be stopped from jumping off a cliff in the belief that he can fly. On the other hand, it is much less justifiable to prevent people who have the capacity to reason and make a decision from smoking or drinking, because once they have been informed about and understand the risks they are exposing themselves to it is up to them to decide whether or not to smoke or drink themselves to an early death.

THE MENTAL HEALTH ACT 1983

Mental health law has an ancient history – the first statute was passed in 1324, giving the King jurisdiction over the persons and property of 'idiots' and those who 'happen to fail of [their] wit' (see Bartlett and Sandland 2000, pp. 15–20 for the roots of the current law). Since then there have, of course, been many other statutes but the Mental Health Act 1983 – which covers the reception, care and treatment of the mentally disordered as well as the management of their property – was passed at a time when patients' rights were treated more seriously than ever before in this century.

When it was enacted the Act was hailed as a liberalizing statute and a revolutionary break with the traditions of the past. This was because, even though it contained many similar provisions to the Mental Health Act 1959, it set limits on the exercise of compulsory powers, established the Mental Health Act Commission and attempted to maintain the civil and social status of patients. But 25 years later few would disagree that the law is in need of radical reform and the Act is unlikely to survive in its present form for much longer. Until new legislation is introduced, however, the 1983 Act remains the governing statute.

It is supplemented by a Code of Practice now in its third edition (Department of Health/Welsh Office, 1999), which makes recommendations and sometimes stipulations for 'good practice'. The Code does not impose additional statutory duties nor is there any legal duty to comply with it, yet, because it contains material supplemental to the legal standards set in the Act, it is supposed to aid practitioners. Whether it does so, however, is debatable. Arguably it only complicates matters further because – as a Japanese proverb says – a person with a clock knows the time; a person with two clocks is never sure (Bartlett and Sandland, 2000, p. 20).

Overall, the Act attempts to balance several considerations, namely, the liberty of the mentally ill, the need to treat them (where treatment is required and can be beneficial) and the protection of the public. How effective the Act has been in balancing these conflicting considerations is, of course, a matter of some debate. Thus many critics, while conceding that protecting patients from self-harm may initially appear attractive, even though they do not know that they are ill and may not seek help, nevertheless argue that the Act's core definitions of concepts like mental disorder fail to clarify what degree of mental 'ill-health' is sufficient to justify compulsory powers. Furthermore even if is accepted that society has a right to protect itself several basic questions remain unanswered, in particular exactly what kind of behaviour can justify depriving patients of their liberty. The fear here is that if the identification of mental illness is a subjective process then there is a real risk that any behaviour that offends society's 'norm', however discriminatory it may be, can be used as a ground for compulsory action.

It is perhaps because of these concerns that the Act makes several distinctions. One of the most important is the distinction between admission and treatment on an informal basis, and compulsory treatment and care. Another focuses on the different criteria that must be met before patients can be compulsorily admitted on a long-term basis for treatment and those that apply for short-term admission for assessment only. But before looking at these distinctions the Act's definitions need to be outlined.

The central concept is 'mental disorder', which the Act defines widely as 'mental illness, arrested or incomplete development of mind, psychopathic disorder and any other disorder or disability of mind'. As we shall see, this broad interpretation is sufficient to justify compulsory admission for assessment (under section 2) but for longer-term compulsory admission for treatment (under section 3) one of the four forms or classes of mental disorder specified in the Act need to be present – mental illness, psychopathic disorder, severe mental impairment or mental impairment.

As was noted earlier, mental illness is not statutorily defined but includes psychotic illnesses and depressive illnesses of all kinds such as reactive depression, postnatal depression and the mental disorders of old age (Fegan and Fennell, 1998, p. 81). Other terms defined in the Act are the following:

- **severe mental impairment** – 'a state of arrested or incomplete development of mind' which includes severe impairment of intelligence and social functioning and is associated with 'abnormally aggressive or seriously irresponsible conduct';
- **mental impairment** – a state of arrested or incomplete development of mind

(not amounting to severe mental impairment) which includes significant impairment of intelligence and social functioning and is associated with abnormally aggressive or seriously irresponsible conduct;

- **psychopathic disorder** – a persistent disorder or disability of mind (whether or not including significant impairment of intelligence) which results in abnormally aggressive or seriously irresponsible conduct.

Not surprisingly, there has been considerable debate on the precise meaning of all these terms (see, for example, Hoggett, 1996, Ch. 2), which are very broad and flexible. They were, however, never intended to have fixed or static meanings – the assumption being that they would therefore more readily respond to changes in medical knowledge and social attitudes as well as advances in psychiatry. Nonetheless, it has been argued that the definition of psychopathy in particular highlights how mental health law can be used as a mechanism of social control. This is because it allows some aspects of behaviour or personality to be defined as illness, without any obvious mechanism to distinguish them from similar, non-ill traits (Bartlett and Sandland, 2000, p. 29).

The various routes into care are as follows.

Informal admission (section 131)

Admission on an informal basis accounts for the vast majority of people (roughly 90%) who receive inpatient psychiatric care. Because they are admitted without the use of compulsory powers they are often referred to, albeit inappropriately, as 'voluntary patients'. The terms are, however, not synonymous and should not be used interchangeably because a significant number of informal patients lack the capacity to make the decision either to enter hospital or leave it and are also subject to various pressures while there (Bartlett and Sandland, 2000, p. 87).

Overall, section 131 encourages admission without any legal formality, similarly, in other words, to the way in which patients enter hospital for physical disorders. The legal status of informal patients is very different from those detained compulsorily because in theory at least they can go (and come) as they please, i.e. leave when they want to go; and reject (or consent to) any form of treatment (psychiatric or otherwise) providing they are competent. Yet despite their 'voluntary' status informal patients are accorded few of the safeguards given automatically to compulsory patients, who have, among other rights, the right to challenge their committal. There is also evidence that informal patients are not treated in the same way as 'ordinary' patients, in particular that their consent is not always sought for minor or routine procedures.

Given the uncertainty about the status of informal patients it is perhaps surprising that it was not until the late 1990s that the lawfulness of their informal treatment came before the courts. However, in the controversial case of *R* v. *Bournewood Community and Mental Health NHS Trust* ex p. *L* [1998] 3 WLR 107, the House of Lords confirmed that people who lacked capacity, e.g. people with dementia or severe learning disabilities, could be deemed to be content with their informal admission providing they did not show signs of wanting to leave or to 'opt out'. This meant that if they were not actively opting out it was lawful to keep them in hospital under section 131 and treat them without sectioning them under the Act's compulsory provisions (under the principle of necessity).

The case concerned a profoundly retarded autistic adult who was admitted for inpatient treatment following an outburst of self-harming behaviour. He was not compulsorily detained as he did not resist admission. As Mason and McCall Smith note in their commentary on the case (1999, p. 510), detaining such patients compulsorily would be a luxury that the system simply could not pay for.

Nevertheless many were dismayed by the decision because of its potential impact on the rights of informal patients who, as was noted above, have fewer opportunities to challenge questionable and controversial decisions made by doctors. But whatever the eventual impact of the case it is clear that women, particularly white women, are much more likely to be informally admitted than men (see, for example, Pilgrim and Rogers, 1993). Whether this is because women are disempowered in current society is, of course, another question (Bartlett and Sandland, 2000, p. 88).

Detaining an informal patient (section 5)

In cases where informal patients can no longer be detained on an informal basis – they may become extremely disturbed, violent or aggressive, for example, and try and leave the ward – there may be no other option but to detain them against their will. In this kind of situation it may be possible to resort to the so called 'holding powers' conferred by section 5 of the Act. The effect of using these powers is that the informal patient's status is converted to that of compulsory detention. But detention is only short-term, usually, although not inevitably, a first step to more long-term compulsory detention under the Act. Under section 5(2) the doctor in charge of an inpatient has authority to authorize the patient's detention for up to 72 hours if the doctor thinks that an application for compulsory admission ought to be made.

Prescribed nurses (i.e. those trained in mental illness or handicap) have similar, albeit shorter, holding powers of up to 6 hours (or earlier if a doctor can attend before then) under section 5(4). This power – which was used on 1505 occasions in 1996/7 (Department of Health, 1998) – can only be exercised when a doctor is not available and in respect of inpatients receiving treatment for mental disorder who, for their own safety or the protection of others, need to be 'immediately restrained'. Detailed guidance is given in Chapter 9 of the Code about how this power is exercised. This stresses among other things the emergency nature of the power, what the nurse should be assessing (e.g. what is likely to happen if the patient does leave hospital) and what reports must be completed. It also stresses how the decision to detain patients is a 'personal one' of the nurse who 'cannot be instructed to exercise the power' (Dimond and Barker, 1996, pp. 27–30).

Compulsory admission

We now turn briefly to the main compulsory powers under the Act that are likely to concern nurses, bearing in mind that only a minority of patients – roughly 10% – are admitted to NHS psychiatric hospitals compulsorily each year. Irrespective of how patients get to be compulsorily admitted and detained (a process that is usually referred to as 'sectioning'), their liberty is restricted in two ways. First, unless they have been granted leave, they are not free to go and come when they please. Second, they may be treated for their mental disorder without their consent.

Admission for assessment (section 2)

Admission for assessment is a short-term measure designed for a very specific purpose, namely an assessment of the patient's condition. This involves carrying out those medical procedures that are necessary to form a diagnosis and devise a treatment plan To be admitted under this provision the patient must be suffering from 'a mental disorder of a nature or degree which warrants detention' and the detention is necessary 'in the interests of his own health or safety' or to protect others. Admission under this section lasts for up to 28 days, although the patient can be discharged before then. Several requirements have to be complied with if the admission is to be lawful, including (among other things) two medical recommendations, one of them from a doctor with 'special experience in the diagnosis and treatment of mental disorder' (i.e. a psychiatrist). Overall, according to Bartlett and Sandland (2000, p. 99) the provisions in section 2 reflect a concern to safeguard the rights of mentally disordered persons from unwarranted compulsory hospitalization. They also mean that a decision to admit should not simply be a clinical, medical one but should also include an assessment of what would happen if the patient was not hospitalized.

Admission for treatment (section 3)

Admission for treatment is a long-term provision, which can last initially for up to 6 months. If further detention is necessary the initial 6-month period can be renewed once for a further 6 months and thereafter for any number of 12-month periods. Overall, admission for treatment is intended for those whose condition is believed to require a period of treatment as an inpatient. The section is complex and the specific grounds are as follows:

1. that the patient is suffering from mental illness, severe mental impairment, psychopathic disorder or mental impairment and his mental disorder is of a nature or degree which makes it appropriate for him to receive medical treatment in hospital; and
2. in the case of psychopathic disorder or mental impairment, such treatment is likely to alleviate or prevent a deterioration of his condition; and
3. it is necessary for the health or safety of the patient or for the protection of other persons that he should receive such treatment and it cannot be provided unless he is detained.

Several points need to be emphasized here. First, given that admission can last for several months, if not much longer, it is not surprising that the admission criteria are more stringent than for admission for assessment; in particular, mental disorder by itself is insufficient to warrant compulsion as it must also require treatment in hospital. This means that if the disorder could be treated in the community detention is not justified. Second, if the patient is suffering from mental impairment or psychopathic disorder then the so-called 'treatability test' must be passed. This 'test' is one of the most controversial aspects of this section as it has not been easy to interpret, despite the efforts of the Court of Appeal in *R* v. *Canons Park MHRT* ex p. *A* [1994] 2 All ER 659, in which a six-point guide to treatability was given. Note finally that the procedures that must be followed under this section are similar to those required for section 2 admission, although there are additional requirements. Further advice on this section can also be found in the Code (Chapter 5).

Which to choose – section 2 or section 3?

Because it is not always easy to determine whether a section 2 or section 3 admission is the most appropriate, the Code (Chapter 5) provides several pointers. Those supporting a section 2 admission include (among others) cases where the diagnosis and prognosis is unclear or where an inpatient assessment is necessary to formulate a treatment plan. Section 3 pointers include cases where a patient has a mental disorder that is already known to his clinical team and has been assessed in the recent past by that team. Finally it is worth noting that, as with informal admission, these sections do not seem to affect all groups equally, in that Afro-Caribbeans, especially men, are statistically over-represented in the detention statistics (see, for example, Flannigan *et al.*, 1994).

Emergency admission (section 4)

Approximately 10% of patients are initially admitted compulsorily under section 4. Because the medical recommendations are much less stringent than the other 'sectioning' provisions – only one doctor (who does not need to be a psychiatrist) needs to recommend admission – this section is one of the most controversial parts of the Act because of the obvious risk that an inexperienced 'panic' diagnosis may result in an overhasty and unnecessary detention (Hoggett, 1996). According to the Code this section should only be used for a 'genuine emergency' when 'those involved cannot cope with the mental state or behaviour of the patient'. But in practice it tends to be used as a 'short-cut' variant of ordinary admission for assessment, to which it can later be converted. Grounds for admission are that there is an urgent necessity for the patient to be admitted and detained under section 2 but complying with that section would 'involve undesirable delay'. Detention can last for up to 72 hours but can be extended by admission under section 2.

Note also other routes into compulsory detention, namely the power of justices of the peace under section 135 and the police under section 136.

Compulsory treatment under the Mental Health Act 1983

Ethical issues

The justification for depriving patients of the right to consent or reject treatment mirrors that for compulsory admission and detention, i.e. even if some patients are not legally responsible for their behaviour, society is entitled to protect itself from conduct that threatens its safety. Compulsory treatment is also justified on the basis of the patients' own interests, i.e. to protect them from self-harm.

The assumption underlying both these justifications is, of course, that treatment will if not cure the patient then at the very least help him/her in some way. But is this so? Antipsychiatrists would almost certainly disagree, claiming that patients labelled mentally ill end up being imprisoned in institutions, which can only do damage by making it much less likely that they can be socially and psychologically rehabilitated. Furthermore, even if it is possible that patients can be helped by treatment and so may ultimately be glad that their wishes were overridden or ignored, their 'thanks' are arguably not enough to justify compulsory treatment since otherwise compulsion in other contexts would also be legitimate. Thus you might be glad that a dentist has taken a tooth out but few would argue that you should therefore be forced to have such treatment against your will if for one reason or another (such as an irrational fear of dentists) you have decided never to go to one (Hoggett, 1996, p. 47).

It is also important to question the moral basis for compulsory treatment because without such an inquiry patients may be denied the right to make decisions, not because their competence has been thoroughly assessed but because once they have been labelled 'mentally ill' they are assumed to be incapable. In addition, some of the non-consensual treatments authorized by the Act are very intrusive and hazardous. Finally, the right of bodily self-determination has long been protected in law as part of 'the free citizen's first and greatest right, which underlies all others' (*Pratt* v. *Davis* [1904]).

Legal provisions

Part IV of the Act contains several provisions that authorize compulsory treatment for mental disorder. It has been suggested that it should be read as a truce between two competing models of psychiatric treatment: as 'medicine' and as 'control'. This is because it 'weaves notions of treatment and control, autonomy and beneficence, rights and their overriding, together in complex and sometimes perplexing patterns' (Bartlett and Sandland, 2000, p. 203). Part IV applies, irrespective of the patient's age, to most detained patients (i.e. those detained under section 2 and 3 but not, for example, under section 4, the section 5 holding powers or sections 135 and 136). Exceptionally one provision (see section 57) also applies to informal patients.

There are four categories of compulsory treatment, all of which are governed by different sections. But first some preliminary points needs to be stressed.

One is the wide definition of 'medical treatment' in the Act, which 'includes nursing, and also includes care, habilation and rehabilitation under medical supervision' (section 145), i.e. a broad range of activities including physical treatment, medication and psychotherapy. Note also that seclusion, although not a procedure specifically regulated by the Act, may in some circumstances constitute medical treatment – for example, as part of a behaviour modification programme, providing that it is given by or under the direction of a 'responsible medical officer' (usually the consultant psychiatrist in charge of the patient's treatment).

The second important point is the requirement that the medical treatment must be given for the patient's mental disorder. In other words, the Act does not authorize treatment for physical disorders that are unrelated to the patient's mental disorder. But as we shall see the distinction between physical and mental disorder can be a difficult one to make in practice as some physical disorders can be either the cause or a symptom of mental disorders.

The four treatment categories outlined here are as follows (for further detail see Dimond and Barker, 1996).

Psychosurgery and surgical implants (section 57)

Treatments regulated by section 57 are the most drastic and intrusive. They include pyschosurgery, defined as any surgery that destroys brain tissue or functioning, and surgical implants to reduce male sex drive. Psychosurgery is reserved for patients with chronic obsessional and depressive disorders but is rarely used – between 20 and 30 are carried out each year, the majority on women (Mental Health Act Commission, 1995) – and only one referral for a surgical implant has been made since 1983. Note that these treatments can only be carried out with the patient's consent, which must be verified by three independent people (including a nurse). As Dimond and Barker note (1996, p. 63), nurses have an important role to play in the consultation process. One of the three (a doctor) must also certify in writing that, having regard to the likelihood of the treatment alleviating or preventing a deterioration of the patient's condition, the treatment should be given.

Electroconvulsive therapy and long-term drug treatment (section 58)

Introduced in the late 1930s, electroconvulsive therapy (ECT) soon became controversial. In the 1950s it was often used as treatment for schizophrenia (Fennell, 1996) and although opinions about it are still divided – in particular, its long-term benefits have been questioned (Farrell, 1997) – it is still commonly used. ECT is now mainly used for patients with depressive illnesses associated with life-threatening complications. Long-term medication – usually referred to as psychotropic drugs – is that which is given to patients for longer than 3 months from the time the patient was given drugs (drugs given before then are regulated by section 63 (see below)).

Both forms of treatment can only been given if several conditions are satisfied. These are either that the patient consents (his/her consent must be verified in writing either by a doctor treating the patient or by a second opinion doctor (SOAD)), or that a SOAD certifies in writing that the treatment is necessary notwithstanding that the patient either lacks capacity or is unwilling to give consent. In reaching any decision, the SOAD has to consult with two other people who have been professionally involved with the patient, one of whom must be a nurse. Note too that consent can be withdrawn at any time even though it has initially been given.

All other forms of treatment (including medication; section 63)

This section allows medical treatment (apart from that covered by sections 57 and 58) to be given without consent to detained patients for the mental disorder from which they are suffering. It has become one of the most controversial treatment sections in recent years because of the courts' willingness to extend its scope well beyond what was originally intended. In fact, its interpretation has been so broad that the section has been described as representing 'a slippery slope that could lead to formally detained patients losing the right to say no to certain forms of treatment' (Davies, 1998, p. 216).

The leading case on the meaning of section 63 is now *B* v. *Croydon HA* [1995] 1 All ER 683, in which the Court of Appeal held the words 'treatment for mental disorder' to include nasogastric feeding of a patient with anorexia nervosa. It reached this decision because it decided that:

1. a range of acts ancillary to the core treatment that the patient is receiving fell within the term 'medical treatment' (as defined in section 145);
2. treatment was capable of being ancillary to the core treatment if it was nursing and care 'concurrent with the core treatment or as a necessary pre-requisite to such treatment or to prevent the patient from causing harm to himself or to alleviate the consequences of the disorder'; and
3. relieving the symptoms of the mental disorder was just as much part of treatment as relieving its underlying cause.

In citing this case, the Code (Department of Health/Welsh Office, 1999, para 16.5) advises that treatment for a physical disorder cannot be given under part IV 'unless it can reasonably be said that the physical disorder is a symptom or underlying cause of the mental disorder'.

Section 63 treatment has also been held to cover the use of reasonable force to deliver a baby by caesarean (*Tameside and Glossop Acute Service Trust* v. *CH* [1996] 1 FLR 762). The case concerned a woman detained because of schizophrenia who believed that doctors were trying to harm her baby. A new drug regime was recommended but, given its potential harm to the fetus, doctors considered that labour should be induced by a caesarean – to do otherwise would jeopardize the patient's health as her well-being depended on the delivery of a healthy baby. They therefore sought the court's permission that the caesarean was lawful. The court agreed on the basis that the procedure was treatment ancillary to her mental health because the birth of a stillborn child would cause her mental health to deteriorate. As this case followed the Croydon case and coincided with other 'forced' caesarean and anorexic cases (see case study below), it has been suggested that the treatment of mental disorder is 'shot through with gender assumptions' (Bartlett and Sandland, 2000, p. 225). That is not to say, however, that they reflect a gendered judicial conspiracy, as Widdett and Thompson have implied (1997).

Urgent treatment (section 62)
In certain circumstances section 62 allows treatment to be carried out without the need to comply with the legal safeguards of sections 57 and 58 (see Dimond and Barker, 1996, Ch. 8). In practice it is almost always used when a patient needs drug treatment the administration of which would otherwise be caught by the 3-month rule. Although intended for genuine emergencies – treatment must be necessary to save the patient's life or, providing it is not irreversible or hazardous, must alleviate serious suffering or deterioration – there is evidence that this provision is all too often misunderstood and seen as providing 'blanket permission to impose treatment upon any patient' (Hoggett, 1996, p. 147).

TREATMENT OUTSIDE THE MENTAL HEALTH ACT 1983 – THE 'BEST INTERESTS' TEST

This section looks briefly at the medical treatment of patients with mental handicap and learning disabilities and those patients, whether detained or informal, who require treatment for physical disorders not related to their mental disorders but who lack capacity. The Mental Health Act 1983 does not cover the treatment of any of these patients, so what justification is there for overriding their autonomy?

Ethical issues

It is not difficult to justify treating without their consent patients whose autonomy is questionable because of incapacity, whether temporary, transient or permanent, on the basis of paternalism (see above and Chapter 2), especially if treatment is necessary to save life. It is, however, less easy to do so when their lives are not threatened or when treatment is controversial. Questions need then to be asked about who should make medical decisions for them and on what basis.

As we shall see below, the law authorizes such non-consensual treatment if it is in the patient's 'best interests'. This too is the test that is adopted in various codes, e.g. *Guidelines for Mental Health and Learning Disabilities* (UKCC, 1998). Yet there is always a danger that nurses will too readily make decisions on behalf of such patients not because they are actually incapable of making a particular decision but because they are simply assumed to be incompetent. In other words, just because patients may lack competence in one context it does not necessarily mean that they are therefore incompetent in relation to all matters. Furthermore, as Rumbold points out (1999, p. 237). even persons who might be judged as being capable of rational thought do make irrational decisions. We may try to change their minds, but ultimately we have to respect their wishes. In this same way we should at least try to respect those whose capacity seems limited and at the very least give them the opportunity to be consulted and make their wishes known.

Legal issues

Until *Re F* [1990] 2 AC 1 (a case involving the sterilization of a 36-year-old mentally handicapped woman), the legality of treating incompetent adults under the common law was very uncertain. In that leading case, however, the House of Lords laid down guidelines on when the non-consensual treatment of incompetent adults would be lawful. These were that patients who were incapable for one reason or another of consenting to treatment could be treated without their consent providing the treatment was in their best interests, i.e. it was carried out either to save their lives or to ensure improvement or prevent deterioration in their physical or mental health.

Although the kind of treatment this could cover was not specified in the case, it was clearly intended to be broadly interpreted and so includes minor routine procedures as well as major surgery. Whether it covers others aspects of a patient's care such as washing and cleaning is another matter, although it would probably not be difficult to establish that such care was broadly in the patient's interests. Nevertheless, nurses will only be deemed to have acted in a patient's best interests if they have followed a responsible body of professional practice (i.e. they have complied with the Bolam test (see Chapter 3). Noteworthy too in *Re F* was how the Law Lords perceived the role of ethical and professional guidelines. These were (1) to assist doctors in taking difficult ethical decisions when treating incompetent adults and (2) to provide doctors with a degree of legal protection (Hurwitz, 1998, p. 97).

Although *Re F* was welcomed at the time for clarifying the law, it soon became apparent that the 'best interests' test begged several questions. What precise values and factors, for example, did it require health professionals to consider, and which were the most important? What interests were to be considered – long-term or short-term – and should they be confined just to medical interests or include social interests too? And should the decision be left to doctors or should others be included in the decision-making process, given that what is at stake are questions of value and social policy (Kennedy and Grubb, 1994)? And what if a nurse disagrees with a doctor's opinion as to the patient's best interests? As McHale points out (1998, p. 66) acting as the patient's advocate she should be able to raise her concerns and take the matter further.

Nor did *Re F* clarify what kinds of procedures the best interests test should cover – was it only treatment that was therapeutic, i.e. intended to benefit the patient in the sense of preventing, removing or ameliorating a physical or psychiatric disorder, or did it include non-therapeutic procedures such as certain clinical trials?

Although the answers to some of these questions will inevitably turn on the facts of individual cases it is arguably unsatisfactory that, because the best interests test is such a value-laden and indeterminate concept, nurses and other health professionals have a very wide discretion to decide in what circumstances treatment should be given. Once the Law Commission's proposals are adopted, however (and in late 1999 the government said that it would implement them as soon as there was parliamentary time), a much more patient-centred approach will be required. Reporting in 1995 the Commission recommended that the following criteria be taken into account in determining 'best interests':

- the ascertainable past and present wishes of the person concerned and the factors that s/he would consider if able to do so;
- the need to permit and encourage the person to participate or to improve his/her ability to participate as fully as possible in anything done for and any decision affecting him/her;
- the views of other people (whom it is appropriate and practicable to consult);
- whether it is possible to achieve the desired outcome in a way that is less restrictive of the person's freedom of action.

For these recommendations to be useful in practice, however, the legal criteria for assessing competence also needs to be clear. But, as was noted in Chapter 2 and despite *Re C* [1994] 1 All ER 819, there are still no fixed legal criteria for assessing competence, not least because the level of competence required varies according to the treatment proposed. Furthermore, even though *Re C* was widely welcomed at the time as an enlightened judgement – because it challenged paternalistic practice and seemed to introduce an unpatronizing and objective capacity test (see Stauch *et al.*, 1998, pp. 119–126) – later applications of it have revealed considerable inconsistencies in the way capacity has been determined. Thus although *Re C* seemed to require **actual** understanding and appreciation of the consequences of giving or withholding consent, the Mental Health Code (Department of Health/Welsh Office, 1999), despite referring to the case, emphasizes the **ability** to understand rather than actual understanding (see Bartlett and Standland, 2000, Ch. 11).

Once the Law Commission's recommendation are enshrined in legislation, however, there should be a more uniform determination of capacity. There will be a statutory definition of incapacity. Thus a person will be deemed to be without capacity if at the time that a decision needs to be taken s/he is 'unable by reason of mental disability to make a decision on the matter in question; or unable to communicate a decision on that matter because he or she is unconscious or for any other reason'. A person will be unable to make a decision by reason of mental disability if s/he is 'unable to understand or retain the information relevant to the decision, or unable to make a decision based on that information'.

CASE STUDY 7.1 **FORCE-FEEDING JANE – A DISCUSSION**

(Refer to the scenario presented on page 171.)

As the Mental Health Act Commission itself has acknowledged (1997), force-feeding has a bad press. Not only is it seen as highly coercive but also 'conjures up images of suffragettes being force-fed in prison'. Nonetheless it claims it can also be an 'act of compassion' without which there would be no alternative but to consider anorexia as a terminal disease for which palliative care only could be provided.

So what moral justification is there for force-feeding Jane? To answer this question it is necessary to determine whether her recent actions, notably her suicide attempt and refusal of food and fluids, are autonomous actions. If they are, if in other words Jane's decision to take her own life is not symptomatic of mental illness or disorder, then health professionals are morally obliged to respect her wishes. Yet it is possible to question whether Jane's choices are truly autonomous. Did her suicide attempt, for example, reflect a genuine intention to die or was it a temporary response to a crisis and thus only a 'gesture' suicide (Fletcher et al., 1995, p. 42). If so and if she was unconscious when she was admitted to hospital then it is certainly arguable that health professionals can justify saving Jane's life, not least because at that time there was unlikely to be any opportunity to find out much about her wishes and intentions.

But what about Jane's anorexia nervosa? Kennedy and Grubb (1994, p. 143) have argued that it may impair a patient's ability to understand his/her condition in so far as it results in a misperception of reality. Is this so in Jane's case? This is a very difficult question, given that some patients with anorexia nervosa may retain the capacity to understand the nature, purpose and likely effect of treatment yet their capacity may be compromised by fears of obesity or denial of the consequences of not eating. In such cases it is plausible to suggest that the patient is not acting autonomously and so paternalistic interventions are morally justified, providing, of course, that they are in the patient's best interests. But this involves, as Lewis (1999, p. 31) points out, finding a balance between saving an anorexic's life and damaging the patient by controlling him/her so that the future prognosis is impaired. In other words, given that there is evidence to suggest that force-feeding can make matters worse in the long run (leading to more life-threatening behaviour, even suicide – Lewis, 1999, pp. 33–34), it should not assumed that force-feeding is always in a patient's interests.

As to the law, what is in issue here are the conditions that must be satisfied before a patient can be force-fed using section 63 of the Act. These are:

1. that the patient is detained under the Act;
2. that what is proposed must count as 'medical treatment'; and
3. the treatment proposed (i.e. force-feeding) must constitute treatment for the mental disorder.

As to the first condition it is now clear – following *Riverside Health NHS Trust* v. *Fox* [1994] I FLR 614; *Re KB* [1994] 19 BMLR 144 – that 'sectioning' of anorexia nervosa patients is a reasonably common occurrence (Orbach, 1986, p. 185) and has been accepted by the Mental Health Act Commission (1997, paragraph 2.2.1). In other words, anorexia nervosa is recognized as a mental disorder under the Mental Health Act 1983.

The second condition, that what is proposed counts as medical treatment under section 145 of the Act, was decided in *B* v. *Croydon HA* [1995] (see p. 185). Here the court said that treatment included 'a range of acts ancillary to the core treatment'. As such it extended it to force-feeding.

On the final issue, it is clear following *Re KB* [1994] (above) that feeding by nasogastric tube does constitute treatment for the mental disorder of anorexia nervosa. As the judge said:

> [A]norexia nervosa is an eating disorder and relieving symptoms is just as much a part of treatment as relieving the underlying cause. If the symptoms are exacerbated by the patient's refusal to eat and drink, the mental disorder becomes progressively more and more difficult to treat and so the treatment by nasogastric tube is an integral part of the treatment of the mental disorder itself.

Note finally that, following *Tameside and Glossop Acute Services Trust* v. *CH* [1996] 1 FLR 762, it is also lawful to use reasonable force in detaining and administering treatment.

Commenting on recent cases, Mason and McCall Smith have said (1999, p. 518) that some of the reasoning in these cases may seem to lean towards sophistry. However they do 'demonstrate a judicial anxiety to save lives when that is possible and some distrust of an autonomy which allows patients to take treatment decisions in circumstances in which their competence to do so is, at least doubtful'.

To summarize, it is clear then that Jane can be treated (i.e. force-fed under section 63) regardless of her competence. Following *Re F* 1990 (p. 187) she can also be treated at common law if she is incompetent (or if she is under 18 regardless of her competence).

CASE STUDY 7.2   STERILIZING ALVA – A DISCUSSION

(Refer to the scenario presented on page 172.)

Few forms of treatment are as controversial as non-consensual sterilization, which not only interferes drastically with a woman's reproductive autonomy but also violates what many consider to be a basic human right, namely the right to reproduce (see Chapter 6). It also raises awkward questions about eugenics and whether the 'real' reason for the procedure is to prevent the patient's condition being inherited, thereby raising the spectre of the compulsory sterilization programme – usually associated with Germany in the 1930s but common in the USA well before then (Meyers, 1970).

So, what justification is there for sterilizing Alva? The principle of non-malficence, the duty to do no harm, and the paternalistic rationale that sterilization is the only effective way to ensure that Alva can lead as 'full' a life as her intellectual capacity allows are the principles that are most likely to be invoked here. In short, sterilization is in Alva's 'best interests'. Yet because sterilization – which is in practice usually an irreversible procedure – represents such a serious invasion of her right to bodily integrity and reproductive autonomy, the concept of 'best interests' (likewise the concept of 'harm') needs to be examined very carefully.

So what exactly are the 'harms' that Alva must be protected from? Typically it is claimed that women like Alva cannot cope with the complexities of contraception and despite being sexually active have no understanding of the relationship between sex and pregnancy. The pain and emotional trauma of childbirth (or an abortion) would also be too great a burden (Rumbold, 1999). Assumptions are also invariably made about their maternal instincts and ability to understand the responsibilities of parenthood. In other words, so the argument goes, it is unlikely that such women could ever care for a child yet they would be traumatized if their babies were taken away from them.

But how compelling are these arguments? In some cases it may well be that sterilization is indeed the best option. But it is all too easy to jump to this conclusion and fail to assess, for example, just how likely it is that patients like Alva will actually become pregnant. It is also important to make sure that Alva is really unable to make an informed judgement both now and in the foreseeable future, bearing in mind that the fact that she may be legally incompetent for some purposes does not mean that she is incompetent for the purposes of the sterilization. In his role as Alva's advocate Basil may be the best person to find out what Alva thinks and whether she does have an informed view about sterilization.

However, even if it is accepted that Alva could not cope with pregnancy and motherhood, these are not in themselves good enough reasons to sterilize her. If they were, then similar arguments could be applied to many other women who, although competent, may be incapable (through drink or drug abuse, for example) of being 'good' mothers. Yet few would seriously suggest that all such women should be compulsorily sterilized. Furthermore, what evidence is there that Alva would be unable to cope with contraception (given that she seems to be able to cope with menstruation)? Her intellectual mental age may be low in respect of certain functions but mental age provides very little guidance about how she could manage a whole range of other tasks. Nor does it tells us much about how Alva might develop in the future, or of her social and emotional development (Bartlett and Sandland, 2000).

Turning now to the law, it is clear that Alva's sterilization is not covered by the Mental Health Act 1983, even supposing that she was being compulsorily detained, which she is not. Nevertheless, as we know from *Re F* [1990] (see p. 187), providing the sterilization is in her 'best interests' it will be lawful (as judged on Bolam principles).

But it was another case, *Re B* [1988] AC 199, that first catapulted non-consensual sterilization into the headlines. B was a 17-year-old girl who was epileptic, subject to mood changes and at times violent and aggressive. She was said to have the intellectual ability of a 5- or 6-year-old but was showing signs of developing sexuality. She could dress and bathe herself and cope with menstruation, but was considered incapable of ever forming a long-term adult relationship or of having maternal feelings. Her carers wanted her to have greater freedom and less supervision. The House of Lords authorized her sterilization but provoked a storm of protest in so doing. The decision was described as 'Nazi-like' and, given the cursory attention paid to B's rights and the inadequacies of the best interests test, little different from neutering animals (Davies, 1998, p. 303; for other comments on the case see Fortin, 1998, p. 275, fn. 9).

One of the main concerns raised by the case was the 'proper' interpretation of the best interests test in this context, in particular whether only medical interests should be considered. Later case law has now clarified the issue – see for example, Re M [1988] 2 FLR 497 and Re P [1989] 1 FLR 182, both of which can be described as authorizing sterilization on social grounds, notably to protect the young women's lifestyles (Mason and McCall Smith, 1999, p. 101). Indeed, given that Re M concerned a girl suffering from genetically controlled fragile X syndrome, it has been claimed that it is difficult to exclude an element of eugenics from the decision (Mason, 1998, p. 84).

It is also clear, according to Practice Note: Official Solicitor: Sterilisation [1996] 2 FLR 111, that court permission would be needed to sterilize Alva. To comply with the practice note, evidence would have to be provided of her capacity, the risks of pregnancy, the consequences of pregnancy and alternatives to sterilization. Court declarations are now much more common than in the past but in practice decisions made by health professionals will usually be endorsed by the courts (see, for example Re W [1993] 1 FLR 381 and Re X [1998] 1 FLR 944 and more recently Re ZM and OS [2000] 1 FLR 523 and Re S [2000] 1 FLR 465). So if the court is persuaded that Alva is incompetent and unlikely to develop sufficiently in the foreseeable future to make an informed decision; that she is fertile and sexually active or is likely to engage in sexual activity; that she would experience 'substantial trauma or psychological damage greater than that resulting from sterilization itself'; and that there is no appropriate reversible method of contraception available; it will authorize her sterilization. On the other hand, if the court considers that the risk of pregnancy is merely speculative, then it might refuse the order (as it did in Re LC [1997] 2 FLR 258 and Re S [1998] 1 FLR 944 (see also Re A 2000 Family Law 150, a case concerning male sterilization that the court refused to authorize).

LAW and ETHICS – a comparison

Few areas of medical law and ethics bring so sharply into focus the conflict between autonomy and paternalism than the compulsory detention and treatment of those who are mentally ill. It is therefore no coincidence that the ethical principles justifying such a drastic infringement of civil liberties are similar to the principles that underpin the Mental Health Act 1983 in so far they seek to balance two potentially opposed interests. These are on the one hand the legitimate expectation that people have the right to run their own lives without interference (as long as they are not harming others) and on the other hand the state's duty to protect society at large. A similar balancing exercise has to be undertaken in order to justify compulsory treatment of those with mental handicap or learning disabilities. Although not many people would deny that such patients are entitled in principle to have their autonomy respected, it is inevitable that sometimes the only way to protect them from self-harm is to override or limit their autonomy.

Looking first, however, at the compulsory detention provisions of the Mental Health Act we see that, although it fails to resolve the difficulties of definition that concepts like mental illness continue to pose, it does, in adopting what is usually called a legalistic model (briefly this is one that places high value on the liberty of the individual and so gives less discretion to professionals), specify in some detail the criteria that must be complied with before detention is lawful (see for example, sections 2 and 3). So, even though the Act is underpinned by paternalistic concerns – i.e. the protection of the patient's own interests as well as the duty to protect those of other people – it spells out very clearly the grounds upon which detention is lawful and also provides safeguards to protect patients' interests (i.e. the Mental Health Act Commission and Mental Health Review Tribunals).

As regards the compulsory treatment provisions of the Act in part IV of the Act it is clear that, although they are again informed by similar broad ethical principles, i.e. paternalism and the duty to protect the community, the law (and the Code, which compliments it) is much more detailed and specifies strict conditions and various legal safeguards that must be complied with before non-consensual treatment can be carried out (e.g. the requirement for a second opinion). Yet despite these provisions the recent very broad interpretation of section 63 (the meaning of 'treatment for mental disorder' now covers caesareans and force-feeding for anorexia nervosa) have arguably left patients with few (if any) legal right to reject treatment they do not want. As a consequence it seems, at least in relation to section 63, that the law allows health professionals very broad discretion to act paternalistically and impose treatment whenever they think it is in the patient's best interests.

It is these best interests that justify treatment for those who lack capacity under the common law. So how does the legal and ethical approach to the treatment of people with mental handicap or learning disability compare? Both certainly rely on the concept of the patients' best interests but it seems that neither are prepared to articulate very precisely how those interests should be arrived at nor what factors should be considered in assessing them. This is so in respect of any treatment that is proposed for those who are incompetent but particularly in relation to sterilization. Here we have seen that, despite the Practice Note, the courts will usually be content to endorse decisions made by health professionals – providing they accord with a responsible body of medical opinion. This is so irrespective of whether they alone are always best placed to make such decisions. In conclusion, then, it is certainly arguable that the courts, despite the rhetoric of rights and the retreat from paternalism that *Re C* [1994] represented, now seeks as much comfort from relying on the ill-defined and indeterminate concept of 'best interests' as does the principle of paternalism.

REFERENCES

Bartlett, P. and Sandland, R. (2000) *Mental Health Law*, Blackstone Press, London.

Bowden, P. (1996) Violence and mental disorder. In: *Dangerous People*, (ed. N. Walker), Blackstone Press, London.

Campbell, T. and Heginbotham, C. (1991) *Mental Illness, Prejudice, Discrimination and the Law*, Dartmouth, Aldershot.

Cavadino, M. (1989) *Mental Health Law in Context: Doctor's Orders?*, Dartmouth, Aldershot.

Cavadino, M. (1991) Mental Illness and neo-Polonianism. *Journal of Forensic Psychiatry*, 2, 295.

Davies, M. (1998) *Medical Law*, 2nd edn, Blackstone Press, London.

Department of Health (1998) *In-patients Formally Detained in Hospitals under the Mental Health Act 1983 and Other Legislation, England: 1987–1988 to 1997–98*, Stationery Office, London.

Department of Health/Welsh Office (1999) *Mental Health Act 1983: Code of Practice*, 3rd edn, Stationery Office, London.

Dimond, B. C. (1997) *Mental Health (Patients in the Community): An Introductory Guide*, Quay Publishing, Dinton.

Dimond, B. C. and Barker, F. H. (1996) *Mental Health Law for Nurses*, Blackwell Science, Oxford.

Farrell, E. (1997) *The Complete Guide to Mental Health*, Vermilion, London.

Fegan, E. V. and Fennell, P. (1998) Feminist perspectives on mental health law. In: *Feminist Perspectives on Health Care Law*, (eds S. Sheldon and M. Thomson), Cavendish Publishing, London.

Fennell, P. (1996) *Treatment Without Consent: Law Psychiatry and the Treatment of Mentally Disordered People Since 1845*, Routledge, London.

Flannigan, C. *et al.* (1994) Inner London collaborative audit of admissions in two health districts: introduction, methods and preliminary findings. *British Journal of Psychiatry*, 165, 734.

Fletcher, N. *et al.* (1995) *Ethics, Law and Nursing*, Manchester University Press, Manchester.

Fortin, J. (1998) *Children's Rights and the Developing Law*, Butterworths, London.

Gomm, R. (1996) Reversing deviance. In: *Mental Health Matters*, (eds T. Heller *et al.*), Macmillan, Basingstoke.

Hoggett, B. (1996) *Mental Health Law*, 4th edn, Sweet & Maxwell, London.

Hurwitz, B. (1998) *Clinical Guidelines and the Law*, Radcliffe Medical Press, Abingdon.

Kennedy, I. and Grubb, I. (1994) *Medical Law: Text and Materials*, 2nd edn, Butterworths, London.

Lewis, P. (1999) Feeding anorexic patients who refuse food. *Medical Law Review*, 7(1), 21–37.

Lindley, R. (1978) Social philosophy. In: *What Philosophy Does*, (eds R. Lindley *et al.*), Open Books, London.

McHale, J. (1998) Consent to treatment II: children and the mentally ill. In: *Law and Nursing*, (eds J. McHale, J. Tingle and J. Peysner), Butterworth Heinemann, Oxford.

Mason, J. K. (1998) *Medico-legal Aspects of Reproduction and Parenthood*, 2nd edn, Dartmouth, Aldershot.

Mason, J. K. and McCall Smith, R. A. (1999) *Law and Medical Ethics*, 5th edn, Butterworths, London.

Mental Health Act Commission (1995) *Sixth Biennial Report 1993–1995*, HMSO, London.

Mental Health Act Commission (1997) *Guidance Note 3: Guidance on the Treatment of Anorexia Nervosa under the Mental Health Act 1983*, HMSO, London.

Meyers, D. W. (1970) *The Human Body and the Law*, Edinburgh University Press, Edinburgh.

Orbach, S. (1986) Hunger Strike: The anorexic's struggle as a metaphor for our age, Faber, London.

Pilgrim, D. and Rogers, A. (1993) *A Sociology of Mental Health and Illness*, Open University Press, Buckingham.

Rosenhan, D. (1996) On being sane in insane places. In: *Mental Health Matters*, (eds T. Heller *et al.*), Macmillan, Basingstoke.

Rumbold, G. (1999) *Ethics in Nursing Practice*, 3rd edn, Baillière Tindall, London.

Scheff, T. (1966) *Being Mentally Ill: a Sociological Theory*, Aldine Press, Chicago, IL.

Stauch, M. and Wheat, K., with Tingle, J. (1998) *Sourcebook on Medical Law*, Cavendish Publishing, London.

Szasz, T. (1970) *Ideology and Insanity: Essays on the Psychiatric Dehumanisation of Man*, Doubleday, Garden City.

UKCC (1998) *Guidelines for Mental Health and Learning Disabilities Nursing*, United Kingdom Central Council, London.

Widdett, C. and Thompson, M. (1997) Justifying treatment and other stories. *Feminist Legal Studies*, 5, 84.

FURTHER READING

Freeman, M. (1988) Sterilising the mentally handicapped. In: *Medicine, Ethics and the Law*, (ed. M. Freeman), Stevens, London.

8 RESEARCH

INTRODUCTION

There can be few people who are not aware of the Nazi eugenics programme of the 1930s and 1940s during which physicians and scientists willingly sterilized nearly 400 000 mentally handicapped and other 'genetically unfit' people. So called 'mercy deaths', including 'euthanasia by starvation' and gassing of those considered 'racially impure' were also routinely carried out at mental hospitals. Equally infamous were the medical experiments carried out on concentration camp inmates and other 'valueless' persons. Camp doctors used inmates to test the limits of human endurance and wholly experimental gynaecological operations were carried out on female victims, usually without any form of anaesthesia. These caused immense pain and suffering, disability and often death. They also provided very little useful scientific knowledge.

It was perhaps not surprising, therefore, that once details became widely known – 20 doctors were tried at Nuremberg for crimes against humanity and four were hanged – a determined attempt was made to ensure that such perversions would never again be repeated (Tusa and Tusa,1983). Thus it was that the most famous and earliest international code on the ethics of research, the Nuremberg code, was drawn up in 1949. Yet the Nuremberg code (and subsequent international and national guidelines) have not eliminated unethical research altogether and in the postwar period whistleblowers such as M. H. Pappworth (1967) in the UK and H. K. Beecher (1966) in the USA have exposed how the systematic violation of the rights of research subjects is not a relic of the past (Brody, 1998). One of the most shocking scandals was the American Tuskegee study involving 400 poor black sharecroppers. The study began in 1932 and lasted 40 years. It was designed to test the degenerative effects of untreated syphilis but was continued long after effective treatments had become available. Although some subjects in the study had consented to participate, many were not even aware that they were involved in the research. Most, however, were discouraged from receiving any treatment and 100 men died (Brody, 1998, p. 33).

Although the most infamous examples of unethical research have involved doctors there is evidence that nurses were involved, not just because they were aware of the research but also because they identified potential research subjects, collected information and so on. It is thus important that nurses are aware of the legal and ethical issues raised by research, especially now that research has become a recognized part of nursing that many nurses incorporate in their daily practice. What then are the aims of nursing research and how may nurses become involved?

It has been suggested that the aims of nursing research are twofold (de Raeve, 1997, p. 139):

- to understand what nursing is;
- to promote good nursing care and understand failures of practice.

As to nurses' involvement, this can take many forms. They can, for example, be undertaking research themselves or be practising in settings where research is to be carried out. Alternatively, they may be in positions of authority where research is to be carried out or be supervising research. (For other research contexts involving nurses and key texts on nursing research see RCN, 1998, section 2 and appendix 5.) But irrespective of how nurses are involved they must practise within an ethical framework and follow the law. This may sometimes – as the following case studies reveal – pose several dilemmas.

CASE STUDY 8.1 | Is Jessica's consent valid?

Jessica is 17 years old. Her baby, Dan, was nearly 8 weeks premature and was delivered by caesarean section. Just as Jessica was coming round from the anaesthetic she was told that Dan was suffering from several congenital deformities and was also likely to suffer serious and irreversible brain damage. There was a chance, however, that his prognosis, which was currently very poor – at most he might live a few months – could be improved if he received an new operation. Jessica was given details of the new procedure, including information about its expected benefits. Little, however, was said about its possible side-effects, in particular that the treatment was more painful than conventional treatment. She was also told that although she was under no obligation to agree to participate, if she did agree she must make her mind up very quickly as surgery had to be carried out by the end of the week.

Jessica agrees to volunteer Dan for the research but the following day she tells Kate, a paediatric nurse, that she is not sure that she has made the right decision. She is also convinced she was never told that the new treatment would be more painful, or at least does not remember.

Kate believes that Jessica was not given enough information and doubts therefore that her consent is valid. What should she do? She is also concerned as to whether it is legally and ethically justifiable to involve Dan in the research.

CASE STUDY 8.2 What role does Valerie have?

Emile is 65 years old and suffers from Alzheimer's disease. The disease has advanced so far that soon Valerie, his wife, will be unable to look after him at home. Last week she was told that it would be a good idea to involve Emile in a research project into the organic manifestations of Alzheimer's disease – a project that would involve continuous testing of Emile's blood and bodily functions. Valerie supports the research but is reluctant to give her consent because of Emile's fear of needles.

Is the research morally and legally justified? Does Valerie have right to decide whether her husband should participate in the research?

CASE STUDY 8.3   MICHAEL'S CONSENT TO A DRUG TRIAL

Michael has been diagnosed with a neurological disorder that is making it increasingly difficult for him to walk. Although drug treatment is currently available, it is not very effective and a randomized controlled drug trial has been set up. Michael is very keen to be involved and has made it very clear that he wants to try the new drug. Pamela, a nurse who is part of the multidisciplinary research team, is aware of his preferences but is so convinced of the merits of the research that she does not fully explain the nature of a randomized controlled trial, leaving Michael with the impression that he will receive the new drug.

What legal and ethical issues does the randomized controlled trial raise?

TYPES OF RESEARCH

Traditionally two distinct types of research have been recognized: therapeutic and non-therapeutic research. Therapeutic research aims to benefit patients by using new methods or procedures, such as, for example, a new operation that is more likely to cure their disease or improve their condition. It combines research with the care and treatment of patients. In contrast, the principal aim of non-therapeutic research is to gain scientific knowledge. Often it involves testing new drugs but whatever form it takes it is unlikely to confer any benefit, unless very long delayed, on the research subjects, who may well be healthy volunteers or existing patients. It may nevertheless provide knowledge that will ultimately benefit other individuals or society as a whole (Mason and McCall Smith, 1999).

The distinction between therapeutic and non-therapeutic research has been questioned in recent years largely because technological advances make it increasingly difficult to distinguish between research – which can be broadly defined as a systematic course of scientific enquiry – and innovative treatment, which is arguably a much more speculative process (Fox, 1998). Note too Smith's point (1999, p. 9) that the fact that a treatment is new or different or has not been properly tested before does not automatically make it research. It only becomes research if, in the words of the Declaration of Helsinki, it is 'formulated in an experimental protocol' and compared in a formal way with other treatments or with no treatment, or if a careful assessment is made of its safety and value to patients.

But even though distinctions can be blurred it is useful to retain the traditional distinction here for several reasons. First, almost all the ethical guidelines and codes covering do so. Second, it is crucial in weighing the risks and benefits of a particular project. Third, the nature of the research can determine the amount of information that has to be disclosed.

Finally it is worth noting another common classification, notably between invasive and non-invasive research. Invasive research is essentially any activity that involves bodily contact, ranging from simple procedures such as taking blood to much more high-risk ones like biopsies. Non-invasive research does not involve any bodily contact and so includes activities such as conducting surveys, observation, researching into medical records and so on. Unsurprisingly, non-invasive research is likely to raise fewer legal and ethical concerns, largely because it is only likely to carry minimal risk. It may, however, raise issues of confidentiality and privacy.

ETHICAL PRINCIPLES

The 1996 UKCC guidelines for professional practice identify several criteria that must be met for research to be 'safe and ethical'. These focus (among other things) on consent, confidentiality and not exposing patients to unacceptable risks (clauses 91–93). More detailed guidance on research ethics from the RCN in 1998 echoes these criteria and also emphasizes the main ethical principles underpinning research: beneficence; non-malficence, autonomy and justice (Evans and Evans, 1996). Although these have been discussed in previous chapters, in the context of research different aspects need to be emphasized.

The principles of beneficence and non-malficence require nurses not just to promote and safeguard the well-being and interests of research participants, in other words to try to do good, but also to try to avoid doing harm. But what are the practical implications of these principles?

First, participants should be protected from harm. In research contexts this is clearly problematic because almost all research carries some risk of harm, however minor. Harm can take many forms, both physical and psychological. Physical harm can include temporary inconvenience or discomfort or involve more permanent injury or disability. Just as damaging is the psychological harm that may result from some research – into sensitive subjects like child abuse or domestic violence, for example. Sometimes the cost of research can be financial – loss of income, for example – or can be more difficult to estimate, such as when it involves loss of privacy or time. Note too that the assessment of harm includes estimating not just the what the harms might be but also how severe and how likely they are to occur. But however harm is defined or estimated there can be little doubt that the principle of non-malficence makes it very difficult, if not impossible, to justify ever using human research subjects, for the simple reason that any intervention, however small, risks generating some harm. On the other hand, failure to carry out any research at all clearly contravenes the principle of beneficence, in so far as patients and society will be denied the knowledge and understanding gained through research.

The second issue, then, is to establish what those potential benefits are. That these are difficult to assess is widely acknowledged (Smith, 1999, p. 96). For patients involved in therapeutic research, benefits – which may be medical, emotional or social – may include improving their physical condition or quality of life or relieving their symptoms. However, often the precise degree and probability of benefit can be hard to predict. Moreover, in many cases the benefits may only become apparent long after the research has been completed and so are unlikely to lead to immediate changes in practice. As to the benefits of non-therapeutic research, these too can be very long delayed and for the participants may only consist of the satisfaction of knowing that they have contributed to the advance of medical knowledge. More controversial is whether research aimed at saving money – which involves cost–benefit analyses – is ethical (see Smith, 1999, pp. 98–101).

Given the inherent conflict between the principles of non-malficence and beneficence it is self-evident that a balancing exercise has to be carried out, in which the risks and potential benefits of research are assessed. This is an exercise that should ensure that any risk of harm is in proportion to the probable benefits (Veatch and Fry, 1987). The concept of risk can be defined in several ways but commonly a distinction is made between minimal and less than minimal risk (Royal College of Physicians, 1990). Thus, risk is minimal if it involves risk of injury or death that is no greater than that encountered in everyday life. This is the only kind of risk to which it is generally agreed that healthy volunteers should be exposed (Smith, 1999, p. 91). An example of an activity involving minimal risk is giving a sample of urine (Mason and McCall Smith (1999, p. 454). Note, of course, that in discussing risk a distinction should be made between adverse events, of which there is a high risk but only minor consequences, and serious adverse events, of which there is a low risk with devastating consequences. As to the potential benefits in the risk/benefit exercise, these, as was noted above, can range from, for example, major improvements in the participant's health and well-being to relatively minor ones. But once they have been assessed the crucial question is: Are the potential benefits from the research sufficient to justify the remaining risks? (See Evans, 1993 for a discussion of the problems of balancing risks and benefits.)

Another important principle is respect for autonomy and the right that individuals have to be treated as self-governing agents capable of making their own decisions according to their own aims and values. Having the right of self-determination means that individuals should be participants in research rather than subjects and so must have the right to decide freely whether to participate or not. They must also have the right to withdraw from the study at any time. In other words, consent to research must be voluntary and free from duress or coercion, implicit or explicit. Care must be taken too to ensure that existing patients are not 'persuaded' to take part in research for fear of reprisals if they refuse, i.e. that their care and treatment may be compromised or that they will be discriminated against in some way.

To make free and rational choices about research, participants also, of course, need to have adequate information on which to base their decisions. They have the right, in short, to be 'informed participants' (see below). The principle of respect for autonomy also means protecting those who because of their youth or mental disability or serious illness are unable to make decisions for themselves. And finally it is worth noting that autonomy raises questions about privacy, in particular the right to confidentiality and anonymity. As the RCN guidelines point out (1998, p. 9), individuals have a right to control access to information about themselves.

The remaining principle, that of justice, is about fairness. In this context it focuses on the selection of participants – in other words making sure that the risks and benefits of research are as fairly distributed as possible so that no particular individual or group is discriminated against or benefits overwhelmingly from the research (Capron, 1997). Applying this principle should ensure that vulnerable and disadvantaged groups – such as the poor and institutionalized – are not selected just because they may be easier, cheaper or simply more convenient to use. Rather, researchers should select participants for reasons directly related to the study in question. Justice in research is not, however, confined to the selection of subjects, since it also requires researchers not to neglect their everyday duties and responsibilities and to treat participants fairly during and after the research has ended by, for example, making sure they have access to professional support and assistance should harmful side-effects occur (Singleton and McLaren, 1995).

ETHICAL CODES AND PROFESSIONAL GUIDELINES

The Nuremberg code (1949) is undoubtedly the most famous international code. Although not as original as is sometimes suggested – the code was partly based on earlier German codes of research ethics – the 10 basic principles it articulated have been very influential (Brody, 1998, p. 33). The code was later supplemented by the Declaration of Helsinki, which was first drawn up in 1964 but has been revised several times since then, most recently in 1996. The modifications made by the Declaration were threefold.

- It introduced a conceptual distinction between therapeutic and non-therapeutic research.
- It advocated the establishment of institutional mechanisms, namely independent committees, to oversee and review research protocols.
- It made express reference to proxy consent by family members when participants in research were incompetent.

Professional guidelines are also a fruitful source of guidance on research. These have been issued by the Royal College of Physicians (1990, 1996); the International Council of Nurses (1996); the British Paediatric Association (1992); the Medical Research Council (MRC, 1991a, b, 1992) and the Royal College of Nursing (RCN, 1998).

The RCN guidelines are designed to help nurses ensure 'that research, from the planning and commissioning stage to the dissemination and utilization of findings, is conducted in an ethically acceptable way, consistent with current statutory ethical guidelines' (1998, p. 11). They apply to nurses undertaking research themselves, whether as principal investigator, as a research student or as a member of a research team.

Three broad areas are emphasized in the guidelines. The first, which deals with the integrity of the researcher, stresses that nurses must possess relevant knowledge and skills compatible with their involvement in the proposed investigation. Other provisions require them to: recognize and make known personal prejudices, biases or conflicts; ensure that arrangements for data management will protect confidentiality; publish or otherwise make available the results of research; and promote the appropriate use of their research findings.

The second section focuses on responsibilities owed to research participants and begins by emphasizing that researchers must be satisfied that the knowledge that is being sought is not already available and could not be acquired equally well by other means. It also reminds researchers that in all studies involving NHS patients or clients the approval of the local research ethics committee (LREC) must be sought (see below). Other provisions focus on confidentiality and also stress that there must be identifiable safeguards to protect participants from harm and that consent must be informed and given freely. The final section focuses on relations with sponsors, employers and colleagues and covers (among other things) issues of competence, resources and the conditions under which research is carried out.

It seems then that there is no shortage of ethical codes and professional guidelines to guide practice. But what is their effect; in particular, do they have legal force? The brief answer is no. This means that breach of the guidelines and/or codes will not automatically give rise to any civil or criminal liability. Nevertheless, they are universally considered as very strong evidence of 'best practice'. Accordingly, any failure to comply with them could result in disciplinary proceedings. Furthermore, should a subject claim compensation for injuries arising from research, it would be difficult for researchers to avoid a negligence claim unless they had a convincing reason for breaching them. In other words, the guidelines are very likely to set the legal standard against which the conduct of research would be judged. This is perhaps why such guidance is often described as 'quasi-law'. These are rules that are not legally binding, although they have some legal force and will in practice determine how people act (Montgomery, 1997, p. 12; for further discussion of the impact of codes and professional guidelines see Hurwitz, 1998).

RESEARCH ETHICS COMMITTEES

Although research ethics committees were first set up in the late 1960s – largely as a response to initiatives by the Royal College of Physicians and the Ministry of Health – it was not until 1991 that more comprehensive government guidelines were issued by the Department of Health (HSG(91)5). These reaffirmed the need for independent review but as before left the responsibility for regulating research to local research ethics committee (LRECs). The guidelines (which were supplemented in 1994 by further guidance on how to ensure that LRECs operated properly in scrutinizing proposals) are fairly detailed and include provisions about working procedures, legal liability and membership. Thus it is recommended that an LREC should have eight to 12 members drawn from both sexes and a wide range of groups such as hospital medical staff, nursing staff (with day-to-day contact with patients in the community or on the wards), GPs and two or more lay persons.

The most important function of an LREC is to advise health service bodies on the ethical acceptability of research proposals taking place within the NHS that involve human subjects. To do this effectively the following matters are expected to be considered:

- the scientific merit of the proposal;
- how the health of the research participants will be affected;
- what distress or discomfort is foreseen;
- whether the investigator is suitably qualified and experienced;
- whether proper procedures for obtaining consent and for monitoring the research are in place;
- whether an information sheet has been prepared (Montgomery, 1997, p. 338).

Once the guidelines had been issued there was an expectation that even although there was still no formal legal obligation to establish LRECs, their practice and procedures would become more formalized, uniform and consistent. But this did not happen. Certainly, LRECs have proliferated in recent years (as has their workload – Nicholson, 1997) but their effectiveness remains questionable. One of the most fundamental problems is that, in the absence of any clear definition of what constitutes an effective research committee, practices vary widely (Neuberger, 1992). The diversity and independence of LRECs – often fiercely defended – also mean that generally they operate in isolation from each other with little or no coordination or formal central or legal framework. There also seems to be little attempt to ensure that research is adequately monitored after initial approval has been given – a significant failing given that most committees approve over 90% of proposals (Fox, 1998). Notable too is that LRECs have no authority to take legal action against researchers who repeatedly violate the terms of approval.

Some of these weaknesses could be eliminated by establishing and maintaining a minimum standard of practice – which could, for example, specify when the committee should meet and what method it should adopt to scrutinize proposals. Other improvements that have been suggested include the establishment of a recognized forum, such as an association, that would improve communication between committees and ensure that new developments in research and their implications for practice could be discussed and debated (Foster, 1993).

Yet even without these improvements there is little doubt that ethics committees have had a major positive impact on the conduct of research in recent years, especially through their insistence on the provision of full and clear information to subjects. Thus, as Foster notes (1993, p. 167), whereas in the past it was common to subsume the needs of a few patients to the good of many future patients it now seems that there has been a discernible shift to a more

Kantian approach – in which any use of people 'merely as a means' is considered unacceptable. Moreover, in the process of assessing and reflecting on ethical practice LRECs have unquestionably encouraged wider public debate on many sensitive issues of research, albeit not always on every 'moral' aspect of research, e.g. aspects that might be considered more spiritual (Smith, 1999, p, 38).

Before concluding it is important to note the latest guidelines issued by the Department of Health (1997; HSG(97)23), which authorize the setting up of multicentre research ethics committees (MRECs). Research is regarded as multi-centre if it is carried out within the geographical boundaries of five or more LRECs. Before the setting up of MRECs large-scale research required approval by the research committee in each area where it was to be carried out. But given the independence and diversity of LRECs this was not necessarily forthcoming. Now, however, once MREC approval has been obtained local committees will still have the opportunity to reject the proposal for local reasons (although they may need to seek amendments that have a purely local application and do not affect the integrity of the proposal).

LEGAL REGULATION OF RESEARCH

Unlike research on animals, which has long been regulated by legislation (first by the Cruelty to Animals Act 1876 but now by the Animals (Scientific Procedures) Act 1986), there is no specific legislation regulating research on humans. The absence of any statutory control may seem surprising but is not difficult to explain. First, as we have seen, many professional and government guidelines have been published in recent years, which, although not imposing any legal obligations nonetheless do have persuasive quasi-legal authority. Second, almost all NHS districts have established LRECs. While these have no statutory backing or any other legal basis they have undoubtedly positively influenced practice.

Yet the most likely reason for the lack of legislation is the assumption that the common law provides sufficient protection for research subjects both from unethical researchers and from those who are negligent. Whether or not the common law does in practice provide sufficient safeguards is, however, far from certain as it is the law of consent that provides the main protective mechanism. (Contract law and the criminal law also have a role, albeit a less significant one, see Dyer, 1992). However, as was noted in Chapter 2, reliance on common law principles of consent is unlikely to guarantee either that subjects' consent will always be genuinely 'free' or that it will be always be 'informed'. The question then arises: If the common law fails to adequately protect patients when they make treatment decisions, how can it be effective in research contexts? In other words, the difficulties that patients typically face in giving or withholding consent in treatment contexts are likely to be repeated, albeit in different ways, when they decide whether or not to participate in research. This is borne out by almost all documented cases of abusive research, in which failure to use adequate consent procedures is the main complaint.

Before looking at those aspects of consent, notably competence and the disclosure of information, that pose special problems in research contexts, the main legal consequences of acting without consent need to be outlined. Briefly these are as follows. If no consent at all is obtained then a researcher could face criminal charges and a civil action for trespass – assuming, of course, that the research involved some kind of physical contact. More likely, however, is a claim by a participant that, although consent was given, it was flawed in some respect – the most likely contention being that it was based on insufficient information. In such cases a negligence action would have to be brought (see Chapters 2 and 3).

Competency

Adults

There seems little doubt – despite the suggestion that a more sophisticated level of understanding or comprehension ought to be required – that the test for competency that applies in respect of medical treatment applies equally to research, both therapeutic or non-therapeutic. In other words, in the absence of evidence to the contrary, the law presumes that adult subjects are competent. As was noted in Chapter 2 the legal test for competency is now a three-stage one (see *Re C* [1994] 1 All ER 819): the subject must be capable of comprehending and retaining information; of believing it; and of weighing up the information. When the research is therapeutic it will, of course, be necessary to take into account factors such as pain, drugs and so forth in so far as they may, albeit temporarily, affect capacity. Note too that in non-therapeutic research the third element of the capacity test will involve balancing the risks not with needs but with other factors, e.g. financial benefits or the satisfaction of contributing to the advance of scientific knowledge.

Children

The assessment of competence in children is more problematic than with adults. There are several reasons for this. The main problem as regards 16- and 17-year-olds is that it is doubtful that the Family Law Reform Act 1969 applies in research contexts. This is because the Act makes their consent lawful (if they are competent) in respect of 'surgical, medical or dental treatment'. Thus it is only if these statutory words are very broadly interpreted to include research that the Act applies at all. And even if it did – which most legal texts doubt – it certainly would not extend to non-therapeutic research.

To be on the safe side, therefore, it is recommended that legal authority for giving consent be found elsewhere, namely the common law. In other words, the 'Gillick test' (see Chapter 2) must be relied on. However in the absence of any English case on whether 'Gillick competency' does actually apply to research it can only be assumed that it does. Also uncertain is the degree of understanding and maturity that young people must posses in research contexts. There is an argument, which is especially strong if the research is non-therapeutic but also arguably even when it is therapeutic, that a higher level of understanding and maturity should be required than is necessary for medical treatment (Hendrick, 1997). Until this is decided in the courts, it is safe to assume that 16- and 17-year-olds can be considered legally competent if they understand the nature and purpose of the research. As such they will be expected to appreciate how the research may benefit them (if at all), what will happen if they agree to participate and, of course, the risks they face.

But what if a Gillick-competent 16- or-17-year-old refuses to participate? In such cases researchers would be ill-advised to rely solely on parental consent but should respect the minor's refusal. Finally, it should be noted that there may be some circumstances, e.g. where there is doubt about competency, when it is wise to get parallel consent from a parent (subject to the minor's prior permission for parents to be informed).

Let us turn now to young people under 16. There is little doubt now that, providing they are Gillick-competent, they can independently consent to participate in research. That said, the more invasive the research the more difficult it will be to reach the required level of maturity and understanding, especially if the research is non-therapeutic and so is unlikely to provide any benefit. It is perhaps because the Gillick test is so difficult to apply uniformly that most of the professional guidelines (likewise Department of Health guidance) recommend complementing children's consent with that of their parents. Note finally that, as with competent 16- and-17-year-olds the refusal of Gillick-competent under-16-year-olds to participate in research should be respected.

As to children who are not Gillick-competent, consent must be obtained from a proxy – usually a parent, anyone else with parental responsibility or a court. A proxy's power to consent is fairly extensive but is not limitless. The limitations will depend on whether the research is therapeutic or non-therapeutic. If it is therapeutic the guiding principle is that proxy consent will be lawful if it is in the child's 'best interests'. Regrettably, however, there is no authoritative legal guidance of the meaning of 'best interests' in research contexts (Brock, 1994). Clearly, however, the concept is not limited to physical benefits but can include psychological, emotional and even financial benefits. But despite the uncertain scope of the term it is widely accepted that it includes any research in which the benefits outweigh the possible risks of harm. No problem arises, therefore if the potential risks are very small. And it may even be lawful to expose a child to more significant risks if the child's condition merits it. It is also worth noting here that, although not legally required, most professional guidelines recommend that researchers should nevertheless obtain the child's assent or agreement. Assent means getting the child's permission. Obviously it does not have the legal force of consent and so can be obtained at a much younger age. If the child refuses to participate, the research is still lawful but whether researchers would ignore a child's views is another matter.

As regards non-therapeutic research, the legal limits imposed on a proxy's consent are uncertain. In the absence of any case law on this issue, two alternative solutions are usually proposed. One is to fall back on the familiar 'best interests' test. However, in this context it is unhelpful, given that research that is likely to benefit a child only indirectly (or will provide no benefit at all) is almost certainly not in the child's best interests, especially if it carries some risk. The other solution is to adopt a broader, less restrictive interpretation of a proxy's duty, namely that consent can be given for any research that is not against the child's interests (Hendrick, 1997). This lower standard is widely accepted – in most legal texts and professional guidelines – but has yet to be tested in the courts. What is means is that a child can lawfully be volunteered for research that carries no greater risks than the risks that reasonable parents commonly expose their children to in ordinary life – or, to put it another way, minimal risk (such as non-invasive physiological monitoring).

Incompetent adults

Research involving incompetent adults is legally problematic because English law does not authorize a proxy system whereby consent can be given on their behalf (unlike children, whose parents can usually act as a proxy, *Re T* [1992] 4 All ER 649). This raises the question as to when, if at all, incompetent adults can be volunteered for research. As yet, no English court has had to decide this specific point. Nonetheless, most legal texts assume that, providing the research is therapeutic, incompetent adults can be involved. The legal authority for this assumption is *Re F* [1990] 2 AC 1, see Chapter 7). Although the case concerned sterilization rather than research, the principle it established – that medical treatment is lawful providing it is carried out in accordance with a responsible body of relevant professional opinion and is in the best interests of the patient – can be extended to therapeutic research. This is because 'best interests' were defined in *Re F* by Lord Brandon as treatment carried out 'either in order to save their lives or in order to ensure improvement/prevent deterioration in their physical/mental health'. In so far as therapeutic research is intended to benefit patients it arguably would be in the participants' best interests even though it may carry some risks. Similarly the Department of Health guidance (1991), despite stressing how research on mentally disordered people requires particular care, does not rule it out because of the 'need to advance knowledge so people with mental disorder may benefit'.

It is also worth noting here guidelines issued by the MRC (1991b) on the ethical conduct of research on the mentally handicapped. These state that, provided the necessary safeguards are in place, the ethical grounds for including mentally incapacitated people in therapeutic research are so compelling that it would be contrary to accepted practice to be deterred by the comparative lack of clarity surrounding the legal position.

Most commentators doubt, however, that even though the *Re F* best interests test has been interpreted very broadly in recent years, it is wide enough to justify non-therapeutic research on incompetent adults (see, for example, McHale, 1998, p. 128; Montgomery, 1997, p. 350). Until such time as the issue is decided it is therefore prudent to seek the court's permission before undertaking such research. In the meantime, the observations of the Law Commission are worth noting (especially as the government has indicated that the many of its recommendations will be incorporated into legislation). In its report (Law Commission, 1995) it recommended that it was justifiable to involve participants who could not consent in non-therapeutic research provided certain conditions were satisfied. These included the establishment of a special committee, the Mental Incapacity Research Committee, which would have to approve the research. Other criteria were that:

- knowledge of the cause or treatment or care of people affected by the incapacitating condition was desirable;
- the research related to the condition from which the patient suffered;
- the object of the research could not be effectively achieved without involving those who could not consent;
- the procedures involved no more than negligible risk and were not unduly restrictive or invasive.

Information disclosure

As we saw in Chapter 2 the question of how much information the law requires health professionals to disclose is controversial. In research contexts it is, not surprisingly, an even more controversial issue. This is because, despite widespread expectation that the law should adopt a higher standard of disclosure, this has yet to be confirmed by the courts. As a consequence there is some uncertainty as to whether health professionals are legally obliged to disclose more information when obtaining consent to research than when obtaining consent to medical treatment. In other words, is consent only valid in relation to research if it is fully informed?

In the absence of any English case concerning either the amount or content of information that the law requires to be disclosed in research contexts, no definitive answer can be given to this question. An additional complication is whether the courts would distinguish between therapeutic and non-therapeutic research. Since non-therapeutic research is unlikely to confer any direct benefit on participants (or if it does do so it is likely to be long-delayed), there is certainly a strong argument that they are entitled to receive more information (McHale, 1998, p. 125). In other words, the law should impose a broader duty of disclosure and require researchers to provide a full explanation.

Notwithstanding the uncertainty of the law, many legal texts assume that if faced with deciding on the appropriate standard of disclosure the courts would probably opt for an 'informed consent' approach (sometimes called 'a duty of candour'; see, for example, Mason and McCall Smith, 1999). Indeed for the courts to do otherwise would mean ignoring all the current guidance available to researchers and thus what is considered 'accepted or responsible practice'.

But what does this mean in practical terms, given that it is widely agreed that a patient's consent must be based on four main lines of explanation? These are:

- the purpose of the research;
- the benefits to the patient and society;
- the risks involved;

- the alternatives open to the participant (Mason and McCall Smith, 1999, p. 463).

In relation to therapeutic research it means making 'full and frank' disclosure – a process that involves not just providing information (as outlined above) but also providing opportunities for questions to be asked (which should be answered fully and truthfully). Note too that patients should be told that the research is being combined with their care and treatment (which means explaining the difference between therapy and research and the meaning of relevant research terms). As to the risks involved, there is a strong argument that a pro-patient subjective test should be the legal standard of disclosure. This would require all material risks to be disclosed, i.e. those that the particular participant volunteering for the research would wish to be informed about, bearing in mind that, because the research has a treatment component it would be lawful to withhold information that might adversely affect the patient (therapeutic privilege). Beyond that, subjects should be told of any other significant consequence of the research. This would include anything that is necessary for them to make an informed decisions, e.g. that they might have to stay in hospital longer or return more frequently for check-ups. Finally, it is almost certain that the courts would endorse the Department of Health guidelines (1991) and require that in the majority of cases an information sheet be provided (which the patient should keep) and that consent be written.

As regards non-therapeutic research, it is widely accepted that full and frank disclosure imposes an even greater legal obligation on health professionals to provide information. This would require researchers not only to provide all the information that they would normally provide in relation to therapeutic research but would also require them to reveal all the risks that the actual participant would want to know. This high standard of disclosure has yet to be confirmed by the courts. Nevertheless, there is persuasive authority for such an approach from the Canadian case of *Halushka* v. *University of Saskatchewan* (1965) 52 WWR 608, in which the court said: 'there can be no exceptions to the ordinary requirements of disclosure in the case of [non-therapeutic] research as there may well be in ordinary medical practice'.

CASE STUDY 8.1   JESSICA'S CONSENT – A DISCUSSION

(Refer to the scenario presented on page 197.)

The main issues raised by this case study are whether Jessica was given adequate information about the therapeutic research and whether her consent was truly voluntary. It also raises questions about the circumstances in which consent on behalf of a minor is valid.

For Jessica's consent (as a proxy) to be informed – which all the ethical guidelines on research either explicitly or implicitly advocate – researchers are expected to provide her with enough information (normally via an information sheet) to enable her to make a reasoned judgement about whether or not to participate. According to the RCN guidance (1998, appendix 3) this includes explaining as fully as possible, in terms meaningful to Jessica:

- the purpose of the study;
- the names and positions of the people who will be carrying out the study;
- the nature of any intervention that will be carried out;
- any risks involved or side-effects that could occur;
- any cost and/or time commitments involved; and
- those from whom further information can be obtained if required.

Note also a user-friendly leaflet produced by CERES (Consumers for Ethics in Research, 1993), which aims to encourage debate about research. Written in a jargon-free style it asks the kinds of question participants typically ask, such as: What will happen to me? What will happen if I say no? and, Do I have to decide at once?

So, has Jessica being properly informed in a way that conforms with the various ethical codes and guidelines? Although she is consenting on her baby's behalf there is no reason to believe that this should have any impact on the nature or amount of information she should be given or on the consent process itself. Yet, although Jessica may well have been told about the purpose of the study and its benefits, some very important information has been omitted, notably the potential side-effects of the new procedure, in particular that it is more painful than conventional treatment. Arguably, then, Jessica's consent was not informed. This is because, even although there is no consensus on which risks and side-effects should be disclosed (Smith, 1999, p. 89), it is doubtful that failure to reveal the known side-effect of pain would be morally justifiable.

Furthermore, no information sheet was provided and consent was not given in writing, which the RCN guidelines (1998) require (as do almost all other ethical guidelines). Other questionable aspects include the fact that Jessica may have been subjected to unacceptable types of persuasion (e.g. fear of giving offence and so on, see Smith, 1999, pp. 64–70).

As to the legal validity of Jessica's consent, although there is no requirement for it to be in writing it should be 'informed'. Given that she did not know of the increased pain, this is therefore doubtful. Legally too there are doubts about whether Jessica's consent is voluntary. To be so it must be free from coercion. Yet she has been put under considerable pressure to volunteer Dan for the research. Not only had she just come round from surgery and an anaesthetic – which raises questions about her competency to consent – but she was given very little time to reflect on her decision, being 'persuaded' instead to make up her mind very quickly. Being pressured to make a quick decision also contravenes the RCN guidelines (1998). That being so, the law would question whether 'good' practice had been followed – unless, of course an immediate decision was necessary because treatment had to be initiated promptly.

But Jessica's consent is that of a proxy. As Dan's mother she is entitled to give consent on his behalf. According to the MRC and British Paediatric Association guidelines (MRC, 1991a; British Paediatric Association, 1992), therapeutic research involving children who cannot consent is only ethical if it is in their best interests and if certain principles are observed. These are:

- that the relevant information cannot be gained by comparable research on adults;
- that all proposals are submitted to an approved LREC;
- that legally valid consent is obtained from the appropriate person (and that those included do not appear to object in either words or actions); and
- that the benefits should outweigh the possible risk of harm (note that if the research is non-therapeutic then it is ethical only if it exposes children to no more than a negligible risk of harm).

The legal position is much the same – that it would be lawful to volunteer Dan for research and rely on Jessica's consent providing that the research is in his best interests. Although this concept has not been interpreted by the courts it is widely accepted as including any research in which the benefits outweigh the risks.

Finally there is the question of what Kate should do. According to the RCN guidelines (1998, p. 21), nurses practising where research is undertaken should act as witnesses that informed consent has been given. In this capacity Kate's doubts are certainly well-founded, given that Jessica's proxy consent was arguably neither informed nor voluntary. So, what should she do? The guidelines recommend that in such cases the nurse should convey her anxieties to the researcher and/or the appropriate person in authority (RCN, 1998, p. 22). Legally too there is a question as to whether Kate may have a duty to intervene. No case has yet decided what duty is owed (if any) in such circumstances but at the very least Kate would be expected to report her concerns to an appropriate person.

CASE STUDY 8.2	INVOLVING EMILE IN RESEARCH AND VALERIE'S ROLE – A DISCUSSION

(Refer to the scenario presented on page 197.)

Two major issues are relevant here: one focuses on whether Emile's participation in the research – which is non-therapeutic – is ethically and legally justified and the other on Valerie's role, in particular what rights she has to act on her husband's behalf. The first thing to establish, however, is whether or not Emile is competent to make a decision. According to MRC guidelines (1991b), many people with mental impairment or disorder will be capable of giving or withholding consent. Similarly, the Department of Health guidance (1991) states that the presence of mental disorder does not by itself imply incapacity. Nevertheless, given the advanced state of Emile's disease, it is probable that he is incapable of understanding the nature of the proposed research and thus cannot give his consent.

This then raises the question as to whether he can be involved in research to which he has not consented. That this is ethically acceptable is acknowledged in the

Department of Health guidelines, although they do state that such research 'will need particularly careful consideration in terms of the balance of benefits, discomforts and risks for the individual patient and the need to advance knowledge so that people with mental disorder may benefit'. The MRC guidelines also support including those unable to consent in non-therapeutic research, claiming in fact 'that there is a strong ethical case' for so doing providing that certain safeguards are observed. These are:

- that the research should relate to their condition;
- that the relevant knowledge cannot be gained by research in persons able to consent;
- that all projects must be approved by the appropriate LREC(s);
- that an informed, independent person must agree that the individual's welfare and interests have been properly safeguarded;
- that those included in the research do not object or appear to object in either words or actions; and
- that those included are placed at no more than negligible risk (defined as not greater, considering the probability and magnitude of physiological or psychological harm or discomfort, than those ordinarily encountered in daily life or during the performance of routine physical or psychological examination or tests such as obtaining blood and urine samples).

It would seem therefore that it would be ethically justifiable to include Emile in the research, providing his fear of blood tests would not result in the risk (to him) being more than minimal. Indeed the Alzheimer's Disease Society (1993) positively encourages such research, arguing that progress in finding the causes and developing new approaches to treatment will only be possible so long as people with the condition and their relatives and carers are willing to participate in research.

As to the legal position, this is more uncertain because it is difficult to argue that non-therapeutic research is in Emile's best interests. Nevertheless, Emile's participation would probably be considered lawful according to the Law Commission recommendations. In its report (1995) it endorsed non-therapeutic research providing certain conditions were met. These broadly repeat those specified by the MRC, with the addition that prior approval should be obtained from a special statutory committee, the Mental Incapacity Research Committee (which has yet to be set up). Again, however, there is one proviso: Emile's needle phobia. This, combined with the fact that his bodily functions would have to be continuously monitored, could make his participation unlawful given the Law Commission's specific 'risk' criteria. These specify that a participant should not be exposed to more than negligible risk and the research should not be unduly invasive or restrictive nor unduly interfere with a participant's freedom of action or privacy.

The other main issue to consider is Valerie's role. According to the MRC, participation in non-therapeutic research of an individual unable to consent can only be ethical if a relative, friend or person acceptable to the LREC and not directly involved in the research agrees that participation would place that individual at no more than negligible risk of harm and is therefore not against that individual's interests. As Emile's wife Valerie would seem to be the ideal person to fulfil this role.

The legal position is different in that the law does not authorize anyone to give consent on behalf of another adult. This means, of course, that Valerie has no legal right to give consent on Emile's behalf. As a consequence, if researchers did rely on her consent her consent would, as a matter of law, be meaningless. The safest course, then, would be to seek the court's prior approval. However, in practice this is not realistic or even practicable, in which case it would be wise to comply with the Law Commission's recommendations, even though these have yet to be implemented. They recommend that this gap in the law be filled by an 'individualized independent check' confirming whether or not the subject should be involved in the research. In most cases the appropriate person to carry out the check will be a registered medical practitioner not involved in the research. The doctor who has had responsibility for caring for Emile should therefore be the one whose 'consent' should be sought, bearing in mind that in practice it is likely that he would at the very least consult Valerie and find out what her views were.

CASE STUDY 8.3   MICHAEL AND THE DRUG TRIAL – A DISCUSSION

(Refer to the scenario presented on page 198.)

Randomized controlled trials (RCTs) are now widely used as a method of testing new drugs as they are an efficient and impartial way of finding out about the impact of a treatment or intervention (Hogg, 1999). In a randomized trial patients are allocated into groups at random – the intention being to avoid bias (conscious or unconscious) in deciding who should be in each group. One group (the treatment group) will be given the new drug; another group (the control group) will be given the conventional treatment or perhaps just a placebo (a sham substance that looks, feels and tastes the same as the new drug being tested).

It is also fairly common for the trial to be double-blind. In this kind of trial neither the researcher nor the subject knows which drug the subject has been given until the trial is completed. Again, double-blind trials are used to eliminate bias. But despite their widespread use, randomized controlled trials are not suited to all clinical research. One reason is that patients are asked to give up their right to chose what treatment they receive – a loss of control that many patients find distressing. Another is that it can be difficult to evaluate interventions such as surgery, psychiatry or complementary therapy, where success depends on the skill of the practitioner and on the attitudes and personalities of patients and clinicians (Hogg, 1999, p. 67).

Arguably the most fundamental ethical concerns in this kind of case, however, are whether it can ever be justifiable to deny the control group taking the standard treatment (or placebo) the potential benefit of the new treatment or existing treatment. In other words, is it ethical to deprive Michael (who, given the random nature of the trial, may only be getting the conventional drug) of the potential benefit of the new drug which might help improve his mobility? If it is clear before the trial starts that the new drug is likely to do this then there can be little doubt that the trial is unethical. Thus only if Pamela does not know which drug is more effective is it ethical for Michael to participate in the trial. Similarly, if there is a conventional drug that can increase Michael's mobility it would almost certainly be unethical to give him only a placebo. Indeed, the so-called placebo effect raises several concerns, in particular the risk that those on the placebo will be harmed by not receiving any treatment (see Smith, 1999, Ch. 10 for a discussion on the ethical issues surrounding the use of placebos).

The other major issue is that of consent. Because the trial is randomized and double-blind it is not possible for Pamela – even if she was being as honest as possible – to give Michael a full explanation of the implications of the trial and the risks he faces. This raises the question as to whether participants in RCTs can ever be informed. A further problem here is that Pamela has not revealed to Michael the nature of the RCA. It would seem very doubtful, therefore, that Michael's consent is valid, especially as he has expressed a very strong preference for the new drug. If that is the case that it would be unethical to enter him into this trial, which, being double-blind and randomized means that he may well get the conventional treatment.

In legal terms too randomization is problematic because of the doubts as to whether Michael can be given enough information to satisfy the legal standard of disclosure. For consent to be legally valid in relation to the therapeutic research there is a very strong argument that consent should be fully informed. This means that the nature of the RCT should be explained to Michael, likewise the purpose of the trial, the benefits it offers over conventional treatment, the risks involved and the alternatives. Yet because of the nature of the trial Michael cannot be given all this information. At most he can be told the purpose of the trial and the fact that subjects are to be randomly allocated. Beyond that he cannot be provided with any useful information, in particular the implications of the trial, what will happen to him and more specifically which drug he will receive – because it is a double-blind trial so neither he nor Pamela will know. Despite this lack of information, however, it is generally accepted that Michael's consent will be lawful if he is given a proper explanation of the trial – which is doubtful in this case – and has accepted that the drug he will receive will be determined by chance (i.e. providing he is aware of what randomization means). But given Michael's expressed preference for the trial drug and the fact that he has been denied a full explanation of the nature of the RCT it is doubtful that any 'consent' would be valid.

LAW and ETHICS – a comparison

Research on human subjects can take many forms. It can be therapeutic or non-therapeutic, invasive or non-invasive. The risks involved may also vary widely. But however research is classified and whatever form it takes, the same ethical and legal issues are commonly raised. As we have seen, these mainly focus on how research should be regulated and controlled; how abuses and mistreatment can be prevented; and how a proper balance can be maintained between protecting the rights of the individual and the advancement of science. That these individual rights – which include the right to self-determination, privacy, confidentiality, fair treatment and protection from harm – are paramount few can doubt. Indeed it is widely accepted that whatever benefits research may confer there can be no justification for treating human subjects as simply a means to an end.

Yet despite the almost universal consensus that the interests of people must prevail over those of society or science, it is self-evident that there is a conflict of interest between researchers and those who participate in research. Although such a conflict may well be inevitable, given that the fundamental aim of all research is to advance knowledge, it also means that the way it is managed – both in legal and ethical terms – must be constantly reassessed.

As we have seen, the law's response is to rely almost entirely on the concept of consent. This is because there is no legislation regulating human research (except embryo research). Several reasons are usually given for this lack of statutory regulation. The most common is that no statute could be sufficiently comprehensive or flexible to accommodate the rapid developments in science and medical technology that now typify research. Another is that if legislation were enacted it would be difficult to enforce, given the lack of public consensus on the scope of research and the resources that should be allocated to it.

But whatever the reason, there can be no doubt that the legislative gap contrasts sharply with the plethora of ethical guidelines – the combined effect of which is to provide fairly detailed and clear criteria on how research should be designed and conducted. These guidelines have been issued both by international bodies (for example the Nuremberg code and Declaration of Helsinki) and professional bodies (such as the Royal College of Nursing and the Medical Research Council). Other non-statutory guidelines have also been issued by the Department of Health that deal with local research ethics committees and more recently multicentre research ethics committees.

On a general level, then, the law's response can be described as minimal in that it has failed to prescribe any specific framework for regulating research and has relied instead on the long-established common law principle of consent to protect research participants.

It is clear too that, compared to the law, ethical guidelines provide much more precise and clearer guidance on several aspects of research. The disclosure of information is one area, for example, where guidelines are far more explicit. It is therefore not surprising that the RCN guidance gives a detailed account of the information participants are entitled to, the assumption being that their consent is not valid unless they are fully informed and so can make a 'reasoned judgement'. In contrast, the law on information disclosure is at best unclear and at worst confusing. Thus, although many legal texts assert that in relation to research (especially non-therapeutic research) patients can expect a fuller explanation than that which is normally given in relation to medical treatment, it cannot be said for certain that the courts would endorse this higher standard.

It is also worth noting that, generally, ethical guidelines draw a much clearer distinction between therapeutic and non-therapeutic research, both in relation to adults and children. As such it is not surprising that they specify the conditions that must be met before each type of research is ethical. This distinction, although implicitly recognized in law, is far less clear. The different legal and ethical approach is perhaps most obvious in relation to non-therapeutic research involving adults who lack the capacity to consent. Hence guidelines from the MRC fully support involving those who cannot consent in such research claiming:

> *that although it cannot be argued that a mentally incapacitated person's participation in non-therapeutic research is directly in his interests there are circumstances in which it is important to gain knowledge which may be of benefit to mentally incapacitated people in general and which can only be acquired as a result of research which involves those who are unable to consent.*   MRC (1991b)

The law's response, in contrast, is more far more cautious, most legal texts suggesting that non-therapeutic research involving mentally incompetent adults is probably unlawful. Yet they also claim that, given the Law Commission's recommendations (which do not rule out such research altogether providing certain safeguards are met), a court might well follow suit.

REFERENCES

Alzheimer's Disease Society (1993) *Volunteering for Research into Dementia*, Alzheimer's Disease Society, London.

Beecher, H. N. K. (1966) Ethics and clinical research. *New England Journal of Medicine*, 274, 1354–1360.

British Paediatric Association (1992) *Ethics Advisory Committee Guidelines for the Ethical Conduct of Medical Research Involving Children*, British Paediatric Association, London.

Brock, D. (1994) Ethical issues in exposing children to risks in research. In: *Children As Research Subjects*, (eds M. A. Grodin and L. H. Glantz), Oxford University Press, Oxford.

Brody, B. A. (1998) *The Ethics of Biomedical Research*, Oxford University Press, Oxford.

Capron, A. M. (1997) Human experimentation. In: *Medical Ethics*, 2nd edn, (ed. R. Veatch), Jones & Bartlett, London.

CERES (1993) *Medical Research and You*, Consumers for Ethics in Research, London.

De Raeve, L. (ed.) (1997) *Nursing Research: An Ethical and Legal Appraisal*, Baillière Tindall, London.

Department of Health (1991) *Local Research Ethics Committees, HSG(91)5*, Department of Health, London.

Department of Health (1997) *Ethics Committee Review of Multi-centre Research: Establishment of Multi-centre Research Ethics Committees, HSG(97)23*, Department of Health, London.

Dyer, C. (ed.) (1992) *Doctors, Patients and the Law*, Blackwell Scientific, Oxford.

Evans, M. (1993) Evaluating risks and benefits. In: *Ethical Review of Clinical Research,*

A Training Conference for Ethics Committees, Delegates Folder (1997), Association of Independent Clinical Research Contractors, London.

Evans, D. and Evans, M. (1996) *A Decent Proposal*, John Wiley, Chichester.

Foster, C. G. (1993) The development and future of research ethics committees in Britain. In: *Choices and Decisions in Health Care*, (ed. A. Grubb), John Wiley, Chichester.

Fox, M. (1998) Research bodies: feminist perspectives on clinical research. In: *Feminist Perspectives on Health Care Law*, (eds S. Sheldon and M. Thomson), Cavendish Publishing, London.

Hendrick, J. (1997) *Legal Aspects of Child Health Care*, Chapman & Hall, London.

Hogg, C. (1999) *Patients, Power and Politics*, Sage, London.

Hurwitz, B. (1998) *Clinical Guidelines and the Law*, Radcliffe Medical Press, Abingdon.

International Council of Nurses (1996) *Ethical Guidelines for Nursing Research*, ICN, Geneva.

Law Commission (1995) *Mental Incapacity, Law Com. No. 231*, HMSO, London.

Mason, J. K. and McCall Smith, R. A. (1999) *Law and Medical Ethics*, 5th edn, Butterworths, London.

McHale, J. (1998) Clinical research and the nurse. In: *Law and Nursing*, (eds J. McHale, J. Tingle and J. Peysner), Butterworth Heinemann, Oxford.

Montgomery, J. (1997) *Health Care Law*, Oxford University Press, Oxford.

MRC (1991) *The Ethical Conduct of Research on Children*, Medical Research Council, London.

MRC (1991) *The Ethical Conduct of Research on the Mentally Incapacitated*, Medical Research Council, London.

MCR (1992) New MRC guidance on research ethics. In: *Bulletin of Medical Ethics*, **84**, 18–23.

Neuberger, J. (1992) *Ethics and Health Care*, King's Fund Institute Research Report, King's Fund, London.

Nicholson, R. H. (1997) What do they get up to? LREC Annual Reports. *Bulletin of Medical Ethics*, **129**, 13–24.

Pappworth, M. H. (1967) *Human Guinea Pigs: Experimentation on Man*, Routledge & Kegan Paul, London.

RCN (1998) *Research Ethics: Standards of Care*, Royal College of Nursing, London.

Royal College of Physicians (1990) *Research Involving Patients*, Royal College of Physicians, London.

Royal College of Physicians (1996) *Guidelines on the Practice of Ethics Committees in Medical Research Involving Human Subjects*, 3rd edn, Royal College of Physicians, London.

Singleton, J. and McLaren, S. (1995) *Ethical Foundations of Health Care Responsibilities in Decision Making*, Mosby, London.

Smith, T. (1999) *Ethics in Medical Research*, Cambridge University Press, Cambridge.

Tusa, A. and Tusa. J. (1983) *The Nuremberg Trial*, Papermac, London.

UKCC (1996) *Guidelines for Professional Practice*, United Kingdom Central Council, London.

Veatch, R. M. and Fry, S. (1987) *Case Studies in Nursing Ethics*, J. B. Lippincott, London.

9 DEATH, DYING AND THE INCURABLY ILL PATIENT

INTRODUCTION

It is perhaps not surprising that many of the most controversial and widely debated legal and moral issues centre on the treatment of terminally or incurably ill patients. The care of such patients has, of course, always raised acute dilemmas, not least because – as has been wryly observed – 'none of us has ever died, and thus euthanasia is the one subject on which it is impossible to say that a given view is right or wrong' (Mason, 1996, p. 161). But decision-making at the end of life is inevitably more difficult than it once was. There are several reasons for this.

First, as Brock has pointed out (1997, p. 364), where once nature took its course and pneumonia was 'the old man's friend', now increasingly someone must decide how long and by what means a life will be prolonged, and when death will come. Yet progress in medical technology and pharmacology that enables patients to live much longer than they would have done in the past can be a two-edged sword (Pace, 1996, p. 76). Thus, although artificial ventilation, feeding and hydration can prolong life – sometimes for many years – they cannot always restore health and reverse disability or disease and so may not always be in a patient's best interests. Is it, for example, unquestionably beneficial to extend the life of a profoundly handicapped baby so that she becomes a 'passive prisoner of medical technology' with no (or very little) hope of recovery or improvement?

Secondly, a steady trickle of much-publicized cases such as the trial of Dr Cox for attempted murder and the case of Anthony Bland, the young man injured in the Hillsborough football stadium disaster, have brought standards and practices once mainly left to doctors out into the open and thus made them more likely to be scrutinized and challenged.

Thirdly, changing medical relationships in a less paternalistic age, especially the assertion of patients' rights and the expectation that they and their families should be consulted, have increased the opportunities for disputes to arise and for court involvement in the process of decision-making (McLean, 1996, p. 50).

For nurses, all these developments have very significant implications, not just because they may be involved in making 'life and death' decisions but because even if they are not they will almost certainly be involved in the consequences of such decisions. In the Bland case, for example, the role of the nurses was repeatedly recognized, with one Law Lord noting that 'the decision to withdraw life support may well have been a merciful relief for almost all concerned except for the nursing staff who will be called upon to act in a way which must be contrary to all their instincts, training and traditions'.

The process of dying and the treatment of those who are incurably ill raise many legal and ethical issues. But this chapter will focus on the most common themes in the 'euthanasia' debate and those that have involved the courts. These include the nature of the legal and ethical duties owed at the end of life; the distinction between acts and omissions, the principle of double effect, 'do not resuscitate' (DNR) orders and advance directives. The chapter begins, however, with the usual hypothetical case studies.

CASE STUDY 9.1 ROGER'S DNR ORDER – IS IT ETHICAL AND LEGAL?

Roger, who is 23 and weighs 32 kg, was born with serious brain malformation and cerebral palsy. For the first 17 years of his life he lived at home but is now mainly cared for in a residential home. Roger has never developed any formal means of communication. He cannot walk or sit upright unaided. He also suffers from a range of other problems, including epilepsy, blindness, deafness and incontinence and operates basically on the level of a newborn infant. After his last discharge from hospital (he has been admitted several times in the last year suffering from recurrent chest infections, fits, dehydration and bleeding from ulceration) his consultant decided that, since he was deteriorating neurologically and physically, it would be unethical to continue treating him. In others words, it would be in Roger's best interests for nature to take its course next time he had a life-threatening crisis. After consultation with his family a 'do not resuscitate' (DNR) order was made. But Julian, a nurse, who has looked after Roger in the past, disagrees. He believes that he knows Roger better than anyone and thinks that he would want to be resuscitated should the need arise.

Is the DNR order ethical? What factors should be considered? What difference would it make if Roger was in a permanent vegetative state? Is a court likely to override the order?

CASE STUDY 9.2 KYLIE'S TERMINAL ILLNESS – CAN TREATMENT BE WITHDRAWN?

Kylie is 16 months old and suffers from the fatal disease spinal muscular atrophy. She is very seriously disabled and her life expectancy is very short. She is in intensive care and on ventilation, which the health-care team considers should be withdrawn so that she can end her life peacefully, i.e. she should not be resuscitated in the event of a respiratory arrest but should be given palliative care only. Kylie's parents refuse their consent to the withdrawal of treatment.

How relevant are the parents' wishes?

Is the withdrawal of treatment in Kylie's best interests?

CASE STUDY 9.3 STEVE'S ADVANCE DIRECTIVE – IS IT VALID?

Steve is in his early thirties and a very keen cyclist. A few days ago he was run down and very badly injured. One leg had to be amputated and there are concerns that the other may have to be amputated also. Steve also suffered irreversible brain damage. Since the accident he has been in a coma and is on life support. Yesterday, his partner Mark showed doctors a 'living will' that Steve had signed several years previously. The will made it clear that if he suffered serious irreversible brain damage he did not want any life-saving treatment and certainly would not want to be kept alive if he could not carry on cycling.

What is the effect of Steve's advance directive? Should life support be switched off?

DEFINITIONS

Euthanasia

Many of the issues examined in this chapter involve, directly or indirectly, the concept of euthanasia. It is appropriate therefore to begin by defining what the concept means, likewise the concept of death and that of medical treatment (which has a special meaning in this context).

Euthanasia, translated literally from Greek, means 'a good, happy or easy death' and was used traditionally in a broad metaphorical sense to describe the 'spiritual state of the dying person at the impending approach to death' (Carrick, 1985, p. 127). Although the term is now more often used to describe the deliberate ending of life, contemporary definitions are much more varied. This is perhaps not surprising, since the euthanasia debate, like that on abortion, has generated an enormous literature but very little consensus. Thus advocates of euthanasia describe it as 'mercy killing' and regard the 'right to die', i.e. to decide the time and manner of one's death, as a legitimate right of self-determination. In contrast opponents of euthanasia see it as immoral and tantamount to murder.

But despite the lack of a comprehensive definition several different types of euthanasia are typically recognized. In **voluntary euthanasia** an individual makes a free decision to end his/her life. If help is requested, it is called **assisted suicide**. In the case of **non-voluntary euthanasia** a decision is taken to end a person's life because s/he is hopelessly or terminally ill. It is non-voluntary because the person cannot be consulted about the decision – s/he may be unconscious, for example, or too ill to make a choice. Finally there is **involuntary euthanasia**. This involves ending someone's life either without regard to their wishes, when they are competent to give them, or against their expressed wishes, supposedly in their best interests.

Another distinction that is commonly made is between active and passive euthanasia. **Active euthanasia** implies that a positive action is taken to end life, e.g. administering a lethal injection. **Passive euthanasia** involves allowing a patient to die by omitting to act, e.g. by withholding (or withdrawing) life-saving treatment such as nutrition or antibiotics. Note that all three kinds of euthanasia – voluntary, non-voluntary and involuntary – can be active or passive (Mason and McCall Smith, 1999, pp. 414–418).

Death

As with so many other areas of medicine, recent technological advances have made what was once a relatively straightforward state to identify and define increasingly complex. Death – which may occur suddenly or can be the final event of a phase of deterioration – is no exception. So, in the past when a person's heart or breathing stopped it was accepted that death had occurred and the person was dead. For most deaths this traditional definition remains adequate but it is not appropriate when intensive treatment has been used to maintain a person's vital functions. It is not uncommon now, for example, for patients to be resuscitated after a cardiac arrest. Similarly, ventilation can be maintained artificially long after a patient has stopped breathing. Artificial feeding techniques are also fairly commonplace.

As such techniques have become well established a different definition of death had to be developed that could be applied to patients on life support machines. This led to a new definition of death, **brain-stem death**, i.e. the irreversible loss of brain function, which was developed in the mid-1970s by the Royal Colleges (Conference of Medical Royal Colleges and their Faculties in the UK, 1976; 1979). Death could be declared once several criteria were satisfied. These were:

1. the patient must be in a deep coma;
2. the patient must be apnoeic;
3. the patient must have irrecoverable structural brain damage; and
4. reversible causes of brain-stem depression must have been excluded (Jennett, 1996, p. 15).

In the absence of any statutory definition of death, English courts have since accepted this definition, notably in *Re A* [1992] 3 Med LR 303, a case involving a 19-month-old infant sustained on a ventilator whom the court held was dead for medical and legal purposes. It was therefore lawful to disconnect the ventilator.

Medical treatment

Case law, notably *Airedale NHS Trust* v. *Bland* [1993] AC 789, has made it clear that artificial nutrition and hydration through the use of nasogastric tubes, intravenous lines, surgically implanted tubes and so forth is a form of medical treatment and thus no different from other forms of treatment. As such it can be both lawful and ethical to withhold and/or withdraw it in certain circumstances. What those circumstances are will be examined below but first the arguments for and against euthanasia need to be considered.

ETHICAL CONSIDERATIONS

Can euthanasia be morally justified?

The most compelling argument used by proponents of euthanasia is the principle of autonomy. As was noted in Chapter 2, in health-care contexts the principle requires nurses and other health professionals to respect the fact that patients have the capacity to reason and to make their own decisions. In other words, as patients increasingly assert their right of self-determination so they expect to be involved in all decisions about their care and treatment. This means having the right to choose, and in particular the right to choose death. As Tschudin notes, this has become known as 'the right to die' (1993, p. 117). Although commonly used to describe an 'end of life' decision, it should nevertheless be noted that the phrase 'right to die' is misleading in that what it really involves is the ability to control, as far as possible, the process of dying.

Yet even if the right to die is redefined in this way it may not always be possible for patients, even those whose claim to autonomy is the strongest – because they are conscious and competent or have previously expressed their wish to die by making a living will – to fully control the process. They may be physically incapable, for example, of carrying out their own wishes or they may ask for help to die. This then raises the question of the kind of obligations respect for autonomy places on health professionals (Lamb, 995, p. 113). Do nurses, for example, have a moral duty to assist?

Whatever the answer to this question it is certainly arguable that cases of voluntary euthanasia are the easiest to justify on autonomy grounds. Less easy to justify on such grounds, however, are instances of non-voluntary euthanasia, unless, that is, a decision to end a patient's life is based on a substituted judgement test. This test is based on what the patient him/herself would have wanted, regardless of what others may think is a 'good' outcome. It can be described as 'autonomous' because it looks at the situation from the patient's point of view rather than the view of others. Yet in practice the substituted judgement approach is rarely taken. Instead, as we shall see, when decisions have to made for those who lack capacity the test which is almost always adopted is the 'best interests' one, i.e. one in which the views of others – usually health professionals – determine the treatment the patient should or should not have.

Another justification for euthanasia is related to the autonomy argument in so far as it is concerned with respecting and maintaining a person's dignity (Johnstone, 1989, p. 255). The implication here is that when death occurs the individual is conscious, not connected up to any tubes, drips, or drugs. Expressed another way, what this means is that, although medicine can now provide the means of staving off death, the cost to the individual may be too high. In other words, what patients think both about the life-sustaining technology itself and their quality of life is very important. Patients may not want, for example, to spend their last days, weeks or months stripped of their dignity but may prefer to approach death as autonomously as possible. What needs to be recognized, therefore, is that even if in most cases the pain of the terminally ill can be controlled what cannot be controlled is the loss of self-respect, personal integrity and self-esteem. These are very individual criteria, which no-one but individuals themselves can comment on.

The other main argument in support of euthanasia is that it is practised anyway. In fact, a surprising number of doctors claim to have taken part in some form of euthanasia (Mason and McCall Smith, 1999, p. 415). Nevertheless, few doctors are prosecuted for murder and those who are almost always treated with great sympathy and usually found not guilty. Given that euthanasia is practised behind closed doors, would it not be preferable, so the argument goes, to discuss it openly and regulate it properly within a coherent legal framework, thereby ensuring that health professionals and patients are protected?

As to the arguments against euthanasia, one of the most popular is the sanctity of life doctrine, which is based on the belief that life is inviolable and only God has the right to take it away (Rumbold, 1999, p. 91). This doctrine will be examined in more detail below but it can be briefly summed up as follows: Human life is sacred and taking it is wrong; Euthanasia is an example of taking human life; Therefore euthanasia is wrong. For many, however, the most persuasive objection to euthanasia is the so-called slippery slope argument.

It is an argument that has many forms (often it is called the 'thin end of the wedge' argument or 'the tip of the iceberg') but in this context it maintains that once we begin to kill others, we will find ourselves sliding down a slope that leads to killings of a kind that no-one wants (Singer, 1995 p. 150). In other words, voluntary euthanasia would escalate into compulsory euthanasia. Thus, although initially strict controls will be in place, ensuring, for example, that only those in uncontrollable and excruciating terminal pain will have their request for euthanasia carried out, gradually those controls will be relaxed. Euthanasia will then be extended not just to those who are incapable of requesting it but also to those who are not terminally or even chronically ill but have simply become too much of a burden for their families. And finally, it will not be long before people will simply be killed because their lives are considered unworthy. In other words, euthanasia becomes a euphemism for murderous practices of many kinds (Tschudin, 1993, p. 110).

Another version of the slippery slope argument claims that, even if it was possible to draw appropriate boundaries and legalize euthanasia, it would never be possible to provide sufficient safeguards to prevent abuse – in which, say, vulnerable people would be forced by unscrupulous relatives into making premature decisions they did not really want or would not be fully informed, and so forth. But whichever version of the slippery slope argument is invoked it basically asserts that, given the predictable long term consequences it is better not to take any risks at all and leave well alone (see Lamb, 1988; Frey, 1998).

Finally, it is worth noting some of the other less common arguments against euthanasia. These include the claim that it has a damaging effect on society, in particular on its moral and social foundation, by eroding the traditional principle that all human life should be respected. It is also discriminatory, because it implies that some lives are of less value than others and so are not worth prolonging (Johnstone, 1989, p. 257). In other words, euthanasia discriminates against those who are terminally or incurably ill by reinforcing the idea that their lives, unlike others, are unimportant. Note also the argument that euthanasia is contrary to medical ethics because it puts health professionals in the role of 'killers' and so will gradually undermine patients' trust – that their well-being is the only factor to be considered when 'end of life' decisions have to be made, rather than economic or other pressures. (For a summary of the arguments for and against euthanasia see Johnstone, 1989; Rumbold, 1999.)

Whatever the merits of the various competing claims about euthanasia it is certain that the debate will continue, as will the debate about the moral principles that should guide decision-making at the end of life. It is to these that we now turn.

What ethical framework should guide decision-making at the end of life?

In 'setting the scene' for decision-making in this context, the British Medical Association (BMA, 1999) builds on its earlier consultation paper (BMA, 1998) and gives guidance on the basic moral principles that should guide practice. These are that:

- treatment of patients should reflect the inherent dignity of every person, irrespective of age, debility, dependence, race, colour or creed;
- actions must reflect the needs of the patient (taking into account such issues as the effect on the family, staff, the hospital and the community as well as resources);
- decisions taken must value the person and accept human mortality.

The guidance also makes clear that the primary goal of medical treatment is to benefit the patient by restoring or maintaining the patient's health as far as possible, maximizing benefit and minimizing harm. If treatment fails, or ceases to give a net benefit, this primary goal cannot be realized and the justification for providing treatment is removed. Unless some other justification can be demonstrated, treatment that does not provide net benefit to the patient may be ethically withheld or withdrawn and the goal of medicine should shift to the palliation of symptoms (BMA 1999, pp. 1–4).

Taken together, the consultation paper and the guidance give rise to several ethical obligations.

The duty to act in patients' 'best interests'
According to the BMA, although in the past this concept was almost always equated with the most positive medical outcome, this is not now automatically the case given that modern technology can extend patients' lives beyond the point at which either they desire it or can benefit from it. In short, the prolongation of life can be harmful. What this means in practice is that much more emphasis should now be placed on the personal and social factors that shape peoples' lives and on assessing what patients themselves want, i.e. their known wishes and values.

Furthermore, if it is accepted that all patients have a right to good-quality and appropriate care, then it must follow that in order to make decisions that are in a patient's 'best interests' both the benefits and burdens of life-prolonging treatment must be continuously assessed. As to the meaning of the term 'benefit'; this means an advantage or net gain for the patient but encompasses more than simply whether the treatment achieves a particular physiological goal. It includes both medical and other, less tangible benefits (BMA, 1999, p. 5). Finally, the term 'burden'; this includes 'treatments which might be regarded as intrusive ones, in circumstances where the patient's capacity to experience life and relate to others is very severely impaired or non-existent'. (BMA, 1993, p. 165).

The duty of care

Generally this means that nurses must do their best not to harm patients and should aim positively to help them. As such, they must take reasonable care to avoid acts and omissions that they can foresee would be likely to injure them. Accordingly they should, where possible, discuss options with patients, listen to their views, respect their autonomy and confidentiality and, when necessary, act as their advocate (UKCC, 1996). Finally, as the BMA guidance makes clear, the duty of care means being mindful that it is not an appropriate goal of medicine to prolong life at all costs, with no regard to its quality or the burdens of treatment. Nevertheless treatment should never be withheld, when there is a possibility that it will benefit the patient, simply because withholding it is considered to be easier than withdrawing it later (BMA, 1999, pp. 1–5).

Is there an ethical obligation to prolong life? – sanctity or quality of life

In answering this question, two approaches that are commonly used in the euthanasia controversy need to be examined, namely the **sanctity of life** doctrine and the **quality of life** approach. The sanctity of life doctrine has a long history in Western thought (see Kuhse, 1987 for an analysis of how the concept has become so central). Traditionally, its roots lie in the Judaeo-Christian belief that human life is valuable and worthy of respect irrespective of its quality or kind. As a gift from God, life is 'on loan' and thus is not ours do what we like with. Only God, therefore, has the right to take life away. From this it follows that any intentional act to end life – which interferes with the will of God – is morally wrong.

The belief that life is sacred and inviolable in a religious sense is of course less tenable in a secular society. Yet there is still a universal acceptance of the principle that it is wrong to kill, which arguably explains why the 'right to life' (which is how the doctrine is often described) is now enshrined in the Human Rights Act 1998. But conventional attitudes towards the sanctity of life doctrine are less straightforward than in the past. Many people, for example, who believe instinctively that it is wrong to take human life do, nonetheless concede that in some circumstances it can be justified – for example, in self defence. On the other hand, others still hold the most extreme view of the doctrine – that being alive is intrinsically valuable and that human life must be therefore preserved whatever the cost and whatever the circumstances.

This representation of the doctrine has, however, been challenged. Keown (1997), for example, claims that even in its strongest form it does not assert that life is an absolute good and therefore one to which all others must be sacrificed. Rather, the core of the doctrine is the principle prohibiting intentional killing. It is that principle, i.e. that life may never be intentionally taken, that is absolute, not that life must be preserved at all costs (both to the individual and society). In other words, life-prolonging treatment is not always an overriding priority, as there may be some circumstances when death can be permitted. If Keown's interpretation – which acknowledges that the value of human life is not absolute – is accepted, then clearly the nature of a person's life, i.e. its quality, becomes a relevant consideration.

What is being suggested, therefore, is that in some circumstances factors other than the preservation of life should be taken into account in deciding whether to prolong a person's life. The difficulty lies, of course, in determining what those circumstances are, since it involves asking a question that is almost impossible to answer: When is a life worth living? There is no universal or widely accepted view on how the notion of quality of life should be defined and used nor what qualities make a life worthwhile. This is because, although most people may well agree, albeit on a very general level, on the basic psychological and physical characteristics that make up a 'good' quality of life, there is likely to be far less agreement once more precise aspects are debated. So, few would disagree that a person's capacity to, for example, function socially, physically and emotionally and to derive satisfaction from so doing are important, but how able must they be in performing those functions, how rational, autonomous and self-aware?

These and similar questions are not easy to answer because different people almost inevitably have different attitudes to them. Furthermore, things that were important once in a person's life may change over time, becoming less or more significant as they age. Quality of life judgements are therefore essentially subjective (Downie and Calman, 1994, p. 190).

Nevertheless once quality of life considerations are accepted – and assuming that some agreement can be reached in individual cases as to whether 'a life is worthwhile' – then it becomes possible to make decisions about whether particular treatments ought to be withheld or withdrawn. But this does not automatically lead to the conclusion that it is morally justifiable to take active steps to end a person's life – to put it another way, that there is no moral difference between killing and letting die. (On the 'quality of life' concept, see also Heap and Ridley, 1996; Singer, 1995; Rumbold, 1999.)

Is there a moral distinction between killing and letting die? – the acts and omissions doctrine

Exhaustively discussed in the literature, the distinction between killing and letting die corresponds in general to the so-called **acts and omissions doctrine**. This doctrine maintains that an action that results in some undesirable consequence is morally worse than a failure to act. Or, to put it another way, it is worse to kill a patient, i.e. to initiate a course of events that leads to death (active euthanasia) than it is to allow a patient to die, i.e. not to intervene in that course of events (passive euthanasia).

The acts and omissions doctrine is a reassuring one because most people intuitively feel less responsible for their omissions than they do for their actions, even if the same undesirable consequence occurs. But is this intuitive response valid in a euthanasia context? Is there, in short, a moral distinction between giving a lethal injection to a patient who is dying and in great pain, and withdrawing or withholding life-saving treatment from such a patient? In all three situations the patient will eventually die, albeit sooner following the lethal injection. And in all cases the behaviour of the nurse involved is intentional and deliberate.

So where does the moral difference lie, if at all, and how should the withdrawal and withholding of treatment be classified? Are these actions really 'omissions' or are they simply defined in that way because such an interpretation is more psychologically comforting for health professionals? Or perhaps the questions here should be reframed so that we focus, as Harris does (1985, Ch. 4), on the ways in which killing might be a caring thing for one person to do for another.

One way of justifying the acts and omissions doctrine and distinguishing between killing and letting die is to say that by giving a patient a lethal injection something is made to happen, i.e. death is caused. In contrast, when treatment is withheld or withdrawn it can be said that nature is being allowed to take its course. Thus death is not being made to happen; instead, the 'omission' consists of merely letting something happen, i.e. letting a patient die from the normal progress of his or her disease (Pace, 1996).

But for many commentators this distinction is unconvincing. One of the most well known attempts to dispute is the following example made famous by Rachels (1975). Smith and Jones will inherit fortunes if their young cousins die before them. Smith drowns his cousin in the bath, making it look like an accident, and gets his inheritance. Jones, on the other hand, has every intention of drowning his cousin but luckily for him as he enters the bathroom the youngster slips, hits his head and slides face down in the water. Although Jones is prepared to 'finish the job' if necessary the cousin manages to drown without any help from him. Jones also gets his inheritance. According to Rachels these imaginary cases prove that, given their motives and intentions and the consequences of their behaviour, Smith's action and Jones's omission were identical. From this he concludes that unless there are some other morally significant differences the distinction between killing and letting die is a specious one.

Superficially, Rachels's example seems compelling. What it fails to acknowledge, however, is that there are different types of 'omission' – some being much more blameworthy than others. Deliberately withholding life-saving medicine in order to inherit money, for example, is far more culpable than omitting to give it through ignorance or negligence. Hence, if Jones's 'omission' had been less culpable he would arguably be less responsible for his cousin's death than Smith. Accordingly, the moral distinction between Smith's action and Jones's behaviour would be more obvious. As Glover notes (1977, p. 95) the acts and omissions doctrine seems much less plausible when the omission is deliberate and the motive is bad.

Also neglected by Rachels's example is that some so-called omissions can actually make something happen (and so are more like positive actions). As such, they are not cases of 'letting something' happen, and can thus be just as morally wrong as an action that causes death. To return to Jones, his inaction meant that no other outcome than his cousin's death by drowning was possible. In other words, his behaviour made his cousin's death happen (Pace, 1996, p. 53).

The difficulties of designating different kinds of behaviour as actions or omissions, in particular classifying the positive decision to withdraw, i.e. turn off, life-sustaining treatment as an omission, have prompted alternative attempts to assess the morality of euthanasia. One of the most popular is the principle of 'double effect'.

Is there a moral distinction between intending and foreseeing a consequence? – the 'double effect' principle

The ethical principle of double effect has a long history going back to the Middle Ages. It was developed primarily by Catholic moral theologians to determine in what circumstances an action that has both good and bad consequences is morally acceptable. When, in other words, is it permissible to do something that is intended to produce a good result but that will also have a harmful effect?

In the treatment of terminally ill patients the principle is used to justify medical treatment, typically pain relief, that may also shorten a patient's life. Justification lies in the fact that, although a patient's death may be foreseen, it is an indirect result of the treatment and unintended. Thus, although an act of killing is wrong in itself it is morally acceptable to allow death to occur if this bad 'side-effect' is not an intended consequence of an act carried out for the sake of a good effect.

Classic formulations of the principle usually require four conditions to be met before any action can be judged morally sound. These are:

- the act itself must be morally good or morally indifferent (e.g. relief of suffering);
- the bad outcome (e.g. death of the patient) must not be directly intended (even if it is foreseen);
- the good outcome must not be achieved by means of the bad, i.e. the bad effect is not a means to the good effect;
- the good outcome must outweigh the bad, i.e. there is a sufficiently serious reason for allowing the bad effect to occur (Keown, 1999, p. 53).

Several of these conditions are contentious, in particular the second, which many claim draws an artificial distinction – which is at best self-deceiving and at worse morally dishonest – between a consequence that is intended and one that is foreseen. How, in short, is it possible to deny that you have 'intended' a consequence that you can foresee is certain, or at least very probable?

Thus if, at the request of a patient who is dying and in intolerable pain, a nurse administers a dose of morphine knowing that the dose will shorten the patient's life, is it really plausible to argue that the nurse did not intend that patient's death but merely foresaw it? To put it another way, foreseeing a bad consequence is no different from intending it because, despite knowing that a bad consequence is pending, the agent deliberately refrains from preventing it (Johnstone, 1989, p. 265).

It is perhaps possible to find a distinction between intended and foreseen consequences but only if the notion of intention – which is notoriously difficult to define precisely – is interpreted very narrowly so as to exclude any effects that are neither desired or wanted (Beauchamp and Childress, 1994). But once intention is interpreted more broadly – in a way that arguably corresponds to how most people intuitively define the term – then it can include a much wider range of consequences, including those outcomes that are foreseen or 'tolerated' despite being neither desired or willed for their own sake. That is not to say, as Beauchamp and Childress point out, that a person necessarily intends all the consequences of any action that is intentional. Thus a man who intentionally pulls a trigger in the effort to kill a snake but instead shoots himself in the foot does not intend to shoot himself in the foot. But if the snake were on his foot and he voluntarily and knowingly shot through the snake's head and into his foot, then he intentionally shot himself in the foot (and intended the consequence of a bullet-impacted foot).

Yet even if it is accepted that the distinction between intended and foreseen consequences is somewhat tenuous, for some nurses it may provide a moral solution. Many, however, may find the principle hypocritical and will rely instead on other ethical principles when administering pain relief, notably respect for patient autonomy, beneficence, non-malficence and justice.

THE LAW AND EUTHANASIA

Does the law allow euthanasia?

Until relatively recently the courts had rarely been involved in 'end of life' decisions. Several high-profile cases, however, particularly the trials of Dr Nigel Cox, a hospital consultant, for attempted murder in 1992 and most recently that of a GP, David Moor, who had disclosed that he had helped 10 patients to die, forced the issue of the law's role in the euthanasia debate into the public domain. But it was undoubtedly the House of Lords' decision in *Airedale NHS Trust* v. *Bland* [1993] AC 789 that treatment could be withdrawn from Anthony Bland, a young man crushed in the Hillsborough football stadium disaster, that highlighted, more than any other previous case, the inconsistencies in the law.

Since Bland a handful of other cases involving patients in a persistent vegetative state (PVS) or 'near-PVS' have reached the courts (see below). Yet none of these have resolved all the legal issues that arise at the end of life nor those most commonly experienced by nurses and other health professionals. Nonetheless, even though the law has developed in a piecemeal way some legal principles have emerged about how decisions should be made and what factors should be considered. These will be considered below after the following preliminary points have been noted:

- The courts will never sanction positive steps to end life, i.e. active euthanasia is unlawful.
- Even though active euthanasia is unlawful, competent patients (or those or have completed a valid advance directive) have the right to refuse treatment, even if that results in death.
- In some circumstances treatment can be withdrawn or withheld – thus legalizing passive euthanasia.
- The administration of pain killing drugs may be lawful even if they have the effect of shortening life.
- Although suicide is no longer a crime, assisting suicide is unlawful and contrary to 2(1) of the Suicide Act 1961.

What legal duties are owed at the end of life?

A duty of care

One of the most fundamental duties that the law imposes on nurses is a duty of care. But what does this mean when patients are dying or incurably ill?

This raises two issues: first, what standard of care must be reached, and second, what actual treatment (or non-treatment) options the law recognizes. As in other health-care contexts the Bolam test will almost always apply. Accordingly, the legal standard of care will be set by professional practice, i.e. nurses must act in accordance with a responsible and competent body of professional opinion. That said, it is now possible, following their recent more interventionist judicial stance (see Chapters 2 and 3), that the courts might challenge clinical judgement more often than in the past. However, they are unlikely to do so very often, if at all (especially in this context) given their well-entrenched deference to the medical profession and the observations of Lord Goff in Bland: 'the truth is that, in the course of their work, doctors frequently have to make decisions which may affect the continued survival of their patients, and are in reality far more experienced in matters of this kind than are the judges'.

As to the treatment the law requires, this is arguably a more difficult and controversial issue. Nonetheless, bearing in mind that the objectives of medical treatment and care in this context are preventing or retarding a deterioration in the patient's condition and the relief of pain and suffering, it is clear that a wide range of options are lawful, including withdrawing or withholding life-sustaining treatment, DNR orders and giving pain-killing drugs that may shorten life.

To act in a patient's best interests – a duty not to treat?

All the cases that have reached the court in this area have involved either handicapped neonates, patients in PVS (or near-PVS) or those who, despite being sensate, are very severely impaired. As a consequence the 'best interests' concept has been invoked to determine what medical treatment they should receive. But this test is notoriously imprecise. More seriously, it can be criticized for simply being a convenient formula that gives decision-makers, notably health professionals, a free hand to provide or withhold whatever treatment they choose –

providing, of course, that it accords with a responsible body of medical opinion. Given that the test is very widely applied, i.e. whenever a patient is deemed incompetent, and usually without any court involvement, this criticism is a significant one, especially in this context, where one of the options which has to be considered is non-treatment resulting in death. How then have the courts defined 'best interests', bearing in mind that ultimately each case will turn on its own particular facts?

First, they have stressed that the test is the same whether the patient is a baby, a child or an adult. Secondly, except when patients are in PVS, a balancing exercise has to be carried out in which the factors that favour treatment are weighed against those that militate against it.

But it was not until the courts had to deal with a series of cases involving dying or incurably ill neonates that the term 'best interests' was defined in more detail. In *Re C* [1989] 2 All ER 782, for example, the court had to decide on the treatment options for a 16-week-old premature baby born with very severe hydrocephalus. C was terminally ill. She was also blind, deaf and had cerebral palsy in all four limbs. Her prognosis was described as 'hopeless' – she would not get better and no medical or surgical treatment would alter that fact. The court had to decide whether life-sustaining treatment such as nasogastric feeding or antibiotics had to be given if, as was inevitable sooner or later, these would be required to keep C alive.

Drawing on the principles established in an earlier case (*Re B* [1981] 1 WLR 1421), namely that there will be cases where the proposed treatment will cause increased suffering and produce no commensurate benefits, the court decided that it was in C's best interests to withhold any such treatment, having concluded that her quality of life was 'demonstrably so awful and the life which treatment would prolong would be so cruel as to be intolerable'. Furthermore, since death was inevitable what was being balanced, 'was not life against death, but a marginally longer life of pain against a marginally shorter life free of pain and ending with death and dignity'. Interestingly, it is worth noting that C was described as 'dying' throughout the case. Yet this was not so, although her life expectancy was very limited. The reason she was described in this way is arguably because the court was more openly endorsing passive euthanasia than in any other previous case.

Just over a year later the court came to a similar conclusion in *Re J* [1990] 3 All ER 930. Baby J, who was born 13 weeks premature (weighing 1.1 kg), had severe and permanent brain damage. Nevertheless, he was neither dying nor near death, although his life expectancy had been reduced to his late teens at most and he was expected to die well before then. Five months old by the time the case came to court, J was breathing independently but had been ventilated twice for long periods. He was described as suffering from almost every conceivable misfortune and his prognosis was very poor. The most optimistic view was that he was likely to develop serious spastic quadriplegia, would be blind and deaf, was unlikely ever to speak or develop even limited intellectual abilities but would feel the same pain as a normal infant.

The central issue before the court was: If J suffered a further collapse did the law require him to be reventilated? It decided that the doctors' duty to act in J's best interests meant that, if he could not continue breathing unaided, there was no legal obligation to reventilate him nor to subject him to all the associated processes of intensive care, unless to do so seemed appropriate to those treating him. The official solicitor (acting on J's behalf) appealed against the High Court's decision, contending that, except in cases of terminal illness or where a court was certain that a minor's life, were the treatment to be given, would be intolerably awful, it could never be justified in approving the withholding of life-saving treatment. The Court of Appeal, however, confirmed the High Court's decision. Given the unfavourable prognosis (with or without treatment), the hazardous nature of reventilation and the risk of further deterioration if J was subjected to it, it was in his best interests that treatment be withheld.

All the judges agreed that treatment should be withheld in J's best interests but it was only Lord Taylor who expanded on the concept. For him it involved judging the quality of life the child would have to endure if given the treatment and deciding whether in all the circumstances such a life would be so afflicted as to be intolerable to that child. The circumstances to be considered would include, for example:

> *the degree of existing disability and any additional suffering or aggravation of the disability which the treatment itself would superimpose. In an accident case, as opposed to one involving disablement from birth, the child's pre-accident quality of life and its perception of what has been lost may also be factors relevant to whether the residual life would be intolerable to that child.*

More recently, Lord Taylor's approach was implicitly applied in *Re C* [1996] 2 FLR 43. In that case the court described the condition of a premature baby as 'almost a living death', and agreed with medical staff that artificial ventilation should be discontinued. C had developed meningitis, was blind and deaf and suffered from repeated convulsions but could live for months or even up to 2 years. Although not in a coma she was said to have 'a low awareness of anything, if at all' (see also *Re C* [1998] 1 FLR 384; *Re D* [1997] 41 BLMR 81). Commenting on these recent cases, Mason and McCall Smith (1999, p. 377) claim that they raise the possibility of a subtle change of emphasis leading to the supremacy of 'quality of life' as a unit of assessment.

Whether or not that is a valid interpretation it is clear that Lord Taylor's approach – which involves judging a patient's quality of life after treatment – has little relevance to patients in PVS, for whom, as one of the Law Lords said in the Bland case, 'it must be a matter of complete indifference whether he lives or dies'. In such cases there is no realistic prospect of carrying out any balancing exercise. Thus, although initially life-sustaining treatment was in the patient's best interests – given the possibility that his condition might improve – once all hope of recovery or improvement had been abandoned 'his best interests in being kept alive also disappeared, taking with them the justification for the non-consensual regime and the correlative duty to keep it in being' (Lord Mustill in Bland).

The legality of withdrawing treatment, however, raises further issues, in particular whether there is a legal obligation to prolong life. It is to this we now turn.

Is there a legal obligation to prolong life?

This question raises a debate discussed earlier in this chapter – the relationship between the sanctity of life doctrine and the quality of life approach. How far, in other words, does the law allow quality of life considerations to compromise a patient's right to life?

The principle of the sanctity of life is a fundamental principle recognized in the Human Rights Act 1998 and internationally, notably in article 6 of the International Covenant of Civil and Political Rights 1966. The principle is one that the courts have repeatedly confirmed – most recently in *Re J* [1990] and *Airedale NHS Trust* v. *Bland* [1993]. But the principle is not an absolute one. Thus even though the law prohibits taking active steps to terminate life it does not require every patient to be resuscitated or put on life support. To put it another way, health professionals do not have to preserve life at all costs as there is no absolute right to life.

In effect, then, the law recognizes a 'qualified' sanctity of life principle (Stauch *et al.*, 1998, p. 644). It is qualified because a patient's quality of life might be such that it is not in his/her best interests to prolong it. As the House of Lords said in Bland: 'The doctor who is caring for ... a patient cannot, in my opinion, be under an absolute obligation to prolong life by any means available to him, regardless of the quality of the patient's life. Common humanity requires otherwise, as do medical ethics and good medical practice. ...'

More recently, this approach has been endorsed in *Re H* [1997] 38 BMLR 11, in which the court authorized withdrawal of treatment from a 43-year-old woman who had lived in a severely brain damaged state for 3 years. It said: '[T]he sanctity of life is of vital importance. It is not, however paramount.'

The law's compromise between the sanctity and quality of life approaches has led to the court's refusing to compel health professionals or a health authority (or NHS Trust) to provide treatment which in the *bona fide* clinical judgement of those concerned is contraindicated as not being in the best interests of the patient. This was evident in *R* v. *Cambridge HA* ex p. *B* [1995] 2 All ER 129 (discussed in Chapter 5) and *Re J* [1992] 4 All ER 614, a case concerning a 16-month-old infant with profound physical and mental disabilities whom the court decided need not be given life-saving measures (see also *Re C* [1998] 1 FLR 384).

It is also noteworthy that in *Re T* [1997] 1 All ER 906 the Court of Appeal refused to overrule the parents' refusal of consent to a liver transplant for their baby, who had a life-threatening liver defect and who would die within a couple of years without treatment. The parents had opposed the operation – which doctors were keen to carry out – because they believed that it was better for their baby to live a peaceful, albeit very short life without surgery than endure the pain, stress and upset that an intrusive operation would bring. The court's decision was that T's future treatment should be left in his parents' hands. In other words, it was not in his best interests to have the operation.

This decision was a controversial one and has been described as 'the nadir of the best interests test' (Davies, 1998, p. 337). This was because T was not a tragic newborn like baby J or C and could lead a 'normal' life with no treatment other than immunosuppression – assuming, of course, that the transplant was successful. Furthermore, although the clinical factors strongly suggested that treatment would be successful, the court chose instead to focus on the social factors (which it considered did not support the transplant). These included the extended period of extensive support that would be required from the mother and the fact that, as the parents were living abroad at the time, if an order was made the mother would have to return and then would have to cope, probably on her own. To many commentators these factors were not very compelling and certainly did not outweigh the benefits of a transplant (Mason and McCall Smith, 1999).

It is clear, therefore, that there is no legal obligation to prolong life at all costs – which means, as we have seen, that life-saving treatment can be withheld. But how can the courts – who have consistently stated that they will never sanction active measures to shorten life – authorize the withdrawing treatment?

Is it lawful to withdraw and withhold life saving treatment?

In some circumstances it is, but two conditions must be met: first, the process of withdrawing treatment must be regarded in law as an omission; and second, there must be no legal duty to provide life-support. Another way of saying this is that health professionals are only legally obliged to continue to provide life-sustaining treatment and care if such treatment is in their patients' best interests. Otherwise they can lawfully withdraw it. In short, a health professional could switch off a ventilator or remove a nasogastric tube – assuming of course, that in the same circumstances a responsible body of medical opinion would have managed the patient in the same way.

The leading case on this issue is *Airedale NHS Trust* v. *Bland* [1993]. Anthony Bland, 21 years old when the case came to court, had been crushed in the Hillsborough football stadium disaster 3 years earlier. Since then he had been in PVS but his brain stem was still functioning. In law, therefore, Tony was still alive. He was able to breath and digest food (but not to swallow it), but he could not see, communicate, hear, taste or smell. His bowels were evacuated by enema and his bladder was drained by a catheter. He was fed through a nasogastric tube and lay in bed with his eyes open and his limbs crooked and taut. He had repeated infections and had also been operated on for various genitourinary problems. With constant care he could be kept in alive for many years but he would never regain consciousness.

The House of Lords decided that discontinuing treatment, including ventilation, nutrition and hydration, was an omission because what health professionals were actually doing by stopping life support was simply allowing nature to take its course. They were not therefore – in law anyway – responsible for causing the patient's death. Yet describing the removal of a nasogastric tube as an omission (likewise denying that doing so was the legal cause of death) has been criticized. Some argue, for example, that it is illogical for the law to allow an omission to treat – which leads to a long-drawn-out death – but not to allow an act (such as a lethal injection) that is intended to bring about the same result more humanely and peacefully. Others say it is a legal fudge in so far as it is plainly 'wrong' to define the process of removing a feeding tube as anything other than an 'act'. This 'ordinary' understanding of the conduct in question was acknowledged by Lord Goff:

> *It is true that it might be difficult to describe what the doctor actually does as an omission, for example, where he takes some positive step to bring the life support to an end. But discontinuation of life support is, for present purposes, no different from not initiating life-support in the first place. In each case, the doctor is simply allowing his patient to die in the sense that he is desisting from taking a step which might, in certain circumstances, prevent his patient dying as a result of his pre-existing condition.*

Note too Lord Browne-Wilkinson's unease about the act/omission distinction, which, he conceded,

> *will appear to some to be almost irrational. How can it be lawful to allow a patient to die slowly, though painlessly, over a period of weeks from lack of food but unlawful to produce his immediate death by a lethal injection, thereby saving his family from yet another ordeal to add to the tragedy that has already struck them? I find it difficult to find a moral answer to that question. But it is undoubtedly the law and nothing I have said casts doubt on the proposition that the doing of a positive act with the intention of ending life remains murder.*

Yet despite the inconsistencies that it is claimed Bland gives rise to (see, for example, Huxtable, 1999), the case did provide clear guidelines as to when life-saving treatment could be lawfully withdrawn in PVS cases. This in effect legalized passive euthanasia. (Note that in law there is no distinction between withdrawing and withholding treatment.) Similarly, the combined effect of the baby cases, *Re C* [1989], *Re J* [1990] and *Re T* [1997], has been to clarify the circumstances in which treatment can be withheld or withdrawn from profoundly handicapped neonates.

However, there is less certainty as to the legality of non-treatment decisions in respect of other patients – those who have suffered a stroke, for example, that has left them irreversibly brain damaged. What too of patients whose condition is terminal but who do not require life support – patients like Lillian Boyes, who was dying from an extremely painful form of rheumatoid arthritis? As we shall see, if a health professional deliberately terminates such a patient's life, s/he is almost certainly going to face a murder charge. On the other hand, prescribing medicines that shorten life may be lawful – providing the 'defence' of double effect can be invoked.

Can a patient be deliberately killed? – the 'defence' of double effect

Prosecutions of health professionals in connection with euthanasia are very rare. Nevertheless, it is beyond question that it is unlawful to terminate life deliberately, whether the patient is dying or not. Killing a patient is murder and any nurse who takes steps that are intended solely to accelerate death is likely to face a murder charge, even though juries have traditionally been very reluctant to convict those who carry out what they regard as 'mercy killings'. Yet despite that reluctance it was almost impossible for the jury to avoid convicting Dr Cox (*R v. Cox* [1992] 12 BLMR 38) for attempted murder.

Dr Cox was charged with attempted murder rather than murder because the patient's body had been cremated, making it impossible to ascertain the cause of death. It is more than likely, however, that sympathy for Dr Cox prompted the charge because a conviction for murder carries an automatic life sentence whereas an attempted murder charge gives the court more flexibility, hence the 1-year suspended prison sentence Cox received. Lillian Boyes, whom Dr Cox had treated for many years, suffered from rheumatoid arthritis that made her hypersensitive to pain – so much so that she was said to 'howl and scream like a dog when anybody touched her'. Unable to relieve her pain, Dr Cox injected her with potassium chloride (Mrs Boyes had repeatedly asked to die). She died within minutes. Even though she was very close to death before the injection, there was little doubt that, given the dose and the fact that it had no curative or pain-killing properties, Dr Cox's conduct 'was prompted solely, and certainly primarily, by the purpose of bringing her life to an end'.

But the verdict in the case would have been very different had Dr Cox used morphine or some other pain-killing drug because his primary 'intention' would then have been to relieve pain. As such his actions would have been lawful under the principle of double effect. The principle was first recognized in the seminal case of Dr Bodkin Adams (*R v. Adams* [1957] Crim LR 365), who was tried for the murder of one his patients in 1957. The doctor had injected an 81-year-old patient (suffering from arteriosclerosis and the results of a stroke) with heroin and morphia but was found not guilty following the direction of the judge, who said:

> *if the first purpose of medicine – the restoration of health – could no longer be achieved, there was still much for the doctor to do, and he was entitled to do all that was proper and necessary to relieve pain and suffering, even if the measures he took might incidentally shorten life by hours or even longer....*

Although the law therefore recognizes the principle of double effect – and so distinguishes between the primary and secondary consequences of an action or course of treatment, i.e. between what is intended and what is foreseen – it can only do so by distorting how the concept of 'intention' has traditionally been interpreted in English criminal law. This has long held that something can be intended however little it may have been desired or hoped for. In other words, intention can be inferred from conduct that the defendant foresees will have a virtually certain result.

| CASE STUDY 9.1 | ROGER'S **DNR** ORDER – A DISCUSSION |

(Refer to the scenario presented on page 219.)

In deciding whether the DNR order is ethical, guidelines issued by the British Medical Association and the Royal College of Nursing – first in 1993 but revised in 1999 – are a good starting point. These provide a framework for determining when cardiopulmonary resuscitation (CPR) should be attempted. The guidelines state:

It is appropriate to consider a DNR decision in the following circumstances:
a. where the patient's condition indicates that effective CPR is unlikely to be successful,
b. where CPR is not in accord with the recorded, sustained wishes of the patient who is mentally competent,
c. where CPR is not in accord with a valid applicable advance directive,
d. where successful CPR is likely to be followed by a length and quality of life which it would not be in the best interests of the patient to sustain.

Although the guidelines were clearly designed to promote uniformity, they have been described as concealing 'a hornet's nest of moral dilemmas' (Mason and McCall Smith, 1999, p. 445). One of the most problematic areas is the meaning of the word 'successful' (in paragraph a). The literature reveals that there is little consensus as to what constitutes 'success'. Hence for some doctors treatment is futile – the word futile is often used interchangeably with unsuccessful – only if the possibility of success approaches 0% (Doyal and Wilsher, 1993) while for others the success can be as high as 13% and still be considered futile (Hendrick and Brennan, 1997). Nor is success conveniently always measured in percentage terms, as, for example, when it is suggested that resuscitation should only be attempted in patients 'who have a very high chance of successful revival for a comfortable and contented existence' (Basket, 1994).

Just as problematic is the concept of 'futility', which has existed throughout the history of medical practice but has similarly so far failed to be consistently defined by health professionals. Perhaps this is not surprising, given the term's mythical roots in ancient Greece. The *futilis* was a religious vessel that had a wide top and a narrow bottom. This peculiar shape caused the vessel to tip over easily, which made it of no practical use for anything other than ceremonial occasions (Schneiderman and Jecker, 1995, pp. 159–160). In practice, futility is generally used as a shorthand way to describe the situation in which a patient demands and health professionals object to the provision of a particular medical treatment on the grounds that the treatment will provide no medical benefit to the patient. But 'futility' is not a neutral term since its interpretation depends to a large extent on who makes the definition. As Mason and McCall Smith note (1999, p. 364), 'one man's futility is another's courageous effort'.

It is also clear that futility can be defined quantitatively or qualitatively. A quantitative approach measures futility according to the likelihood of resuscitation succeeding. It assumes (falsely) that there is a consensus as to what constitutes success. It also appears, again misleadingly, to be based on objective clinical criteria. But a qualitative approach is also difficult to apply in practice because it tends to be linked with the equally imprecise 'best interests' test. As such it is said to be measurable only if a balancing exercise is carried out in which the factors that favour treatment are balanced against those that do not. (On 'futility', see also Mason and McCall Smith, 1999, Ch. 15; Lamb, 1995; Schneiderman and Jecker, 1995.)

But it is not just futility that is a problematic term since even if the focus shifts to paragraph d of the guidelines – where 'quality of life' is the determining factor – it is not possible to avoid a subjective approach. As the BMA guidance notes (1999, p. 2), 'quality of life' may be an ambivalent term but it is unavoidable. It further suggests that an important factor in its assessment is whether the person is thought to be aware of his/her environment or own existence, as demonstrated by, for example:

• being able to interact with others;
• being aware of his/her own existence and having an ability to take pleasure in the fact of that existence; and
• having the ability to achieve some purposeful or self-directed action or to achieve some goal of importance to him/herself.

Yet despite this guidance, 'quality of life' emerges as a very broad and indeterminate concept that consists of several 'qualities' the relative importance of which remain unspecified (see above for further discussion).

So, given the uncertainty of the concepts that are typically used in this context it is not surprising that Julian may have different views as to Roger's quality of life. But certainly his views should be sought. As the latest guidance from the BMA (1999, p. 45) notes, all health professionals involved in the care of the patient have an important contribution to make. It further states that 'nurses often have a particular insight into the patient's wishes and may have spent considerable time with the patient and the patient's relatives'. Ultimately, however, responsibility for making a DNR order rests with the clinician in charge. (See BMA, 1999, pp 43–49 for ethical factors to be considered when making decisions for adults who lack the ability to make or communicate decisions.) That said, it should nonetheless be noted that, according to the DNR guidelines (BMA, 1999, para, 7), a record in the nursing notes should be made by the primary nurse or the most senior member of the nursing team, whose responsibility it is to inform other members of the nursing team.

As to whether a court would override the order, the answer would turn again on quality of life considerations and the issue of medical futility, i.e. that treatment is likely to be 'unsuccessful'. But given the traditional deference to medical opinion it is unlikely that a court would often (if at all) challenge clinical judgement. It is thus not surprising that in the only case to reach the courts concerning the best interests of a critically ill incompetent adult, namely Re R [1996] 2 FLR 99 – on which this case study is modelled – the court endorsed the DNR order. It did so on the basis that the order was in R's best interests. In other words, it accepted the opinion of those caring for him that further treatment was futile not least because his quality of life would be 'so afflicted as to be intolerable' (as defined in Re J [1990] and Re C [1989], above). Furthermore, given his frailty, CPR would be a dangerous operation that might cause R to suffer further brain damage. The court also agreed that antibiotics could be withheld but that a gastrostomy could be carried out.

Finally, what if Roger was in PVS? In such cases, guidance issued by the Royal College of Physicians (1996) should be followed (see also guidance issued by the BMA (1996). These specify how PVS should be diagnosed and managed. It is also clear that the termination of artificial feeding and hydration of patients in PVS (or in near-PVS) will, in virtually all cases, require the prior permission of the court. This requirement was established in the Bland case and has been followed in several cases since then (e.g. Frenchay v. S [1994] 2 All ER 403; Re G [1995] 3 Med LR 80; Swindon and Marlborough NHS Trust v. S [1995] 3 Med LR 84; Re H [1997] 38 BLMR 11; Re D [1997] 38 BMLR 1). Interestingly, even though not all the patients in these cases fitted the diagnostic criteria of PVS they were nevertheless described as in a state of 'living death'. As such they were 'effectively' in PVS (or near-PVS) and so could have life-sustaining treatment withdrawn or withheld if it was no longer in their best interests. Note finally that the practice and procedure to be followed in seeking a court's declaration is set out in a Practice Note on PVS [1996] 2 FLR 375 (by the end of 1998, 18 such cases had been considered by the courts).

CASE STUDY 9.2   SWITCHING OFF KYLIE'S VENTILATOR – A DISCUSSION

(Refer to the scenario presented on page 219.)

The issues raised by this case study are in many ways similar to the previous one in that they focus on autonomy, respect for the sanctity of life and the relevance of quality of life considerations. Rights too are important, in particular the right to dignity and to have access to the highest obtainable standard of health. These and other rights are acknowledged in guidelines issued by the Royal College of Paediatrics and Child Health (1997). The guidelines aim to provide a framework for practice in five situations where withholding or withdrawal of curative medical treatment might be considered: the brain-dead child, the PVS child, the 'no-chance' situation, the 'no-purpose' situation and the 'unbearable' situation.

Kylie is terminally ill. She therefore fits the 'no-chance' situation in that life-saving treatment 'simply delays death without significant alleviation of suffering'. According to the guidelines, the decision to withdraw treatment is ethically the same as withholding treatment. Nevertheless they acknowledge that emotionally and psychologically they can be 'poles apart'. That said, the decision to withdraw ventilation from Kylie should be based on several principles. These are:

- **A duty of care and the partnership of care**. The duty of care is not an absolute duty to preserve life by all means. There is thus no obligation to provide life-sustaining treatment if (1) its use is inconsistent with the aims and objectives of an appropriate treatment plan and (2) the benefits of that treatment no longer outweigh the burden to the patient. There is nevertheless an absolute duty to comfort and cherish the child and to prevent pain and suffering.

- **Best interests**. In fulfilling the obligations imposed by the duty of care the health-care team and parents will enter into a partnership whose function is to serve the best interests of the child.

Applying these principles to Kylie, who is dying, would mean that it would be appropriate to switch off the ventilator – assuming of course, that such a decision would accord with a responsible body of medical opinion. But what about her parents' wishes? Because Kylie is incapable of exercising autonomy, decisions have to be made on her behalf. Normally that means that those who have parental responsibility can act for their child. But in this case Kylie's parents and the health-care team do not agree. Whose view should therefore prevail? According to the guidelines, if parental dissent cannot be resolved it is advisable to consider seeking the court's involvement. Nevertheless, ultimately the final responsibility remains with the consultant in charge of the child's care.

In legal terms the central issue is whether it is in Kylie's best interests to withdraw treatment, bearing in mind that what is essentially being measured is the quality of the process of dying rather than the quality of living. In other words, in this case the best interests test is concerned with maintaining dignity and the relief of suffering at the end of life (Davies, 1998, p. 340). Given Kylie's illness, the very poor prognosis and cases like Re J [1990]; and Re C [1996] 2 FLR 43 (in which the court authorized the withdrawal of treatment from a very severely handicapped 3-month-old baby with at most 2 years to live), it is therefore almost certain that withdrawing artificial ventilation from Kylie would be lawful.

It is worth noting that it has been suggested that recent case law on incurably or terminally ill children raises the possibility of a subtle change of emphasis in which 'quality of life' considerations seem to be emerging as the supreme unit of assessment in life and death decision-making (Mason and McCall Smith, 1999, p. 377).

Finally, how would the law deal with the wishes of Kylie's parents? The most recent case in which parents opposed the withdrawal of treatment was Re C (Medical Treatment) [1998] 1 FLR 384. It concerned a severely disabled baby suffering from a fatal disease. Her life expectancy was very short – a few months at most. The hospital authority sought the court's approval to withdraw artificial ventilation and to withhold resuscitation if C's heart were to fail. It also wanted the court's approval for palliative care to ensure that the end of her life was as dignified and comfortable as possible. Because of their religious convictions – they believed that their daughter's life should be preserved at all costs – C's parents opposed the termination of treatment. The court, overrode their refusal, reiterating yet again that the child's best interests were the paramount consideration, not the sanctity of life. The court also cited the guidelines issued by the Royal College of Paediatrics and

Child Health in support of its decision that the withdrawal of treatment was in C's best interests and therefore lawful.

CASE STUDY 9.3 STEVE'S ADVANCE DIRECTIVE – A DISCUSSION

(Refer to the scenario presented on page 219.)

The issue in this case study is Steve's advance directive (also called an advance statement or 'living will'). Although the terminology is unclear in the UK (Docker, 1996, p. 180), advance directives, if not universally welcomed as yet, are increasingly being recognized as a legitimate expression of autonomy and the right of self-determination. But despite the rhetoric, only a small minority of people presently have sufficient confidence to commit themselves about future choices (Sommerville, 1996, p. 46).

One reason is that there is evidence that they make little or no difference to treatment of the seriously ill. In other words, no significant differences exist between those with and without advance directives in terms of patient satisfaction, general well-being and length of survival (Sommerville, 1996, p. 43). There is also the concern that patients may change their minds. As Dworkin notes (1993) a person who drafts a living will and the incompetent who benefits from it are, effectively, different persons and the one need not necessarily be empowered to speak for the other. Nevertheless, as a way of extending choice for patients in relation to medical care, the House of Lords Select Committee on Medical Ethics (HL Paper, 1994) was keen to encourage them. In response the BMA published a code of practice (1995) giving detailed information about advance statements about medical treatment. This was followed by the Law Commission report (1995), which recommended that the legal effect of advance directives should be recognized by new legislation.

An advance directive is a document made when a patient is competent that indicates his/her preferences about medical treatment and care in the event of becoming incompetent. Advance directives can take several different forms and can be very general – providing a kind of biographical portrait – or more specific, in which case they typically state in what circumstances, such as when the patient is diagnosed with PVS or any other state of irreversible deterioration, life-sustaining treatment should be withheld or withdrawn. Alternatively, an advance directive may operate as an advance refusal of a particular treatment or treatments.

In several cases, notably Re T [1992] 4 All ER 649 and Airedale NHS Trust v. Bland [1993] the courts have made it clear that health professionals have a duty to respect anticipatory refusals of treatment made by competent adults even though they do not consider such refusals to be in their best interests. But advance refusals are only legally binding if several conditions are met. These are, first, that the patient was competent at the time of the refusal; secondly, that the refusal was applicable to the current circumstances, i.e. the patient had contemplated the situation that later arose; thirdly, the patient had not been unduly influenced by anyone, i.e. the decision was an autonomous one, and finally that s/he had been informed in broad terms of the nature and effect of the treatment that was being refused, i.e. the consequences of non-treatment (BMA, 1995).

Although Steve's advance refusal seems to be rather brief there appears nothing to suggest that it does not fulfil these conditions. Health professionals must therefore respect his decision and withdraw treatment. Note, however, that if Steve had requested a lethal injection, this would not be lawful. Nor would health professionals have to comply with a refusal of basic care (according to the BMA guidance, 1995). 'Basic care' means those procedures essential to keep an individual comfortable. The administration of medication and the performance of any procedure that is solely or primarily designed to provide comfort to the patient or alleviate that person's pain, symptoms or distress are facets of basic care. The term also includes warmth, shelter, pain relief, management of distressing symptoms, hygiene measures and the offer of oral nutrition and hydration (BMA, 1999, p. 6).

Finally, it is worth noting the most recent government proposals about advance statements. It believes that the guidance contained in case law, together with the code of practice issued by the BMA (1995), provide sufficient flexibility to enable the validity and applicability of advance statement to be determined, if necessary, by the courts, without the need to introduce specific legislation.

Law and Ethics – a comparison

It is perhaps appropriate that this book should end with a chapter in which law and ethics interact more closely than in any other health-care setting. This is not, however, surprising given the impact of modern technology on the care and treatment of those who are terminally or critically ill and the progress that has been made in saving and improving patients' lives. Yet these advances have consequences not just for patients and their relatives but also for nurses and other health professionals. In particular, more than ever before, very difficult and sometimes tragic choices have to be made – about whether someone should live or be allowed to die. Inevitably these 'life or death' decisions have exposed the inadequacies of existing legal and ethical frameworks. These have been slow to respond, first, to the fact that modern medical science has irrevocably changed the picture of death and, second, to the changing (and less paternalistic) relationship between patients and health professionals.

As they have struggled to adapt it was almost inevitable that the courts would become increasingly involved in the decision-making process. In the absence of any specific legislation on euthanasia it is also not surprising that, in edging slowly towards a more open endorsement of passive euthanasia, the courts have been tempted to use professional guidelines – in PVS and near-PVS cases, in the treatment of terminally ill neonates and in the case of sensate but severely impaired adults – to make decisions.

But the close relationship and interdependence between law and ethics is not confined to the law's use of professional guidelines. It is also reflected in the fact that the main concepts and concerns in the euthanasia debate – autonomy, the sanctity of life doctrine and the quality of life approach – underpin all decision-making in this context. In so doing they pose similar dilemmas for the courts, lawyers and ethicists, especially when decisions have to be made on behalf of those who lack the capacity to make choices for themselves, i.e. when the 'best interests' test has to be applied. Thus it is no surprise that in interpreting this concept the legal and ethical approach is very similar.

Hence case law and professional guidelines have both concluded that there are circumstances when life is not preferable to death. To put it another way, there is no absolute legal or ethical duty to prolong life at all costs and by all means. Similarly, the legal and ethical frameworks that guide the practice of withdrawing and withholding treatment (and making a DNR order) have much in common in that they both recognize that, even though there is something special about human life (so that active steps to terminate it can never be sanctioned), nevertheless quality of life considerations are relevant in making decisions about ending life.

This is a conclusion that the courts have reached in a number of recent cases, albeit on a case-by-case basis. That this has led to the law developing in a piecemeal way (McLean, 1996, p. 50) is therefore not surprising and is echoed by the continuing ethical debate, which continues to focus on the relatives merits of the sanctity of life doctrine and the quality of life approach.

The convergence of law and ethics has also been particularly obvious in controversial cases when, in making very difficult decisions, the courts have explicitly invoked ethical principles – cases like Bland, for example, when the distinction between acts and omissions was recognized in law. Yet the distinction could only been achieved by describing the process of removing artificial hydration and nutrition in a way, i.e. as an omission, that understandably made the judges feel uncomfortable. That the courts nevertheless recognized the distinction suggests that, whatever the philosophical merits of the debate, the distinction is nonetheless a functional one that forms part of the framework in which we lead our moral lives, and one, moreover, that has strong legal resonances (Mason, 1996, p. 200).

Similarly, reliance on the principle of double effect in 'mercy killing' cases so that health professionals can avoid murder charges when they prescribe medicines that shorten life may do much to highlight the close relationship between law and ethics and their interdependence. Nevertheless, it also means that the flaws in the principle, in particular the dubious distinction between intended and foreseen consequences, are incorporated into the law, thereby making this area of the law not just irrational but impossible to reconcile with other aspects of criminal law (Watson, 1999, p. 864).

In summary, it would seem therefore that the legal and ethical approach to end-of-life decisions and the principles that guide practice have much in common. Whether they will continue to develop policy and practice in the same way remains to be seen, however, and will only be clearer once legislation on euthanasia is on the statute books.

REFERENCES

Basket, P. J. F. (1994) The ethics of resuscitation: a statement by the chairman of the European Resuscitation Council. In: *The ABC of Resuscitation*, 3rd edn (1995), (ed. T. R. Evans), BMJ Publishing, London, p. 55.

Beauchamp, T. L. and Childress, J. F. (1994) *Principles of Biomedical Ethics*, 4th edn, Oxford University Press, Oxford.

British Medical Association (1993) *Medical Ethics Today: Its Practice and Philosophy*, BMA, London.

British Medical Association (1995) *Advance Statements About Medical Treatment*, BMA, London.

British Medical Association (1998) *Withdrawing and Withholding Treatment: A consultation paper from the BMA's Medical Ethics Committee*, BMA, London.

British Medical Association (1999) *Withholding and Withdrawing Life-prolonging Medical Treatment: Guidance for Decision Making*, BMJ Books, London.

British Medical Association, Resuscitation Council (UK) and Royal College of Nursing (1999) *Decisions Relating to Cardiopulmonary Resuscitation*, BMA, London.

Brock, D. W. (1997) *Death and Dying*. In: *Medical Ethics*, 2nd edn, (ed. R. Veatch), Jones & Bartlett, London.

Carrick, P. (1985) *Medical Ethics in Antiquity*, D. Reidel, Dordrecht.

Conference of Medical Royal Colleges and their Faculties in the UK (1976) Diagnosis of death. *British Medical Journal*, ii, 1187–1188.

Conference of Medical Royal Colleges and their Faculties in the UK (1979) Diagnosis of death. *British Medical Journal*, i, 322.

Davies, M. (1998) *Textbook on Medical Law*, 2nd edn, Blackstone Press, London.

Docker, C. (1996) The way forward? In: *Death, Dying and the Law*, (ed. S. McLean), Dartmouth, Aldershot.

Downie, R. S. and Calman, K. C. (1994) *Healthy Respect*, 2nd edn, Oxford University Press, Oxford.

Doyal, L. and Wilsher, D. (1993) Withholding cardiopulmonary resuscitation: proposals for formal guidelines. *British Medical Journal*, 306, 1593.

Dworkin, R. (1993) *Life's Dominion*, Harper Collins, London.

Frey, R. G. (1998) The fear of the slippery slope. In: *Euthanasia and Physician-Assisted Suicide*, (eds G. Dworkin, R. G. Frey and S. Bok), Cambridge University Press, Cambridge.

Glover, J. (1977) *Causing Death and Saving Lives*, Penguin, Harmondsworth.

Harris, J. (1985) *The Value of Life: An Introduction to Medical Ethics*, Routledge, London.

Heap, M and Ridley, S. (1996) Quality of life after intensive care. In: *Ethics and the Law in Intensive Care*, (eds N. Pace and S. McLean), Oxford University Press, Oxford.

Hendrick, J. and Brennan, C. (1997) Do Not Resuscitate orders: guidelines in practice. *Nottingham Law Journal*, 6, 24–46.

HL Paper (1994) *Report of the Select Committee on Medical Ethics*, HMSO, London.

Huxtable, R. (1999) Withholding and withdrawing nutrition/hydration: the continuing misadventures of the law. *Journal of Social Welfare and Family Law*, 21(4), 339–353.

Jennett, B. (1996) Brain death and the persistent vegetative state. In: *Ethics and the Law in Intensive Care*, (eds N. Pace and S. McLean), Oxford University Press, Oxford.

Johnstone, M. J. (1989) *Bioethics: a Nursing Perspective*, Baillière Tindall, London.

Keown, J. (1997) Restoring moral and intellectual shape to the law after Bland, *Law Quarterly Review*, 113, 481.

Keown, J. (ed.) (1997) *Euthanasia Examined: Ethical, Clinical and Legal Perspectives*, Cambridge University Press, Cambridge.

Keown, J. (1999) 'Double effect' and palliative care: a legal and ethical outline. *Ethics and Medicine*, **15**(2), 53–54.

Kuhse, H. (1987) *The Sanctity of Life Doctrine in Medicine*, Clarendon Press, Oxford.

Lamb, D. (1988) *Down the Slippery Slope: Arguing in Applied Ethics*, Routledge, London.

Lamb, D. (1995) *Therapy Abatement, Autonomy and Futility*, Avebury, Aldershot.

McHale, J. and Fox, J., with Murphy, J. (1997) *Health Care Law: Text, Cases and Materials*, Sweet & Maxwell, London.

McLean, S. (1996) Law at the end of life: what next? In: *Death, Dying and the Law*, (ed. S. McLean), Dartmouth, Aldershot.

Mason, J. K. (1996) Death and dying: one step at a time? In: *Death, Dying and the Law*, (ed. S. McLean), Dartmouth, Aldershot.

Mason, J. K. and McCall Smith, R. A. (1999), *Law and Medical Ethics*, 5th edn, Butterworths, London.

Pace, N. (1996) Withholding and withdrawing medical treatment. In: *Ethics and the Law in Intensive Care*, (eds N. Pace and S. McLean), Oxford University Press, Oxford.

Rachels, J. (1975) Active and passive euthanasia. *New England Journal of Medicine*, **292**, 78–80.

Royal College of Paediatrics and Child Health (1997) *Withholding or Withdrawing Life Saving Treatment in Children*, RCPCH, London.

Rumbold, G. (1999) *Ethics in Nursing Practice*, 3rd edn, Baillière Tindall, London.

Schneiderman, M. D and Becker, N. (1995) *Wrong Medicine: Doctors, Patients and Futile Treatment*, Johns Hopkins University Press, Baltimore, MD.

Singer, P. (1995) *Rethinking Life and Death*, Oxford University Press, Oxford.

Sommerville, A (1996) Are advance directives really the answer? And what was the question? In: *Death, Dying and the Law*, (ed. S. McLean), Dartmouth, Aldershot.

Stauch, M. and Wheat, K. with Tingle, J. (1998) *Sourcebook on Medical Law*, Cavendish, London.

Tschudin, V. (1993) Euthanasia. In: *Ethics: Aspects of Nursing Care*, (ed. V. Tschudin), Scutari Press, London.

UKCC (1996) *Guidelines for Professional Practice*, United Kingdom Central Council, London.

Watson, M. (1999) A case of medical necessity? *New Law Journal*, **149**(6891), 863–864.

FURTHER READING

Keown, J. (2000) Beyond Bland: A critique of the BMA guidance on witholding medical treatment. In *Legal Studies*, Vol. **20**, No. 1, March 2000, 66–84.

Rachels, J. (1986) *The End of Life*, Oxford University Press, Oxford.

INDEX

Cases and statutes have not been indexed, see separate lists on pages ix-xv. Page references in *italics* indicate figures.